ANATOMY
OF AN EPIDEMIC

ANATOMY
OF AN EPIDEMIC

Gordon Thomas and
Max Morgan-Witts

DOUBLEDAY & COMPANY, INC.
GARDEN CITY, NEW YORK
1982

Library of Congress Cataloging in Publication Data
Thomas, Gordon.
    Anatomy of an epidemic.
    Bibliography: p. 354
    Includes index.
    1. Legionnaires' disease—Pennsylvania—Philadelphia.
I. Morgan-Witts, Max.   II. Title.
RC152.7.T48   616.9'2
AACR2
ISBN 0-385-14371-0
Library of Congress Catalog Card Number 81–43273

This has been called the epidemic of the century. We have been witness to one of the most intensive and extensive epidemiological investigations in modern medical history . . . and we shall ask the witnesses to refrain from offering a step-by-step account of possible methods of killing large numbers of people.

> John M. Murphy,
> Chairman of Congressional
> Subcommittee Hearings into the cause
> of legionnaires' disease,
> November 23, 1976

With each passing day, the chances that the cause of Legionnaires' Disease will be uncovered dwindles. We need desperately a major breakthrough by the scientific community.

> Leonard Bachman, M.D.,
> State Secretary,
> Pennsylvania Department of Health,
> November 23, 1976

The outbreak has produced a number of unusual and complex features. And it has run counter to our expectations that contemporary science is infallible and can solve all the problems that we can confront.

> David J. Sencer, M.D.,
> Director, Center for
> Disease Control, Atlanta,
> November 24, 1976

Extreme remedies are most appropriate for extreme diseases.
Hippocrates

This strange disease of modern life.
Persius

Contents

Personae   xi
Introduction   xiii

ORIGINATION

1 Premonition   3
2 Preparation   19
3 Expectation   36
4 Convention   48
5 Separation   70
6 Valediction   82

INVESTIGATION

7 Interrogation   101
8 Correlation   125
9 Interpolation   151
10 Interruption   168
11 Proliferation   187
12 Obliteration   210
13 Coarctation   229

ISOLATION

14 Collaboration   251
15 Concentration   270
16 Realization   294
17 Resolution   310

CONTINUATION

Aftermath   341

APPENDIXES

Special Thanks   351
Acknowledgments   352
Bibliography   354
Index   355

PERSONAE

Some of the persons prominent in the story:

The Medical Investigators

Federal Center for Disease Control (Atlanta):

David Sencer, M.D.	Director
David Fraser, M.D.	Chief, Special Pathogens
Charles Shepard, M.D.	Chief, Leprosy and Rickettsia
George Mallison, M.P.H.	Assistant Director, Bacterial Diseases
Joseph McDade, Ph.D.	Research Microbiologist
James Beecham, M.D.	Epidemiologist
Robert Craven, M.D.	Epidemiologist
Mark Goldberger, M.D.	Epidemiologist
Philip Graitcer, D.D.S.	Epidemiologist
Walter Orenstein, M.D.	Epidemiologist
Stephen Thacker, M.D.	Epidemiologist
Theodore Tsai, M.D.	Epidemiologist

Pennsylvania Department of Health (Harrisburg):

Leonard Bachman, M.D.	Secretary of Health
William Parkin, D.V.M.	Epidemiologist

Health Department, City of Philadelphia:

Lewis Polk, M.D.	Acting Health Commissioner
Robert Sharrar, M.D.	Chief, Acute Diseases Control

The Legionnaires

Joseph Adams	Commander, American Legion, Pennsylvania

Edward Hoak   Adjutant, American Legion,
                                 Pennsylvania
Richard (Dicko) Dolan   Commander, Post 239,
                                 Williamstown
George Chiavetta   Legionnaire
James (Jimmy) Dolan   Legionnaire
John Bryant (J.B.) Ralph   Legionnaire

The Hoteliers

William Chadwick   Managing Director
Harold Varr   General Manager
Frank Castelli   Executive Chef
Anna Taggart   Chief Elevator Operator

The Politicians

Frank Rizzo   Mayor, Philadelphia
Albert Gaudiosi   City Representative, Philadelphia
John M. Murphy   Congressman, New York

Introduction

It continues to kill.

To silently claim victims, to leave death and panic in its wake, to defy the most sophisticated techniques for detecting and destroying it.

It seems to be everywhere, to steal effortlessly from continent to continent, mysteriously and easily crossing vast oceans and deserts, striking at large cities like New York, Los Angeles, Washington, Cardiff, Naples, Munich, and Toronto and small towns like Kingston and Corby in England and Benidorm in Spain. It has claimed vacationers in Europe and hospital patients in California, felled South Africans in Johannesburg and Australians in Sydney. During Christmas 1980 it brought fear to the Welsh valleys when its presence was discovered among coal miners working hundreds of feet belowground; at the same time, its ugly specter surfaced a thousand miles away in one of the world's pleasure spots, the Algarve in Portugal. And just as unexpectedly it was found in another of Europe's famed resort centers, the Adriatic Coast of Italy.

Recent research suggests that in the United States alone it now kills over 70,000 people each year. Nobody has yet put a figure to the total number of deaths annually around the world. It might well be many hundreds of thousands. One thing is clear: no human is safe from it.

It might have gone on forever killing anonymously. But then a set of circumstances occurred that were both extraordinary and memorable.

In 1976 the United States celebrated its Bicentennial. There was well-founded pride throughout the country in what America had achieved during its first two hundred years. There was also much unhappiness to forget, if only temporarily. The strain on the nation's tolerance, particularly in recent years, had been considerable. Sometimes forbearance had snapped and the names and places that exhausted patience included Richard Nixon, Watergate, Attica, Kent State, Joe McCarthy, Mylai, and Cambodia. They were part of a lengthy list which stained the pages of American history but which, in this year of celebration, could be exchanged for a roll of honor that featured among others the names of John F. Kennedy, Martin Luther King, and Neil Armstrong.

The Bicentennial was not only an opportunity for Americans to reaffirm public pride in their nation. Private and personal feelings went deeper, touching a strong yearning in those wishing to renounce the present and find restoration in their glorious past. Putting aside a collective pain that their involvement in foreign conflicts for a third of a century had produced, the people of the United States looked inward once more, seeking comfort in their heritage, remembering all they had given to the world: music, literature, and technology, and of course medicine and science. No other country could rightfully claim to be more innovative or to have made a bigger contribution to the detection and treatment of disease. Regular medical breakthroughs pioneered by American researchers were saving lives all over the globe. Many of the great plagues of yesteryear had been tamed because of their skills. The United States also had the world's best-equipped "medical detective" agency, the Center for Disease Control* in Atlanta, an organization specifically charged with the investigation and prevention of disease. CDC laboratories and scientists provided support for state and local health departments within the United States and, increasingly, to any country that asked for assistance. Because of such facilities, Americans were probably the best protected, in a medical sense, of any people. It was comforting facts such as these which contributed to a national euphoria that reached its intended peak in July—the very month the deadly disease struck.

This is a story of fear: of the familiar becoming a source of sudden terror; of ordinary, everyday aids to modern living—air-conditioning units, refrigerators, even chemically treated tap water—taking on a totally unexpected connotation. And like the plague, the dreaded Black Death of medieval times that even now is not yet completely eradicated, the outbreak brought to the surface primeval emotions thought to be extinct.

A few of those who were afflicted or who lost loved ones asked for—and were given—guarantees that their identities would be suitably protected for professional or personal reasons: because their jobs or marriages could be put at risk, because they might be shunned by their friends, or because the reminder of the experience still traumatizes them. Almost everyone sharing in the scientific search gave us total co-

* Now renamed the Centers for Disease Control.

operation amid busy and demanding day-to-day duties. To them, in particular, we express genuine gratitude; without their help our task would have been impossible.

The time frame of the story they tell encompasses a strange period, somewhere between recent history and fading memory. As well as the usual research tools—official records, memoranda, a wide variety of published and private material, and our own personal observations—our main resource, as with our previous works, has been people. Most of the interviews conducted for this book were with eyewitnesses who had not been questioned before or who felt they could now speak more freely because a decent interval had elapsed. And because this story is authentic, often there can be no simple explanation for the way those people behaved. Theirs, though, is the truth of honest recall.

ORIGINATION

1

Premonition

By early July 1976 David Fraser, M.D., hoped that a suitable epidemic would soon appear in the United States.

His definition of "suitable" was quite specific: the outbreak would have no known cause; it could present a serious threat to human life and might even have claimed some victims, thus providing the corpses for all-important tissue samples. With every day that passed, his need for that epidemic grew more urgent. He cast his net wide for news that somewhere between Alaska and the Mexican border a mysterious malady had surfaced. He made sure he was never far from a telephone. And when he went home to his wife, Barbara, and their two children, Evan, aged seven, and Leigh, aged five, and was embraced by the close family atmosphere, part of his mind still wondered whether a suitable epidemic would come in time.

Fraser saw nothing unusual in his attitude. The tall and rangy thirty-two-year-old doctor—with a wickedly handsome lived-in face that made him look remarkably like the late President Kennedy—had a considerable scientific intellect that sometimes threatened to swamp his basic sensitivity toward people and situations. Fraser never suffered fools gladly and possessed an analytical mind capable of swiftly digesting a mass of varied information. He was demanding and dynamic, qualities that early in his career singled him out as a potential leader. Some found him cold and distant; they wondered whether it was anything to do with his Quaker background. He would maintain it was not, although his deep-seated pacifism made him withdraw from any involve-

ment with the military and with killing; his first two years at the CDC
had provided a convenient alternative to serving in the armed forces.

Others might well have wondered about the motivation behind his
hope that a suitable epidemic would soon materialize. In fact Fraser
was neither a closet ghoul nor a physician with a twisted sense of medical ethics. He was simply a dedicated professional totally preoccupied
with the immense challenges of his work, of which epidemics of a very
special kind formed the core.

The shaggy-haired, raw-boned Fraser, who had a penchant for wearing desert boots and an open-neck shirt to the office, was far removed
from the traditional image of a doctor. While fighting disease was very
much his business, his concern was not to treat patients—though eventually their lives could depend on his skills. His interest was in illnesses
that few family doctors had ever confronted. That was why this outstanding graduate of the Harvard Medical School—who had gone on
to work in two of America's better teaching hospitals, the University of
Pennsylvania in Philadelphia and the Mayo Graduate School of Medicine in Rochester, Minnesota—now spent his working days in a world
far removed from emergency rooms and operating theaters. At a moment's notice he could be plunged into some jungle swamp or parched
desert, a tree-lined city suburb or the concrete heart of a vast metropolis. Word could come suddenly, at any hour of the day or night, usually
by telephone.

As July advanced, Fraser increasingly wished, through a succession of
stiflingly hot and humid days, that the telephone in his cluttered and
windowless CDC office would bring news of some enigmatic epidemic
that did not fit into the pattern of the thousand or so outbreaks that
occur annually in the United States. Such an epidemic would allow
him to test in the field the newly acquired epidemiological skills of the
two young doctors who were about to join his Special Pathogens
Branch. The unit was part of the Bacterial Diseases Division at the federal Center for Disease Control, sometimes described as the Scotland
Yard of medical detection.

Within the carefully planned hierarchy of the CDC, the Special
Pathogens Branch was a relative newcomer: a small, elite unit responsible for the surveillance and detection of bacterial diseases that did
not conform to those in any other known category. It was always fas-
cinating and sometimes dangerous work, in which personal lives and
safety were frequently subjugated to the call of humanity. Partly because of this, and partly because of Fraser's own high reputation, there
was a certain glamour in being attached to Special Pathogens. It
offered the challenge of the unknown, a chance to delve deeper into
that sinister subvisible microbic world. Fraser suspected such thoughts
lurked in the minds of the two doctors about to join his unit. Only

after the most careful consideration had they been chosen; presently
the pair were attending an intensive course in the principles and
methods of epidemiology. He did not know the men well, but he was
fairly sure they had the potential, the rare ability to combine their
medical knowledge with the skills of a homicide detective, to build a
cast-iron case only on hard evidence, to convict only when the facts
were beyond dispute. To confirm that they really possessed these and
many other qualities, Fraser wanted to send them on an outbreak as
soon as they arrived in his unit. It was typical of the man.

Inside the restless, thrusting, ambitious, and sometimes ruthless
confines of the CDC, because of his considerable record in the field
and the volume and quality of his published work—his name had already appeared on twenty-five major papers in some of the world's leading scientific journals—Fraser was flagged by some as a future CDC director. Many of his colleagues thought that, given time, he could be an
ideal choice: he had a natural flair for investigation combined with all
the makings of a tough, no-nonsense administrator, capable of steering
the agency through the troubled waters in which it frequently wal-
lowed.

During these July days, waiting for his "good outbreak," Fraser entertained no such long-term ambitions. He was just "eternally grateful"
that so far he had managed to avoid becoming involved in the repercussions following the CDC's most controversial decision in its entire
existence. The agency's director, the urbane and not easily panicked
Dr. David J. Sencer, had, on a mass of complicated and sometimes esoteric evidence, concluded there was a very real danger swine flu could
sweep the United States in the coming months, perhaps producing a
pandemic as lethal as that of 1918–19. Then almost 500,000 Americans
had died from the fever. Sencer had persuaded President Gerald R.
Ford to approve a $135 million campaign to inoculate virtually every
man, woman, and child in the country, a preventive program never before attempted. The proposal had become an issue that continued to
embroil the CDC in both politics and the mores of big business. Fraser
suspected that Sencer was laying his job on the line; the director's professional future depended in part on the findings of a small CDC surveillance team standing by to move at the first sign of swine flu's appearance. That team was ensconced in Auditorium A, five floors below
Fraser's cubbyhole in the CDC's impressive headquarters. Despite their
spacious workplace, Fraser did not envy them. Swine flu, as such, did
not interest him, except to make him ensure that his own staff was not
dragged in on a program that had ground to a halt. That team, too,
was awaiting an epidemic before springing into action.

Both Special Pathogens and the swine flu unit were well placed to
hear quickly of any outbreak. Since 1961 the CDC monitored and re-

ported the nation's patterns of illnesses and deaths as they occurred day by day, week by week, month by month, year by year. Computers helped compile the totals, representing hundreds of thousands of individual medical dramas, in an attempt to reduce the infectious and respiratory diseases that annually produced in the United States some 140,000 deaths, 885 million days of sickness, 145 million days of missed school, and 130 million lost workdays.

Fraser was familiar with such statistics, just as he knew that of his fellow 3,600 CDC employees about half were based, as he was, at the Atlanta complex in a wooded suburb ten miles outside the city, the remainder scattered through the United States—either at CDC field stations or attached to state and city health departments—or on secondment abroad. All were associated in one way or another with a sustained program of research into the diseases that yearly produced such crippling figures.

At the very center of this campaign worked a select group of physicians, nurses, veterinarians, statisticians, biologists, dentists, engineers, demographers, anthropologists, and microbiologists. Drawn from such a variety of disciplines, and from all walks of life, the members of the group had one common bond: they had each been hand-picked during a highly competitive selection process before being admitted to the world's most sophisticated medical detection unit, the CDC's Epidemic Intelligence Service—the EIS—the far-reaching and all-embracing investigative arm of the agency.

Among the group, Fraser was looked upon with uncommon respect and, at times, awe. His work in such diverse areas as Parkinson's syndrome in neurogenetics, parenteral narcotics, bacterial meningitis, leptospirosis, and Lassa fever were regarded as textbook investigations. He was the epitome of what the media had long popularized as a "disease detective." Fraser did not altogether like such labeling, preferring instead to see himself as just one of a team, another of the CDC's more than two hundred epidemiologists who continued to tackle some of the world's most dangerous and spectacular epidemics.

Long ago, in the rote and example of epidemiologic fieldwork—reporting, investigating, collecting, evaluating, discovering, recommending, and preventing—Fraser had learned the value of dividing up aspects of a study, of surveillance, of comparing notes with colleagues to analyze what had been learned. And even though the isolation of the actual agent causing an outbreak was usually the work of a single investigator—a scientist who had never left the laboratory—the on-site epidemiologic investigation to establish the agent's niche and mode of spread was almost always solidly based on team effort. As in any well-run police detective bureau, seasoned CDC investigators such as Fraser were much less interested in personal glory than they were in successfully, collectively cracking a mystery. And it was agency policy for its staff to keep a low profile when working away from their Atlanta headquarters. That was one way of reducing the time-consuming involvement of CDC staff in local medicopolitics.

Recently, and with the minimum of publicity, CDC teams had tackled typhoid fever and anthrax in Florida, cholera in Texas, malaria in California, relapsing fever in Arizona, bubonic plague in New Mexico, and hepatitis in South Carolina. Abroad, four years ago, Fraser had been one of the CDC epidemiologists who risked his life helping to solve an outbreak of Lassa fever in Sierra Leone. Currently, CDC staff were investigating hemorrhagic fever in the Sudan and Zaire.

Fraser could imagine the intense pressure those men were experiencing thousands of miles away in Africa. On the one hand, they would be exercising great care to miss no clue; on the other, racing the clock, knowing that with every minute that passed without a solution the lethal fever could be spreading. Early on they would have assessed the geographic focus of the epidemic by pinpointing every reported case on a map of the area. Trained to regard a wide range of factors as possible causes for the outbreak, they would be eliminating each one only as their accumulating data proved conclusively it was not relevant. It was like this in every case: there were few alternatives to patient routine, and there was little scope for intuitive guesswork to ease what was often hard, unremitting drudgery.

And, as Fraser had frequently experienced, even these meticulous techniques did not always work. He had just returned, still baffled, from an investigation in North Carolina into the cause of a mysterious infection that had afflicted patients recovering from open-heart surgery in local hospitals. Try as he could, the facts he collated failed to complete the epidemiologic jigsaw puzzle. Surveillance would continue in the hope that a solution would emerge. And perhaps, if all else failed and no suitable epidemic materialized, he could assign his two trainees to part of this work. They would undoubtedly find it more appealing than sitting at their desks writing replies to questions from doctors and the public; important though this was, Fraser knew it was no way to sustain the understandable enthusiasm for fieldwork the newcomers were bound to display. Fresh from their EIS course, they would doubtless be anxious to get out and prove their worth.

Increasingly Fraser realized that if his telephone didn't ring soon with news of an epidemic, he might well find that his fledgling epidemiologists had been whisked away as part of the swine flu watch —joining the team waiting impatiently beside its computer for signs of an impending pandemic. And as so often happened with outbreaks, Fraser knew there was a real possibility that by the time the computers helped confirm a coming disaster, the first deaths could have already occurred.

Doris Fetterhoff watched the hearse traveling along the road. The black car gleamed, its glass sparkling in the summer light. She knew it belonged to Dale Hoover: no other undertaker in Dauphin County, Pennsylvania, kept his car so waxed and polished. She wondered who had died. A death was always an event in the Williams Valley, a remote area scarred with derelict coal mine workings some one hundred and twenty miles northwest of Philadelphia. A funeral, as much as a christening or a wedding, was an occasion for the people of the small towns and hamlets in the valley to gather and catch up with one another's lives.

Beside her, James Dolan, Jimmy, coughed; another of his summer colds seemed to be developing. Doris wondered whether she could use that possibility to stop his going to Philadelphia. She was worried enough to try anything. She had come to believe their future together depended on whether or not he went to the city.

The issue had been there from that day a month ago when Jimmy had returned from work and said he was going to the American Legion State Convention in Philadelphia with his older cousin, Richard (Dicko) Dolan, and John Bryant (J.B.) Ralph, and a dozen others, all members of Williamstown's Post 239.

Doris and Jimmy lived together in the small town, a collection of buildings beside a disused rail track parallel to the road along which the hearse was traveling. Williamstown's 1,917 inhabitants were content, on the whole, to exist within an orderly framework: to work, hunt and fish, watch television, and attend social and school functions and meetings of the Chamber of Commerce, Jaycees, and Scouts. And to speculate endlessly about the very special relationship between Doris and Jimmy.

From where they were now sitting, in a secluded dell high up on the side of the valley, the couple looked down on the old mining town, its church spires and towers rising above the squat ugliness of AMP, the electronics factory and main source of local employment. From this distance the sagging porches and peeling paint on the two-story colonnades and fake brick trim of the grander houses were not discernible. On this hot afternoon of July 18 Williamstown was gripped in its usual Sunday torpor. Nothing moved in the vicinity except the funeral car.

Doris was twenty-seven years old, a devout Roman Catholic, a divorcée and the mother of three small children. She had fair hair and skin that glowed with energy from a healthy diet and regular exercise. There was something earthy and immediately sexy about her.

Jimmy was a thirty-nine-year-old six-footer weighing 220 pounds, all muscle except for a thickening waist. He had an open face, deeply tanned like the rest of his body, and a slow easy smile that matched his gentle and inquiring way of speaking. During his life he had fulfilled the highest expectations, as a sportsman, a student, and later a cryptographer in the U. S. Navy, handling sensitive coded material. His military hitch over, he now worked at Fort Indiantown Gap, a U. S. Army base twenty miles from Williamstown. Jimmy's work was classified Top Secret; he liked to add to the mystery by claiming he was "involved" with the CIA.

The couple, and Doris' children, had lived together for the past five years in a small apartment on Williamstown's Market Street. The arrangement had been disapproved of from the start by the majority of the town's older folk, steeped as they were in traditional values and morality. But nowadays everyone in Williamstown was agog with *how* Doris and Jimmy actually lived together under one roof.

In a community where the last sensation had been a year before, when local high school students had entered the Guinness Book of World Records after playing basketball nonstop for forty-nine hours, the titillating story of the couple's pact this past twelve months was, local wags felt, worthy of another entry in the record book. For 365 days Doris and Jimmy had lived together without once making love.

Both freely admitted to friends they had entered into this demanding relationship at the request of Father Thomas Simpson, their pastor at the Church of the Sacred Heart of Jesus. Doris, in particular, told an intriguing tale: after questioning her about her sexual life with Jimmy, the avuncular priest had said that "all this has got to stop" before they got married. He went on to say he would only consent to the couple continuing to live together if they each remembered "the sacraments must come before sex." If that celibate situation was maintained, then Father Simpson would view the relationship as no different from the one he had with his own housekeeper.

Speculation was rife over not only *how* but *whether* Doris and Jimmy had managed to maintain their vow of celibacy.

While not concerned by the gossip, Doris was nevertheless anxious to regularize her relationship. Being a Catholic and keen to remarry in church, she knew that was only possible if the hierarchy formally recognized her civil divorce. That, Father Simpson had also explained, would need the approval of the Apostolic Delegate to the United States and, perhaps, even the sanction of the Vatican.

Doris had been prepared to wait patiently, until Jimmy announced he was going to the Legion convention with Dicko and J.B. Then sudden anger had surfaced. She bitterly accused Jimmy of letting Dicko and J.B. run his life; neither of his friends, she added, approved of her and she was certain they would try, while Jimmy was with them in Philadelphia, to persuade him to leave her.

The three men had been inseparable pals all their adult lives; their hell raising had earned them in some quarters the nickname of the "terrible trio," but in the rough-and-tumble of local life they were looked upon with affection, and their antics as being merely boisterous. By consent, Dicko was the leader. J.B., the son of Mildred Ralph, the widowed owner of the town's funeral home, and Jimmy were enthusiastic followers, ready to tackle anything, or anybody.

Until Doris entered Jimmy's life, the trio moved as a cohesive unit through the area, with their cry of "one for all and all for one." Doris had changed that, setting about "taming" Jimmy, an experience he had surprisingly come to like. Dicko and J.B. resented her interference. The seeds of conflict were sown, and they were nurtured through a dozen small incidents, after each of which Jimmy's companions made their feelings clear to Doris. In turn, she harbored the growing suspicion that Dicko and J.B. would "do anything" to end the affair. She consequently saw the forthcoming visit to the Legion convention as "the ideal place for them to work their devilment on my Jimmy."

She did not suspect that the reason he wanted to go to Philadelphia had nothing to do with her. There was growing talk at work that the convention could be disrupted by a terrorist act. The usually restrained Legion *Journal*, a magazine of the veterans, had just published a lengthy article suggesting that subversive elements were "stalking" the Bicentennial. Philadelphia, the very core of the national rejoicing, might be a prime target. The prospect of trouble produced a strong reaction in Jimmy: although not a violent man, he was deeply patriotic and felt almost irresistibly drawn to Philadelphia, to be on hand to help deal with anyone who threatened his fellow legionnaires.

Not wishing to worry her, he kept these thoughts from Doris. And until this Sunday the matter of their marriage had not been mentioned for some time. Then, after breakfast, when the children were settled down watching television cartoons, Doris casually mentioned she might soon have some good news about the annulment.

Jimmy had swept her into his arms as she explained that Father Simpson expected to have an answer within "a month or so." They talked of being married before the fall, a white wedding with a large reception afterward; later he could carry her over the threshold and they would make love, "like it was for the first time."

With that exciting prospect still in his mind, Jimmy had left the apartment and walked the short distance to the Legion post for his regular Sunday morning drink.

Soon afterward, because of what had occurred there, he had returned home, collected Doris, and driven her here, "to our place," this dell in the woods where they sometimes came when they wanted to be alone.

At last, when the hearse finally disappeared around a bend in the road, Jimmy had turned to Doris and spoken.

Even now, a full hour later, she felt the deep hurt in his voice as he had described the brief conversation with Dicko. He had asked his cousin to be best man at their wedding. Dicko refused, adding bleakly that he could never approve of such a union. At that, Jimmy had walked out of the post.

Doris sat up and looked carefully at Jimmy, at his mop of dark hair the attractive length her mother called too long, his mouth set resolutely, his eyes revealing his troubled mood.

She would always remember how they sat and stared at each other, "both of us aware the crisis had probably come." There was no question now of using Jimmy's developing cold as an excuse for keeping him away from Philadelphia. Things had gone beyond that.

Jimmy finally spoke: they would still get married, "the very day after the annulment comes through and without one other Dolan being there."

She started to pull him toward her. He held her off, anxious to complete what he had to say: if it would please her, he would not go to the convention.

Doris interrupted: he must go. As she spoke, she also thought to herself: *We are going to get married, nothing else matters. Jimmy's given his word and there's nothing Dicko and J.B. can do. Not now.*

She spoke softly and quickly, the way she always did when she had something important to say. He owed it to himself to go; besides, on the neutral ground of Philadelphia he might yet be able to persuade Dicko to change his mind, to make him realize how much they loved each other.

Jimmy had a question: if he somehow found the money, would she come with him?—maybe a relative could look after the children.

She smiled and said he wasn't to be foolish. They would need every penny for the wedding. What was important was that he went. Not to do so would be a mistake, a decision he would regret; as far as she was concerned, there was no more to be said.

He looked at her, realizing there were depths to Doris he had never before suspected.

She kissed him gently. It was her way of closing the episode.

Doris did not tell Jimmy that her decision to let him go to Philadelphia was all the more remarkable because it conflicted with a vague but disturbing feeling of unease. She could not explain the feeling. But it was there.

Throughout Sunday afternoon a regular rumble came from behind a closed door within the headquarters of the Williamstown branch of the American Legion, Post 239, an imposing three-floored building at one end of Market Street. The handful of drinkers around the large horseshoe-shaped bar on the ground floor paid no attention. The sound was familiar to them. It was the voice of the post commander, Dicko, talking on the telephone.

For sixteen years Dicko had been Williamstown's very agent of rescue, falling upon ordeals like an appointed angel. There were few crises Dicko had not helped his neighbors overcome. They still remembered how, when in 1972 Hurricane Agnes roared through the valley, he had turned the post into a shelter for 286 people driven from their homes by the worst floods in recent local history; they remembered with gratitude the campaign he had spearheaded, bombarding the state's representatives in Washington with letters that finally resulted in the ugly burning tips of coal dust around the town being bulldozed. Dicko was also a renowned conqueror of other people's personal problems: he knew how to cut through the state and federal bureaucracy that impinged upon the lives of so many veterans; the strength of his will was a sword to anyone in need. He was always among the first to visit the bereaved family of a legionnaire. He was also a net for those rumors which swam in the shallows of gossip, catching them before they could grow. He was the keeper, too, of other and darker secrets: whose wife was a daytime drinker, which husband was being unfaithful, who was dying of some unmentionable disease like cancer or multiple sclerosis, and who was "going away for a spell," the sheltering expression used by relatives for a loved one about to receive psychiatric help.

Dicko also continued the tradition that for the past fifty-five years had made the post the center of civic and social life in the town. The post sponsored Boy and Girl Scout troops, midget and junior baseball leagues, and a drum corps, provided money for instruments, uniforms, and flags for the high school band, supplied disabled veterans and their families with coal through the winter and food all year round, organized transport for ex-servicemen to and from the hospital, paid their domestic bills, bought the town a new fire truck, launched the Williamstown Military Band, turned the derelict Geist Hotel into apartments, refurbished the old Durbin Mill to provide more local jobs, purchased the ground on which AMP built a factory employing two hundred townspeople, donated a plot for the state National Guard to erect an armory, ran a free home delivery service of essential medicaments to any bedridden veteran in the valley, and published a monthly newsletter that regularly took proper pride in all Post 239's achievements.

There was not a person at the post bar this Sunday afternoon who did not realize his life was constantly being influenced by decisions Dicko Dolan made. Each also knew nobody could match his drive, his dedication, his patriotism, or even the stern tone of his voice, still rumbling on from behind the closed door of what was affectionately known as "Dolan's Hole."

Dicko was forty-three years old, well over six feet tall, sharp and suspicious, ruggedly handsome, and bearing a striking resemblance to one of the men in the famous photograph of the marines raising the flag on Iwo Jima in 1945. A huge enlargement of that picture hung in the post bar, as did others depicting incidents from all the major wars fought by Americans in this century.

For weeks Dicko had spent his free time in the confines of his cramped and cluttered office, tucked away in a corner of the post, either on the telephone or working at the battered desk placed against one wall. In addition to his other responsibilities, two all-important impending events demanded his attention: Williamstown's 150th birthday, to be celebrated in just a few weeks, and the Legion's fifty-eighth state convention, now only three days away.

The convention posed the most pressing problems for 239's commander. It was never easy deciding which candidates to support, which resolutions to oppose. There was the usual spate of calls for pledges from contenders for the various Legion offices and from fellow post commanders wishing to push through particular resolutions. Dicko knew Williamstown's six hundred votes were important to the callers. He replied now to this one as he had to all the others, and as he did each year at this time: he would not commit 239's votes until he had taken "soundings" in Philadelphia.

No sooner had he put down the telephone than it rang yet again. This time it was a barman at a roadhouse some twenty miles away: J.B. had just left, "looking one helluva sight." The man refused to elaborate, tantalizing Dicko with "Just you wait 'n' see."

Dicko wondered what J.B. had done now. His stunts were legendary. Dicko had lost count of the times J.B. had drunk too much and talked himself into and out of scrapes. One of the more memorable was when he and Jimmy had borrowed the town's hearse. Jimmy put on the derby he usually reserved for St. Patrick's Day and got behind the wheel. J.B. daubed flour on his face and stretched out in the back. As Jimmy drove slowly along the mile length of Market Street, J.B. repeatedly sat up and lay down, scaring the wits out of everybody in sight. Some people had wanted him prosecuted for blasphemy.

Dicko had learned to forgive J.B. and his cousin almost anything. An exception was Jimmy's relationship with Doris. Dicko realized he had hurt Jimmy by refusing to be best man. But there was no way he would ever accept Doris.

For a start, she reminded him of his own past.

Dicko was born into the depression. He had felt hunger at a tender age, heard talk of men losing their jobs at Williamstown Colliery, up on Big Lick Mountain overshadowing the town, and seen families pack up and leave. Finally silence—the total, enveloping, and eerie silence of poverty—settled over the area. It was a memory Dicko never forgot, forgave, or wanted ever again to experience. The grim years of his childhood were a time of mendicancy that ended only with Pearl Harbor and the subsequent wartime prosperity, strong enough to carry most Williamstown families forward through three decades of uneasy peace. Doris' family were an exception. They remained "poor church mice."

There were other reasons Dicko rarely mentioned, even to his second wife, why he was so utterly opposed to the affair. These were bound up in the complex currents flowing beneath the placid surface of Williamstown that shaped the mores of everybody living there. Jimmy and Doris had "swum against the tide"; living "in sin" in a deeply religious community, they made a mockery of marriage by regularly attending mass, making their confession, and taking Communion. There were many people who prophesied the couple would be "punished": a vengeful God and hellfire religion were powerful totems in Williamstown.

Finally there was Doris herself. It was not just her family background: Dicko had to admit she had tried to rise above her poverty. Neither was it the fact she was a divorcée: he had himself been divorced. Nor could he fault her as a mother or for lacking in attention to Jimmy. There was something else, some indefinable quality in Doris, that stopped Dicko from warming to her, let alone accepting her into the close-knit Dolan clan, an aggressively Irish-American middle-class family with considerable social influence in the valley.

For a long time Dicko had wondered how best he could persuade Jimmy to end the affair and "find himself a nice Irish girl."

Now, after the incident with his cousin this morning, Dicko suspected the convention was the only hope he had of getting Jimmy involved with that "nice Irish girl." Once Jimmy returned from Philadelphia and Doris received her annulment, there would be no way Dicko could stop the wedding.

He was interrupted in his thoughts by another telephone call, from a counter hand at a diner, asking whether he had seen J.B.

This time the caller was slightly more specific, adding before hanging up, "It's J.B.'s head."

Dicko slammed down the phone, leaped out of his chair, yanked open the door of his office, and shouted at the men around the bar that J.B. had done something to his head.

J.B. had decided to do it on the spur of the moment. At one point he had been cruising along in his car with no such thought in his mind. Then he made the decision. He parked the car, walked into a barbershop in Pottsville, and told the assistant to completely shear and then shave his skull. J.B. had a striking head of hair, strong and wavy; it was one of his most attractive features.

That had been yesterday afternoon. Afterward he played some pool, ate a steak dinner, went to a night spot, drank a great deal, slept late at a motel. For him it was a typical weekend. From time to time he wondered what effect his baldness would have on his mother, his friends, and his enemies. Nowadays he frequently felt there was little left in his life except to shock, anger, or amuse people. His mother, he was certain, would react first with a quick disbelieving shake of the head, then a forgiving smile. Virginia Anne, he guessed, would be upset. His sister always admired his hair. Nevertheless, on balance he was glad his scalp was now almost as smooth as the day he was born forty-one years earlier.

He pulled into a roadhouse. The bartender greeted him warily; barmen within a fifty miles' radius of Williamstown had learned to handle J.B. cautiously. The slightest thing—a too frivolous greeting, too much ice in his whiskey, or a beer too quickly poured—could bring either a smile, through teeth strong enough to crack walnuts, or a flow of abuse that left staff rooted to the spot.

Later, when J.B. was safely gone, the man had made that tantalizing first telephone call to Dicko.

A few miles along the road, J.B. stopped at a diner. He was known here, too. These days he preferred to eat junk food in an attempt to kill the memory of the excellent cook his ex-wife, Carol, had been. He had swallowed a sandwich and left the diner; immediately the counter hand had made the second call to Dicko.

Now, at last heading for home, even sitting behind the wheel of his car J.B. looked enormous. In this lonesome area which bred huge men, he was a massive figure with a huge neck, a barrel of a chest, and bulging biceps. Yet in spite of his physical appearance, he was not a fit man: he suffered from chronic emphysema, which left him prone to crippling attacks of bronchitis, had high blood pressure, and, at 250 pounds, was well overweight. A medical examiner had just recently judged him 50 pounds too heavy and a poor insurance risk. J.B.'s broad shoulders and hard, aggressive jaw were all that remained of his youth, of those days at Duke University where he was not only an outstanding student but also a fine football player.

On this humid Sunday evening there was nothing sartorially to suggest he had gone on to become one of the area's most respected citizens, editor and publisher of the small but thriving *Echo* newspaper in Elizabethville, a tiny community eleven miles from Williamstown. In those days, before he suddenly sold the paper, he wore $200 Brooks Brothers suits, and his shirts, ties, and shoes came from New York's Saks Fifth Avenue. Now he dressed in denim pants, a worn check shirt, and scuffed loafers. He looked like a farmhand and spoke with a country-boy twang. His formerly smooth and modulated accent had been deliberately eradicated.

People said he was making a determined effort to remove every trace of his recent past, that he was driven by some raging inner compulsion to destroy himself. J.B. knew it was true.

He drove across Interstate 81 and onto the winding road leading into the Williams Valley. He reduced speed to avoid hitting the potholes and being stopped by any highway patrol cruising the area. He was certain that, given the slightest provocation, he would be booked for speeding or even drunken driving. He believed "somebody" had passed the word to harass him, perhaps one of those state officials in Harrisburg that Carol now mixed with. He thought it would be typical of his ex-wife to attack him by using other men.

J.B. sometimes wondered whether, if Carol had been more like his mother, things would have turned out differently. His mother showed tact, understanding, and forbearance, virtues he had never found in Carol. Nowadays his mother never mentioned his ex-wife except in relation to the children; since the divorce his two young sons lived with their mother, making monthly visits to see him.

He drove on through one small hamlet after another. These were places where church affiliations decided social status and where the majority of voters were right-wing Republicans. There were no blacks. J.B. passed abandoned refrigerators and washing machines and automobile graveyards: in his time he had dumped several cars onto these ugly heaps of rusting metal, adding to the spoilation of a valley where, a century before, Indians roamed and the only debris was their burned-out cook pots.

Beyond Tower City, J.B. approached the Milk Barn, a bar-diner with a few chalets out back. He had often brought Carol here and later, just once, soon after his divorce, Didi, a black go-go dancer. When he and Didi walked in, they had been greeted by embarrassed looks and a stunned silence from the regulars, white to a man. They had a drink and left, setting off on a tour of all the bars in the valley, J.B. relishing the offended looks he received at each; it was another way of being "different." At the post, Didi offered to give a performance. Instead, J.B. took her to a motel where they spent a week together. Then he tired of her and returned home. That night he received an anonymous threatening telephone call. He never again brought a black to the valley.

J.B. reached the outskirts of Williamstown. He pulled off the road, parked beside the Sacred Heart cemetery, and just sat. He was, he would later tell his mother and Dicko, trying to make some sense of his life, hoping to rationalize the anger and pain within himself. He recognized he had always tried to be "different." At school, at the university, and in the Army he had equated conformity with boredom. That was why he had decided not to enter the family funeral business. Instead he used his savings to purchase the *Echo*; within a year he substantially increased its circulation. From then on, his mother encouraged him to be as "different" as he liked.

Carol was also "different." She was seven years old when she arrived in Williamstown; by her teens she had developed a haunting quality that attracted every man in the valley—that, and her shiny blond hair, marvelous long legs, winsome smile, and skimpy dresses.

J.B., thirty years old and the wealthiest bachelor in town, fell in love the moment he saw her. He courted her passionately, showering gifts and taking her to the most exclusive night spots in the state. Months later, he persuaded her it would be "different" to elope. They drove several hundred miles to be married in a city where nobody knew or cared about them.

The elopement created a scandal throughout the valley. As J.B. expected, his mother quickly forgave him; it took her a while longer to accept Carol.

The newlyweds set up house in a small apartment below the embalming room in the Ralph Funeral Home. J.B. frequently made jokes about what went on above their heads. It was yet another way of showing he was "different": that the hum of the suction pump, the rattle of steel pails, and the gurgle of mortuary fluids held no horror for him.

Carol bore him two boys. Later the family moved to a palatial residence in Elizabethville so that J.B. could be near the *Echo*.

Then one day the marriage was over and done with, dead, killed not so much by one great act of violence or cheating, although both had played their part, but by an accumulation of petty issues that were allowed to fester in the long periods of punishing silence that fell between a succession of bickering rows: fights over her clothes, his drinking habits, her fondness for dancing with other men, his explosive flares of temper, her bitter, sweeping rages. The divorce in 1970 was a relief for them both.

Carol quickly remarried. Automatically J.B. resumed his bachelor ways, but from then on he sought only women who could never begin to touch him emotionally. Sometimes he brought them back to the big, empty house in Elizabethville; most nights he slept alone. During those nights, he told his mother, he had sometimes, in the depths of sleep, flung his arm across the empty expanse of mattress as he unconsciously reached out for Carol.

Eventually he could stand it no longer. He sold the Elizabethville house and moved back to Williamstown to live with his mother and sister. They could do nothing to remove the frozen feeling inside him, a feeling so uncomfortable at times he felt he was choking.

Not long ago, Carol had written saying she proposed to change the boys' family name to that of her new husband. J.B. read the letter several times. It was like a defilement. For a moment dark anger simmered. Then he buried his face in the pages, pressing them tightly against his eyes. It was so many years since he had cried that for a time he was unaware of what he was doing. His mother found him sobbing in the kitchen. She comforted him and together they planned what to do; they hired a lawyer to prepare the legal ground to resist Carol. A few days ago the attorney had telephoned J.B. and warned him the court might deny the motion.

That was why he had gone away for the weekend, to escape the sadness in his mother's eyes. That, he at last admitted to himself, was also why he had ordered his scalp shaved in Pottsville; he no longer cared what he looked like because his life had lost both purpose and direction.

J.B. drove up Williamstown's main street, parking outside the post. He walked down its narrow entranceway and pushed open the door to the ground-floor bar.

Every eye in the crowded room stared at him, at his skull, gleaming whitely in the overhead lights.

From the bar Dicko uttered a long Indian war whoop. It was quickly taken up by the others.

J.B., playing his part, looking suitably savage, moved slowly among the tables, hand upraised as if clutching a tomahawk, a brave on the warpath.

He stopped at the table where Jimmy sat with Doris and made a joke about encountering the barber of Seville in Pottsville.

Everybody howled with laughter. Nobody noticed that J.B. did not join in the mirth.

2

Preparation

At precisely eight-fifty, as he did six mornings a week, wet or fine, apart from a rare day of sickness or his vacations, Frank Castelli emerged from the subway into Broad Street. The twelve-mile-long avenue was one of the major arteries of Philadelphia, a metropolis firmly wedged between two rivers—the Delaware and the Schuylkill—making it not only America's fourth largest city but also the world's largest freshwater port.

The first day he came to work in Philadelphia, Castelli was given three further facts by a well-meaning citizen: the city was founded by Quakers, Benjamin Franklin once lived there, and Broad Street was the "longest straight street in the world." Ever since school Castelli had accepted the first two as fact; being a careful and cautious person, he checked the third. The longest straight street in the world was Chicago's Western Avenue, almost twice the length of Broad Street. It gave him an invaluable insight into the psychology of the people among whom he worked.

Ignoring its slums, industrial muck, sprawling dinginess, and lack of a redeeming skyline—such as New York's seen from the harbor or Boston's viewed from across the Common—Philadelphians preferred to point out historic old houses lovingly restored, wide plazas, and secluded gardens, and to state, never mind what Chicago might claim, that Broad Street was still the longest straight thoroughfare in the world.

Castelli now understood, accepted, and supported such civic pride. Although it was not yet a year since he first emerged into the street at this hour, he felt as if all his life he had been carried along by the tow of the morning rush. His brisk, confident stride cut a man's-man figure, suggesting an outdoor occupation. Castelli was fifty-five years old, in peak physical condition, and his firm, unlined face retained a healthy youthful glow. Few strangers guessed his job.

This Monday morning, July 19, he was thinking: of Spanish omelettes, of aspic glazing for cold turkeys, of how many dollars tomato wedges would deduct from the already tight profit on five hundred green salads. He nevertheless could appreciate the colorful scene around him. Broad Street, like the entire downtown district, was garlanded with bunting and flags to mark Philadelphia's position at the heart of the Bicentennial.

Queen Elizabeth of Britain had just bestowed a royal accolade by delivering a suitable birthday greeting in the city. Gerald Ford, beset by the hundred and one problems any U.S. President faces—his included the fury over his pardon to Richard Nixon, the prospect of a new war in the Middle East, the growing political threat at home from Georgia's Governor Jimmy Carter, and the controversy surrounding the swine flu campaign—had still found time to make a keynote bicentennial speech in Philadelphia, one which Castelli felt properly reflected the renewed confidence of millions of his fellow Americans in their country. He only wished the President would stop mentioning the immunization program; alarming headlines about a possible coming epidemic could only have an adverse effect on the flow of visitors from all over the world to Philadelphia. Castelli's livelihood depended in part on satisfying some of their appetites.

He paused at the corner of Broad and Walnut, as he did most fine mornings, to contemplate a massive granite-faced edifice—he felt "building" was an altogether inadequate word—that stood on the opposite side of the intersection. In a city of idly spaced flat-topped modern skyscrapers set amid extravagant late-Victorian architecture, this craggy gray structure enthralled Castelli; over each of the imposing twin entrances, one on Broad and the other on Walnut, hung the Stars and Stripes, the only external concessions to America's 200th birthday. Castelli felt such decorum entirely appropriate. His mind still toying with culinary matters, he entered the building through a door discreetly marked EMPLOYEES ONLY.

And so, on his 327th day in its employ, the executive chef of the Bellevue Stratford Hotel arrived for work. Walking quickly through the staff area, responding to deferential greetings, Castelli's eyes and nose keenly observed and sniffed, a reflex reaction for the highly experienced hotel man. Nothing disturbed him. All around were the comforting sights, sounds, and smells of a grand old hotel beginning another day.

Born of two hotels—the Bellevue and the Stratford—it had opened its doors on September 20, 1904, owned and managed by George C. Boldt, the legendary steward of Philadelphia's Clover Club. Boldt's high connections had enabled him to raise $8 million, an almost unheard of amount to spend on a hotel in Edwardian times. Boldt set out deliberately to make the hotel a mecca for the very rich or famous. He catered for their every whim and need, keeping a double-sized cup for President Theodore Roosevelt's breakfast coffee, a supply of black stogies for Amy Lowell, polished cuspidors for Rudyard Kipling, crystal goblets for J. Pierpont Morgan, writing tablets for Mark Twain, and a tuner for those days when Sergei Rachmaninoff's personal grand piano arrived just before the maestro swept into the lobby. The Bellevue Stratford quickly became another Philadelphia institution, first choice as headquarters for such events as the Democratic and Republican national conventions and the Army-Navy games. Every American President since it opened had stayed there, a record no other hotel in the country could equal.

Money was lavished on its plush interior: exquisite French period pieces complemented rare Chinese and Japanese artifacts, hand-carved tables from Bavaria supported Meissen china, Dresden statues stood beside long-case clocks from England.

Nobody quite knew when its high reputation had started to slip, when the hotel's 22 public meeting rooms were not constantly in demand, its 3 main restaurants not totally filled for every meal, when many of its 754 guest bedrooms went unlet and room service no longer regularly served champagne breakfasts at dawn and candlelight suppers at midnight. Although this was hardly noticed at first, by the early 1970s many believed the Bellevue, as the hotel was commonly called, was not what it had been. Nevertheless, it still had class.

Some weeks the depressing trend stopped; the hotel would be fully booked and a sprinkling of famous new faces—movie stars, television talk-show hosts, and astronauts—would check in. Then long-serving staffers spoke nostalgically of a resurgence of the "good old days." But a few days later the room clerks and headwaiters would report that trade was once again slack. And so it had gone on through recent years, a slow, steady falling away of custom.

The Bicentennial had dramatically halted the decline. From the spring of 1976 onward the Bellevue had been almost full; the old hectic times seemed to have really returned. The hotel, which only a year ago appeared doomed to a lingering fate, looked now, in the eyes of many employees, to be gaining enough strength to survive into a new century. They spoke of the "old lady of Broad Street"—as the hotel was affectionately described—getting an expensive face-lift, becoming rejuvenated, returning to the splendid glory of her youth.

Castelli guessed that any refurbishing would be unlikely to include the subterranean warren of storerooms and pantries he was walking past. In the basement of the Bellevue there was little reason to paint or to conceal the pipes that heated, cooled, and watered the hotel. And any evidence of the presence of mice or of cockroaches, Castelli knew, did not present a serious health hazard. The hotel waged a relentless war against all vermin and passed the regular checks by City Hall inspectors, who seldom, if ever, complained about rust spots on pipework or rodent droppings.

A distant roar reached the chef's ears. It was the incinerator in the subbasement, one floor below. Castelli did not envy those who worked in the torrid, odorous room sifting refuse before shoveling it into the furnace, trying to spot silverware, unbroken wineglasses, and returnable bottles that had been dumped into the trash carts by careless maids, waiters, and busboys. Annually the garbage detail saved the hotel thousands of dollars in recovered items.

With the city gripped at present in a partial refuse collection slowdown and garbage piling up in the suburbs, a blight that had already caused some distinguished bicentennial visitors to wrinkle their noses in disgust, the Bellevue was totally unaffected by the demand for more money by the sanitation workers. Almost all the hotel's waste was disposed of through the furnace; food slops were taken away by a private contractor.

Castelli did not know that the incinerator was now being operated improperly by a new employee. Nevertheless, he suspected that if the garbage workers' slowdown spread, it might create a public health problem that would soon affect the hotel. Common sense told him the hot weather—cloudy and humid, with highs in the eighties—could quickly rot the accumulating refuse and attract hordes of rats from the city's sewers.

Rats worried the fastidious chef. He had read that bubonic plague was on the increase throughout the world, and he knew rats carried the disease. In the seventy-two-year life-span of the Bellevue there had been fourteen small epidemics of plague within the United States. Recently medical experts had warned it might be only a matter of time before another outbreak occurred that could spread the dreaded Black Death of medieval times. Castelli had "no darned idea" what plans, if any, City Hall had for dealing with such a contingency, but he "sure as hell wished the garbage foul-up would go away."

The chef reached the cold storage area where sides of prime beef, lamb, and pork hung. The refrigeration equipment would be hard pressed to keep the chilling rooms as cold as was needed, and the twenty-year-old air-conditioning system would also be stretched to cool the eighteen-story building.

Like the prospect of rodent-borne plague, the air-conditioning system made the chef uneasy. It was less than perfect. The two centrifugal refrigeration machines were housed in the hotel's engine room, next door to the incinerator. The units were manufactured and installed in 1954 by the Carrier Corporation of Syracuse, New York, a leading manufacturer in the field. One chiller unit had an 800-ton capacity, the other 600 tons. Either machine could comfortably cope with normal climatic conditions. Only on an exceptionally hot day were the chillers used in tandem.

It had already irritated Castelli that in this, of all years, the larger machine had repeatedly "played up." In May, Carrier servicemen stripped down the unit to repair its compressor, mend an oil line, and look for a leak of the machine's potentially dangerous refrigerant, R-11. When the work was completed, the chiller was recharged with the 1,400 pounds of R-11 that had been in the machine before repairs began. Early in June, Carrier was called in again. The servicemen this time detected a leak in the shaft seal of the same unit. Although the leak was considered excessive, the hotel management decided that, since the unit was still operable and the hot summer days were yet to come, any major repairs should be postponed. The Carrier employees added 400 pounds of R-11 to the machine and departed. On July 6 they were back, this time to carry out running repairs to the purge system of the faulty machine.

The possibility of further malfunctions nagged at the chef. In this weather a major breakdown in the hotel's cooling equipment could empty the Bellevue of guests and turn his kitchens into "Calcutta's Black Hole."

Castelli reached the staff locker room. As with much else in the basement, it could have benefited from painting. Yet the chef thought whatever money was available would be better spent on the public areas; here, in a world no guest ever visited, "a fresh lick of paint was not that important."

He changed into starched whites—trousers and jacket fresh daily from the hotel laundry—donned his matching white executive chef's hat, and walked into the main kitchen area. He paused, as he did every morning, to take a long, careful look at the activity before him.

Castelli commanded a hierarchy in which every man knew his role, and jealously guarded his reputation. When the executive chef was absent, the sous-chef, his chief assistant, ran the kitchen. Castelli could see him now, standing with the chef who was in charge of soups, vegetables, and egg and pasta dishes. The men were in animated discussion beside a double row of soup caldrons. Beyond, by the banks of ovens, the *rôtisseur*, the chef responsible for roasts and their garnishes and fried food, was stacking ribs of beef onto trays, which his assistants placed in the ovens. Along one wall the *poissonnier* and his staff were cleaning fish and preparing stocks and sauces.

On the other side of the kitchen, in a large area next to the bakery, the *pâtissier*, a man who had spent a lifetime pastry cooking, was overseeing his staff preparing desserts, ices, petits fours and pastry for all dishes. The *pâtissier* was the oldest man in the kitchen; age had taught him to be calm and unhurried. In contrast, the *saucier*, the chef with special responsibility for stocks, *roux*, and sauces for meat and other entrees, was as usual urging his assistants not to rush while at the same time telling them to work faster. The chef in charge of larders and produce, preparing raw food for others to cook and making pâtés, stuffings, cold sauces, and aspic, was supervising a team at the cold-collations station. For him, how a dish looked was just as important as how it tasted.

Castelli remembered one of the problems he had pondered walking down Broad Street. He would speak to the man in a moment. In the meantime he continued to watch, aware that his presence had been noted but equally conscious that this unhurried scrutiny afforded him the one overview he would get before he plunged into action.

For years these kitchens had satisfied the appetites of gourmets and the standards of some of the great chefs of Europe. Legend had it that Escoffier himself had helped to design the layout. In 1954, when the air-conditioning plant was installed, a substantial amount was spent on modernizing the kitchen. It was extended to cover virtually the entire width of the hotel; around its walls, doorways led off, to the five staff dining rooms, to the Bellevue Room buffet, to elevators serving the twenty-six banqueting suites, the ballroom, and the roof garden on the eighteenth floor.

The executive chef allowed himself a moment longer to savor the sound of a thousand meals under way: banging, chopping, and sawing; the clash of metal against metal, the rattle of stockpots, the unmistakable swish of blades being sharpened and of water pouring into great caldrons. And above it all, the crisp voice of the chef at the cold-collations station cutting through the broader accents of the men working there.

Castelli strode to the station and instructed the chef to include tomato wedges with those five hundred green salads; it would add a fraction to the cost of each plate, but the profit margin would still be acceptable.

He moved on through the kitchen, pausing by the bubbling crucibles of soup, sniffing and approving and listening to the increasingly animated discussion between the sous-chef and his colleague. Both were temperamental perfectionists with decided views on what made a good soup. Sometimes they clashed, their voices soaring above the kitchen clatter. When Castelli judged an argument had gone far enough, he interceded. Now there was no need for him to do so. The men were heatedly discussing the merits of various members of the Phillies baseball team.

Smiling broadly, Castelli continued his tour of the kitchen, pausing to watch the last tray of beef ribs stacked in an oven. The *rôtisseur* was already consulting with the *saucier* about the amount of gravy and other sauces he would require; the *saucier* relayed requests in an urgent voice to his assistant, the *commis-saucier*, who in turn barked out orders to *his* assistants. The nervous tension the *saucier* exuded was an acceptable part of the ambience that made the kitchen hum.

Castelli reached the fish preparation station. The *poissonnier*, a man trained to the standards of Prunier, had left his post to discuss with the *pâtissier* the quantity of pastry needed for the day's fish dishes. Castelli watched a couple of trainees at work. He noticed that in the absence of the *poissonnier* their speed dropped. He stepped forward, took up a spare knife, and with quick slashes topped and tailed a fish, cut it down the middle, and deftly scooped out its innards. The operation was done in half the time taken by the trainees. There was no need for Castelli to say anything. The youths began to work with new vigor. He moved on.

For the next thirty minutes Castelli observed lamb cutlets being trimmed and Spanish omelettes being prepared, tasted several sauces, watched the first of the *pâtissier*'s handiwork being loaded onto the dessert trolley, held a brief conference with the wine cellar steward, and told the *commis-rôtisseur* to check the temperature in the quadruple-unit deep fryer: if the fat became overheated, anything dipped in it would be spoiled.

In these and other ways Castelli showed his staff of ninety he was an excellent judge of their culinary capabilities. Further, he produced the sort of dishes that made the Bellevue's food superior in the city and probably the equal of that of any hotel in America. In the harshly commercial and often corner-cutting world of professional mass cooking, Castelli was a rarity. His only concern, never spoken of in his domain, was how much longer he would be allowed to practice his artistry unhampered.

A lifetime of experience in some of the best hotels in the country had taught the chef more about the business than most people in the industry. He now believed that at the Bellevue Stratford matters were more "delicately poised" than anybody "upstairs" cared to admit. "Upstairs" was the world of assistant managers, night managers, banquet managers, front-desk managers, advance reservations managers, cost account managers. Collectively they were known as "management," a team of smartly dressed men and women who answered directly to the hotel's general manager, Harold Varr, who in turn reported to William Chadwick, the aloof managing director of the hotel. Castelli respected both men, but he doubted he would ever really come to know Chadwick. Chadwick could distance himself from people. The perceptive chef suspected this was a defense mechanism, a means of concealing from everyone that Chadwick felt his hotel was walking the knife's edge between making a healthy profit during the Bicentennial and, afterward, with business falling off to what it had been before, being forced to sell out and become just another unit in some chain of hotels. That seemed the only explanation for the policy the managing director had ordered adopted.

Until recently, "upstairs" kept its collective nose out of Castelli's kingdom. One of the rules for successfully managing any large hotel was never to interfere with "downstairs," the cloistered world Castelli controlled with a firm and steady hand. This rule had recently been broken. Junior management had arrived unannounced asking for some economy or other. Castelli had so far politely rejected such requests. He did not, however, oppose the suggestion that a trainee be stationed to intercept all unused butter returned from the dining rooms: this perfectly good butter could still be used for cooking. The practice was common in most hotel kitchens. But Castelli saw the suggestion as another small but significant pointer, part of a steady cutting back, an extension of a policy of saving money where it was unnoticed, at least by the public.

The chef well understood the ever-increasing pressures that created the need for economies. Throughout America establishments like the Bellevue were losing ground to the big hotel chains. With their bulk buying and standardized service, the chains were able to hold down prices, operate on lower profit margins, and advertise more widely. Jealous of a reputation that placed it in the same category as the Plaza in New York, the Stanford Court in San Francisco, the George V in Paris, and the Savoy in London, to maintain standards the Bellevue had increased room rates and the price of its food and beverages. Rather than introduce further increases, Castelli suspected management would continue to "nibble back of house." That worried him: it could not be long before requests for economies in the kitchen changed into demands. Then what would he do?

Having checked the progress in every department, he now turned to his office. Completely glass-walled, it was a raised command post from which he could observe and intercede at once. As usual, this morning there was a pile of invoices for him to examine. Even the sharpest accountant was no match for Castelli; only after the most thorough examination did he pass a bill for payment.

He noted that prices were up a dime here, a cent there. It was the same almost every week, part of a growing inflation for which there seemed no answer. In the quantities Castelli ordered, these minuscule increases amounted to quite considerable sums. The fact was sure to attract attention "upstairs." He worked steadily through the pile, his eyes regularly pausing to look down on the kitchen. He saw nothing untoward. Finally he pushed aside proof copies of the luncheon menus, which had just been run off on the hotel's printing press. For the moment he could relax. Sipping another of the mugs of coffee that sustained him through the day, he pondered on what he had come to call "our mystery": why the Bellevue was finding it difficult to attract top-of-the-market conventions. Such conventions were the lifeblood of a hotel; the competition to capture them was fierce and often cutthroat. In the past the Bellevue had rarely had to tout for their business. If a topflight convention came to Philadelphia, it had been almost axiomatic it would be headquartered at the hotel. But while Philadelphia continued to attract its share of doctors, lawyers, accountants, and realtors' conventions, these gatherings now often gave the Bellevue a miss.

Castelli preferred not to think about the convention due to start in just two days' time, which would be headquartered in the hotel.

Virtually every available bedroom and hospitality suite had been booked by the American Legion. But except for a few small or basically "fast-food operations"—a continental breakfast for the delegates, a simple luncheon for the Legion chaplains—the veterans did not require the skills of the chef or his staff. More galling to Castelli, management had conceded to other of the legionnaires' demands. The veterans would be allowed to bring into the hotel their own food and cut-price liquor. They would not even require room service staff to run their hospitality suites; for the duration of the convention, legionnaires would act as unpaid, untipped barmen. Apart from keeping the hotel full—at the drastically reduced room rates the legionnaires also demanded—the Bellevue seemed set to gain little from this particular convention. Castelli felt management had, by booking it, made a serious mistake.

The possibility of a mistake of a far different kind was being pondered by Chinese-born Theodore Tsai in a near-silent room. He was sitting at a wooden desk in Auditorium B, the CDC's largest, surrounded by some thirty would-be epidemiologists like himself. Most were men and most were physicians, as he was. Each had completed at least one year of postgraduate training before being accepted for the EIS course. They were there to learn the principles of epidemiology, an inexact science based on a fundamental assumption: that diseases do not occur by chance and are not randomly distributed in the population. Already Tsai had learned that, above all, epidemiology required a special *way* of looking at illnesses. Therefore, after training, it could be practiced successfully not only by doctors but by engineers, statisticians, nurses, and even veterinarians. Many were represented in Tsai's class.

He turned again to a file, working steadily through it, aware that two of the many requirements for success in his new field were patience and perseverance. The twenty-seven-year-old from Nanking was well endowed with both. Perhaps he inherited such qualities from his father, who, when only a few years older than Tsai now was, had been a full general fighting alongside Chiang Kai-shek against the Communist take-over of China. By a strange quirk of fate, Tsai's father had grown up in the same village as Lin Piao, who later become one of the country's leaders. Tsai's father and his family were fortunate to escape from China alive; most of his near relatives who stayed behind had been killed.

A career in the military, which both his father and his great-grandfather, an admiral, had chosen, held no appeal for the younger Tsai. He had opted instead to fight disease. Here, at the CDC, he and his fellow students were now studying a number of actual case histories of past epidemics, learning through the experience of others, attempting to find fault with what previous investigators had done. Each of the files contained, amid a wealth of other material, two basic documents, known as EPI-1 and EPI-2. The first was a memorandum written to the CDC's director at the beginning of every outbreak investigation, briefly outlining the problem. EPI-2, a much fuller document again addressed to the center's director, was prepared a few months after each investigation was over and described in detail the findings of the epidemiologists.

Among the various outbreaks Tsai was looking at, one of the more intriguing was that dealing with Lassa fever, which had helped establish the reputation of the man he was going to work for, David Fraser. He knew it would be hard to pick holes in Fraser's fieldwork.

Tsai barely knew the senior epidemiologist, but Fraser's style of investigating seemed to be stamped on the outbreak: there was the careful way he and his colleagues collated and studied the data, analyzing it for relationships that suggested the likeliest source of the epidemic, and then the disciplined scientific methodology to confirm, or reject, a hypothesis. More than once their efforts had been frustrated; they had gone back and tried again, seeking for new clues, for confirmation of the theory that the virus causing the outbreak was carried by an animal —and if so, which? At each crucial stage of the investigation, it was clear from the file, Fraser had never lost his essential sense of balance, proportion, and objectivity.

Even now, in the air-conditioned comfort of the CDC lecture theater, Tsai could sense the danger and tension Fraser and his fellow epidemiologists had faced in that lonely Catholic hospital deep in the

African forest, working in dark and sodden conditions resulting from the hundred or more inches of rain that fell in the area each year. It was all there in the neatly typed case history, a supreme story of medical detection and personal bravery. When Fraser arrived in Sierra Leone, the highly contagious fever was on the rampage: of the sixty-four cases in one hospital, twenty-three persons had already died agonizing and fearful deaths. With great courage, working sixteen-hour days, Fraser and the other researchers were sometimes out tramping the rain forest as part of their potentially dangerous rodent-trapping attempts; sometimes seeing patients, when they would always be surgically capped and gowned; sometimes in the laboratory, where they wore hot, clammy respirators over their mouths to protect them from the lethal virus. It was feared that if the outbreak was allowed to spread, it might decimate the population of an area the size of Britain or even the southern states of America.

The investigation took Fraser and a colleague away from their African base to London, to carry out tests on missionaries who had once worked in Sierra Leone. Suddenly Fraser's friend, a young doctor Tsai's own age, was taken seriously ill with symptoms of Lassa fever. The contingency plan the CDC had formulated for just such an emergency was put into action; a USAF transport jet flew to London carrying the Apollo moonshot isolation capsule, originally designed to prevent an astronaut's returning to Earth with some deadly alien virus from space. Close to death, the patient was placed inside the module and flown back across the Atlantic to Columbia Presbyterian Medical Center, New York City, then the only hospital in the world with the necessary experience to treat Lassa fever.

While his colleague recovered, Fraser continued to study the former missionaries from Africa as part of the epidemiological search for the fever's vector—the carrier of the disease.

Tsai was stirred not only by the sheer drama of the story; the politics of medicine—to be observed in Africa as everywhere else—required that considerable diplomatic skill be demonstrated by Fraser and the others as the CDC team followed trails that led them through the African bush, to Britain, and eventually back to the center's laboratories in Atlanta. There, in the "hot lab"—a maximum-security laboratory in another part of the huge complex in which Tsai now sat—the Lassa fever virus was at last isolated in tissue cultures from a particular species of rat that had been trapped by the CDC team in Sierra Leone and shipped to the center. Later came the long, involved process of developing a vaccine.

News of the breakthrough had flashed across the medical world. Even now, three years later, Tsai could only marvel at the triumph. In many ways it was a classic investigation, which demonstrated all the epidemiological skills that he was spending this July acquiring. Even in high school, Tsai had wanted to be a disease detective; he was drawn to the CDC because of a growing idealistic desire to serve in public health. His years at medical school, the tough period after qualification as an intern, when he had learned more about real decision-making than during all the time he had spent poring over textbooks, had been preparation for the point where he now was.

Tsai's excellent medical qualifications made him a promising CDC candidate. And back in April, after the highly competitive selection process for the EIS course, Tsai was flattered when Fraser chose him for one of the sought-after places in Special Pathogens.

The EIS course was proving as tough and demanding as Tsai had expected. There was no room for second-guessing, taking a flier, or relying on some gut reaction to suggest treatment, as physicians in private practice were sometimes prone to do. The way Fraser and his colleagues had worked on Lassa fever in the field showed how it must be done: in part, by utilizing a combination of the biological sciences—chemistry and biology allied to some psychology—and the behavioral sciences—sociology, social psychology, and anthropology. A sound knowledge of mathematics and calculus had also been helpful for the statistical evaluations.

Tsai was quietly confident that his own qualifications—a good degree in chemistry and two years of medical internship and residency at the demanding Johns Hopkins Hospital in Baltimore—provided a solid base for a future in epidemiology.

But only in these past two weeks had Tsai come to appreciate fully the many other demands of the job.

One after another, veteran EIS officers had lectured the class on such diverse subjects as rabies, venereal diseases, cancer and birth defects, zoonoses (diseases transmitted from animals to humans), enteric diseases. There had also been seminars on the structure of the World Health Organization and the Food and Agriculture Organization of the United Nations; the CDC worked closely with both agencies. There had been talks on how to handle the media, state and city health departments, private doctors and nurses—almost anybody who might have a stake or emotional interest in an outbreak. Warnings had been given about the pitfalls of becoming involved in regional hospital politics, of siding with one faction against another. There was a lecture on how to operate abroad, how to persuade an African or Arab medical practitioner, steeped in local lore, that the judgment of a CDC epidemiologist as to the source, means of spread, and method of coping with an outbreak was sound. And implicit in every lecture was the reminder that theirs was sometimes highly dangerous work in which hardship was routine and expected.

Try as he might, Tsai found it difficult to fault the various steps followed in the Lassa fever investigation. It perfectly exemplified the description of epidemiology as a thought process, a special way of looking at something baffling and deciding what was normal and what should be considered out of the ordinary.

Tsai also learned that the CDC took a pragmatic approach to the broad role it assumed; highest priority went to problems that appeared capable of cure or prevention. Perhaps that was the reason the swine flu team was still on full alert four months after the National Influenza Immunization Program had been launched—and run into flak. Nowadays the CDC was filled with talk about the calculated gamble its director, David Sencer, had taken in selling hard the idea that the United States, and possibly the world, was threatened by a second great pandemic. Tsai could not know whether Sencer was right, but he had a sneaking suspicion that if he himself was somehow swallowed into the program, his work after the course would be pure drudgery.

At the moment, that seemed unlikely to happen. Just as Tsai had been singled out for Special Pathogens, two others on the EIS course had already been earmarked for swine flu surveillance. One, a dentist from Philadelphia, Philip Graitcer, stood out in the class because of the plaster cast on his foot; he had broken it July 4 while running in Atlanta's annual Peachtree road race.

Although similarly athletic in build—Tsai moved with catlike agility despite shoulders that seemed much too wide for his slim frame—he was far too busy is his off-duty hours to take part in outdoor sports. Married less than a month ago, he and his young American bride, Sherry, a pretty red-haired nurse whom he had met at Johns Hopkins, had just moved into their new home in Atlanta. Tsai's every spare moment was spent helping to clean and decorate the house. In the evenings, as he carefully brushed on coats of emulsion, he could not but ponder how long it would be after he joined David Fraser before he was called away from home; most CDC epidemiologists spent an average of a week away every month and considerably longer when on overseas assignment.

Tsai had chosen a career which, a senior EIS officer warned, was hard on domestic bliss. It was also hard on the leg muscles. That was why, at the end of the course, Tsai could expect to receive a diploma bordered by worn-out shoe soles—the insignia of the elite corps he would be joining. It would be his passport into a world few outsiders realized existed.

What Tsai did not know was that David Fraser was still as far away as ever from finding an outbreak for him to work on. It was becoming almost as big a headache for the chief of Special Pathogens as some of the problems he had faced with Lassa fever.

J.B. awoke late on Monday, hung over from the long night at the Williamstown post. After his war dance there had been a good deal of horseplay during which somebody had written on his skull in lipstick: KOJAK. The letters were smeared but still readable when he looked in the bathroom mirror. He soaped his head and began to scrub them off, rubbing so hard he made the skin bleed. He poured after-shave on the cuts. When the pain eased he inspected his scalp. The lipstick was gone but he noticed hair bristles were sprouting. He lathered and shaved his head, cutting himself in several places. He poured on more lotion, causing him to yell loud enough to bring his mother hurrying to the bathroom. She rubbed soothing cream on his skull until it glistened like a pinball.

Later, in the kitchen, she reacted as he knew she would: she carefully examined his shaven head, then gave him a smile that was puzzled yet forgiving. She offered no criticism over what he had done.

Instead, she quietly suggested he telephone Carol in a last attempt to persuade his ex-wife to let their sons accompany him to the convention. The matter had not been discussed for some days, but it was still uppermost in his mother's mind. She reminded him again of the time and money he had already expended: there were the stand tickets he had bought for the Phillies game on Wednesday night, the suite in the Holiday Inn he had reserved for the boys and himself, the sightseeing tours he had planned to Valley Forge and other historic landmarks and museums. He had done everything, she insisted, to try to be a good father. He must not give up, not now. He should call Carol.

J.B. hesitated. He remembered what had happened a couple of weeks previously when he unveiled all these preparations to his sons. They had stood awkwardly on the doorstep of Carol's new home in Harrisburg; after listening politely the boys declined to go to Philadelphia, saying they already had other plans. He pressed them hard to explain what could possibly be more important. Carol had suddenly appeared, her eyes brushing past him with dislike. She reacted sharply, saying the children had made their decision. J.B. did not realize until then just how much real hatred remained beneath the surface in Carol.

His mother maintained there was nothing to lose. He should still telephone Carol.

J.B. gave in.

Together they considered what he would say. Occasionally she prompted him, making sure he did not neglect any point in his favor. He smiled at her then, and she blushed with pleasure, as she always did when he showed her affection.

He reached Carol late in the afternoon, trying to sound calm and relaxed and to keep the tightness from his voice. Carol was distant and

factual. The boys had not changed their minds. She would not interfere. J.B. felt left with nothing to say. His mother whispered reminders
of the points they had so carefully rehearsed.

He began again, remembering those times when Carol had matched
him in vocal strength, delivering stinging verbal, and sometimes physical, blows. He told her he just wanted his sons to come with him to
Philadelphia. They would enjoy it.

She repeated they were not going.

J.B. felt the blood suffusing his skin. Carol's voice—as with so many
of his thoughts, he shared this one later with his mother—reminded
him of all the rejections that had helped destroy their marriage. He responded in the only way he knew: he began shouting. It was the excuse
Carol wanted.

She hung up.

J.B. looked at the telephone, thinking of everything he should have
said. He hated himself for his loss of self-control.

His mother stared anxiously at him. She was not given to displaying
emotion. People spoke of her dignity, her resolve, her fortitude. Never,
not even at the funeral of her husband, had she been seen weeping
openly. Mrs. Ralph wanted to cry now, to release the sorrow dammed
up inside her. No one, not even her beloved J.B., knew the pain she
felt, the effort she had made since his divorce to try and reorder his life.
Often she wanted to tell him that Carol had always been like this, but
that he had been so much in love, and perhaps still was, that he could
not see her as she was, could not spot those "little differences" which
finally doomed their marriage. Instead she merely took his hand and
held it between hers, squeezing it maternally, the way she had done
when he was a child.

J.B. was silent. His spirit was broken. He finally had to accept that
he would not have his boys with him in Philadelphia. He began slowly
to pull himself together. He would not go to the convention. He would
cancel the hotel suite and give the baseball tickets away. Still in
thought, he left his mother and walked the short distance to the door
leading to the "professional" part of the house: the mortuary. The
sight that met him as he opened the door brought his mind abruptly
back to the present. Stretched out on a cart was the body of a
woman. Mortician Dale Hoover was at work on the corpse, preparing it
for viewing.

Hoover was a big, bluff man, fortyish, with surprisingly lively eyes for
a person who made a living handling the dead. He saw himself as a
grief specialist and memorial counselor, an undertaker who used the
very latest in technology and know-how to help him create a more lifelike appearance in corpses than did most other funeral merchants.

He paused in his work to give J.B. his full attention. Along with a firm handshake and sincere voice, his look of concentration was a Hoover characteristic, instilled in him well before he graduated from a college of mortuary sciences. He had also learned there that bald men presented a special problem for an embalmer because their scalp skin often wrinkled after death, creating what was known in the trade as a "gnomish syndrome." Purely from a "professional standpoint," Hoover thought J.B.'s scalp was the "sort of mess" even an expert would find challenging. He wondered what had prompted J.B. to remove his hair. Hoover knew better than to ask; long ago J.B. made it clear their friendship did not give the undertaker the right to probe. When J.B. explained the purpose of his call was to offer the baseball tickets, Hoover politely refused them, explaining he had a number of funerals to prepare, and then resumed shampooing the hair of the woman lying on the preparation table. Within easy reach were the jars of Avon cosmetics which over the years Hoover had found gave the best results for the "healthy sleeping look" that had helped to make his local reputation.

J.B. walked out of the funeral home and offered the tickets to the first person he met. The man said he couldn't afford to go to Philadelphia just to see a ball game.

J.B.'s pent-up emotions finally broke through. He tore the tickets in pieces, scattering the bits on the street, stamping on them, all the time cursing Carol.

That was when Jimmy saw him. It was early evening when he drove into town, his cold still bothering him in spite of the proprietary medicine Doris insisted he took whenever he developed a sniffle. Normally Jimmy returned from work much earlier, but this time he had stopped in Pottsville to purchase two new suits, a brown and a blue, with shirts and ties to match. He planned to wear the brown suit to the convention and keep the blue worsted for his marriage to Doris. The shopping spree had been her idea; she had virtually ordered him to withdraw $200 from his savings to make the purchases. Jimmy had used some of the money to buy her a present, a bottle of perfume, and toys for the children. And on impulse, he had also bought J.B. something. The day had been a particularly happy one because Jimmy had patched up his argument with Dicko over Doris. While his cousin had not actually gone so far as to say he would be best man at the wedding, he had agreed to reconsider the question after the convention. Jimmy had been satisfied and listened noncommittally while Dicko spent the rest of their lunch break at the Fort Indiantown Gap army base, where Dicko worked as an administrator, talking about the "exciting time" a bachelor could have at the convention. On the long drive home Jimmy wondered how he could convince Dicko he did not want an "exciting time" in Philadelphia, that he had all the excitement he wanted in his

relationship with Doris. The sight of J.B. shambling in the dust interrupted his thoughts. He gunned forward the car and moments later
was listening gravely to J.B.'s reason for his behavior.

When J.B. had finished, Jimmy solemnly handed him a small gift
box. Inside was a button. Printed on its face was: BALD IS BEAUTIFUL.
EVERYBODY LOVES YOU.

They laughed. J.B. put on the badge and got into the car. Still laughing, Jimmy drove them to the post.

Dicko was already at the bar, relaxed and cheerful, glad the rift with
Jimmy was healed and privately optimistic that the convention would
produce at least one "nice Irish girl" able to attract his cousin's attention. When J.B. said he would not be going, that he was canceling his
rooms at the Holiday Inn, Dicko quickly interrupted him, saying he
could stay with Jimmy and himself in the post's official suite at the inn.
During the convention the suite would be a "command center," the
place where Dicko and the other Williamstown delegates would make
their final decisions on how to cast the post's six hundred votes. It was
going to be like old times, enthused Dicko, all three of them under one
roof, politicking and making whoopee.

J.B. was carried away by Dicko's enthusiasm. He would go.

The harmony they all now felt was not only over the prospect of
what lay ahead, but also within themselves. The three men had never
been closer to each other than they were on this night.

It was Jimmy who introduced a sobering note. He said a man in his
section at work had learned from a friend in the FBI office in Philadelphia that both the Bureau and "spooks from the CIA" would be
keeping the convention under surveillance in case of attacks by
members of the counterculture. According to Jimmy's source, guerrilla
units from a Puerto Rican "liberation" organization and sympathizers
from the Palestinian Liberation Organization were among those said to
be converging on Philadelphia.

Unknown to anyone, a far deadlier enemy was already in the city.

3

Expectation

When the bedside telephone rang on the morning of Tuesday, July 20, William Chadwick knew it was precisely seven-thirty.

Barring some emergency that the night manager could not have handled alone—a fire, sudden death, or robbery—the chief executive of the Bellevue Stratford was awakened every weekday morning at this time in the master bedroom of the spacious staff apartment he and his wife, Pat, had lived in for the past five years. It was on the hotel's eighth floor and provided Chadwick with panoramic views of a city he loved almost as much as his wife and children.

He was sixty years old, with an expression that reminded people of Jack Benny. Broad-jowled, high-colored, with receding hair, he almost always looked gentle, like a person who enjoyed seeing others happy— which was true. He appeared rather bland only to those who did not notice that the eyes behind his glasses were invariably alert and penetrating; rival hoteliers regarded him as one of the shrewdest managers in the industry.

Chadwick was equally honest, stubborn, and uncompromising. He disguised these and other strong traits behind the kind of face that made it easy for him to smile. It was a useful prerequisite for all the positions he now held.

As well as supervising the Bellevue Stratford's operations, he was vice-president of the hotel division of Bankers Security, the corporation that held a controlling interest in the Bellevue and Philadelphia's other large luxury hotel, the Benjamin Franklin. Chadwick was also vice-president of the local council for tourism, president of the city's hotel association, a director of the Convention and Visitors Bureau, chair-

man of the Civic Center, and a member of the International Hotel
Greeters Association, the Friendly Sons of St. Patrick, and the Cardinal's Committee on the Laity. In addition he somehow found time
to be chairman of the Philadelphia Catholic Charities division and to
preside over the city's Catholic Philopatrian Literary Institute.

In a city of transient managers of chain hotels, he was a likable, old-
fashioned innkeeper, maintaining a high profile, mixing at all levels,
and ever vigilant for the opportunity to steer business his way.

Asked once by a fawning columnist for the secret of successfully coping with such a variety of interests, he replied: an accurate wristwatch.
Like all *bons mots*, it contained a good deal of truth. Chadwick was a
stickler for punctuality. Proper timekeeping, he would firmly inform a
new assistant manager or dining room captain, helped uphold the hotel's high reputation. And proper timekeeping included on-time wake-
up calls.

Years before, Chadwick discovered a file containing numerous complaints from guests saying they were awakened at the wrong time. For
some reason nothing had been done to remedy the situation. He spent
several early mornings in the hotel's telephone exchange, which was
tucked away in a corner of the seventeenth floor, its door—numbered
1708 as though for just another bedroom—kept locked as a precaution
against any amorous guest seeking to put a face, or body, to one of the
dulcet-voiced operators. The women who worked the graveyard shift—
the lonely stretch from midnight until 8 A.M. when the hotel was at its
quietest, the switchboard disturbed only by occasional demands for
room service or by businessmen making calls abroad—were suddenly
plunged into activity between seven and eight o'clock, the time
requested for 80 percent of wake-up calls. Expert though they were, the
women often fell behind schedule; to try to keep up, they called some
rooms earlier than ordered. Even then, by the end of the shift, some
guests had still not been roused. Chadwick immediately solved the
problem by adding an operator during the crucial period. It increased
the overall wage bill, but it also protected the hotel's reputation, of
which he was fiercely and almost boyishly proud.

This morning there was not enough work to keep the switchboard
women busy. Once more the Bellevue was less than full.

The operator informed Chadwick it looked like being another hot
day. He knew that meant the air-conditioning system would have to be
kept running continuously. He just hoped there would be no more
breakdowns. He already had enough problems. Nobody would have
guessed as much; it was second nature for Chadwick to present a
relaxed front. It was both a strength and a weakness.

If Chadwick was the very visible apex of a management team that
executive chef Castelli collectively called "upstairs," then Harold Varr,
the immensely experienced and capable general manager, was the firm

—although not always velvet-gloved—hand on the daily pulse of the hotel. Varr had been at the Pierre in New York, where he acquired a sharp eye for the food and beverage reports. At the Bellevue Stratford he watched over some thirty separate departments as well as chairing sales meetings, food forecast meetings, room forecast meetings, payroll meetings, and staff meetings. He also handled the unions and the leases for the hotel's concessionaires—Eastern Airlines, the newsstand, gift shop, and hairdressing salons. When he wasn't taking a meeting, he was scrutinizing daily expenditure on a dozen fronts: bed linens, food, drink, towels, light bulbs, flatware, napery, paper, radios, television sets, uniforms, cleaning fluids; he approved work schedules for the squads of staff carpenters, upholsterers, seamstresses, and painters who ran the continuous hotel maintenance program.

Chadwick appreciated Varr's painstaking thoroughness. It left him time to plan overall strategy for the hotel's future. Yet, unexpectedly, in one area this led to disagreement with Varr. It arose over a point of fundamental policy: advance bookings.

Months before, Varr had urged adoption of the policy of "book everything" as far ahead as possible. Chadwick differed, arguing that in this bicentennial year it was preferable to keep a number of rooms vacant for last-minute bookings by "people of the nation" come to visit their country's birthplace of independence. Chadwick thought this not only a patriotic duty but good public relations: it would bring return business.

Varr, a veteran of the 1964–65 World's Fair in New York, maintained that a similar policy had been tried then by Manhattan hoteliers —and failed because the predicted number of visitors to the city did not materialize.

Chadwick had remained confident he would be proved correct. But in fact the Bellevue's July takings were 15 percent below expectations. Even so, the hotel looked set to make a healthy annual profit for the first time in years. Its future and that of its five hundred employees did not depend on Varr's "book everything" policy but more on a different strategy—one the energetic Varr entirely approved of. The Bellevue Stratford was going after convention business as never before.

Already fifty conventions had registered for this fall, and a further one hundred and fifty were scheduled for 1977. Chadwick suspected that, unlike Varr, not all the staff would look upon this with favor. Conventioneers, especially those who attended gatherings in the summer, were often poor tippers; many delegates were on fixed incomes and preferred to eat out in one of the fast-food cafés in the area rather than spend a large portion of their weekly salary dining in the hotel's Stratford Garden restaurant or Burgundy Room.

Equally, Chadwick knew, if the hotel was to prosper, an average of six hundred rooms a day must be let; a regular flow of conventions would ensure this happened. The fact the hotel was now linked to Hilton's international reservation system had created unease in those staff who saw the move as part of a plan to sell out. No amount of denials from Chadwick could stifle the rumor. A stream of conventions would be seen in those quarters as a further sign that the hotel was going deliberately mass-market, in preparation for the day when it would be absorbed in some chain and become just another ship in a quality-controlled fleet of hostelries where everything, including the service, was kept to a conveyor-belt minimum: just enough to satisfy, never to excel, where profits and politeness were uneasy bedfellows.

Accepting the American Legion had not made it easier for Chadwick to convince doubters about the desirability of conventions. But his decision to allow the veterans to run their own hospitality suites and bring in their own food and liquor was a pragmatic one. He had carefully weighed the financial return from a guaranteed full house for three nights against the legionnaires' demands. Yet even Castelli, in Chadwick's opinion the best chef the hotel had employed for many years, was reproachful over the coming convention. The chef disguised his feelings with a wry joke about giving the kitchen staff a vacation during the time the veterans were installed. Chadwick just smiled.

Now, on this Tuesday morning, he could be forgiven if he hoped a further opportunity would soon present itself for him to explain to Castelli why the legionnaires were so important. After putting on one of the smart summer-weight suits that made him possibly the best-dressed hotelier in Philadelphia, Chadwick paused, as he did every morning, to catch the national news headlines on "Today."

President Ford was still under attack for pardoning President Nixon. In spite of opposition, the Administration was going to sell enriched uranium to India. A new sex-in-politics scandal had broken in Washington. The kidnapping and underground entombment of twenty-six California children and their school bus driver continued to attract attention. The local TV news showed mounds of garbage bags piled up in Philadelphia's streets. The slowdown was in its twenty-third day. A reporter standing before one rotting heap of refuse stated that if the dispute was not resolved quickly, there could be a hazard from disease-carrying rats. Chadwick feared that such scary reporting not only would keep tourists away but could be disastrous for the hotel: he doubted anybody would want to stay in a $50-a-day room—let alone the $175-a-day Presidential Suite—and risk running into rodents on the sidewalk.

As he listened to the news, he could be thankful for one thing. There was no mention of an alarming report the house detective had picked up from his contacts in the Philadelphia Police Department. During the Legion convention, plainclothes officers planned to keep the hotel under observation in case of any terrorist action. The local

FBI office would also have agents on hand and, it was rumored, the CIA had men available to point out foreign subversives.

Worrying though the prospect was of an attack by the counterculture, Chadwick was not surprised by the idea. Since the end of May the city's colorful mayor, Frank Rizzo, a tough-talking former policeman and political ally of Nixon's, had been issuing dire warnings on the danger. Rizzo had even requested that President Ford put 15,000 armed troops in the city for the Fourth of July weekend to "help deter and defuse the violence which may occur." Rizzo had claimed that "leftist radicals" were planning an outrage in the city and that his police commissioner had "extensive documentation which includes the magnitude of the threat."

Philadelphia's City Representative Albert Gaudiosi—the former Pulitzer Prize–winning journalist credited with masterminding Rizzo's rise to power—had insisted this was not another of Rizzo's headline-grabbing stunts.

After the FBI office in the city made urgent inquiries, the Justice Department refused to send in the troops. And Pennsylvania's governor, Milton Shapp, no friend of the mayor, rejected Rizzo's appeal to mobilize the National Guard.

The Fourth of July had passed without incident.

But the fear in City Hall that "radicals" might still strike remained as strong as ever.

On the eve of the Legion convention, it took on a new guise. Around the mayor's office, people reminded each other that back in May a supply of poison gas was reported stolen from a Maryland army depot. A strong rumor surfaced that "if you're going to hit America, you hit apple pie and Mom, and what's closer to Mom than the American Legion? If you're antiwar and antimilitary, who else to hit but veterans?"

That disturbing thought spawned another. It would be simple to introduce poison gases—invisible and odorless—into the presence of the veterans: it could be fed through the air-conditioning system of their hotels; it could be sprayed from innocent-looking fly-swat aerosols.

The possibility of such an attack was another worry to add to all the others that now beset Chadwick.

Yet as he breakfasted with Pat, he gave no sign of concern. Long ago, when they were first married and before the children were born— two sons and three daughters—he made a firm rule that breakfast was "family," a time for domestic chitchat when the cares of running a grand hotel could be forgotten for a period. But by eight-thirty, exactly on schedule, they returned. It was time for Chadwick to go to work. He kissed Pat good-bye and stepped out of the apartment. It might be midnight before he came back.

Far below the carpeted corridor along which Chadwick was walking, in the noisy and cavernous subbasement of the hotel that he rarely visited, an employee he had never met was on the verge of setting into motion a sequence of events that Chadwick would not learn about for some days.

The Bellevue's air-conditioner repairman was checking in for work. In the well-ordered hotel hierarchy, the twenty-six-year-old repairman was near the bottom. His duties were to adjust thermostats in rooms, check the air-conditioning units on each floor, and occasionally clean them with aerosols filled with petroleum distillates and chlorinated hydrocarbons. He had worked at the hotel for four months, was married, with two small children, aged four and three. Apart from that, nobody knew much about him.

Unlike many of the legionnaires who would soon be in the hotel, the repairman had seen active service in Vietnam; in 'Nam he had witnessed how effective America's chemical warfare agents had been in poisoning the countryside.

Such thoughts were undoubtedly far from his mind this particular morning. He was feeling increasingly unwell; he had a headache, body aches, a cough, a feeling of oncoming sinusitis, and a fever.

In some ways his symptoms fitted swine flu. To a doctor they might still have been vague enough only to suggest the beginning of a more common flu. But in the basement there was no physician on hand to order him to bed or to attempt to determine what exactly made him feel so sick. Instead the young repairman began his day's work.

Most mornings Anna Taggart, the hotel's chief elevator operator, arranged for her cage to reach the eighth floor just as Chadwick pressed the request button. It was a running joke they both enjoyed.

This morning he smiled but said nothing as Anna sent the elevator ascending to the eighteenth floor at the rate of seven hundred feet a minute. A reporter once calculated she traveled close to sixty miles between floors on a busy shift. Judging by today's traffic, she guessed she would be lucky to have covered twenty miles by the end of her stint.

Anna Taggart was sixty years old and had spent forty-two of them working in the hotel. She had been in charge of the elevators since 1941 and had met more celebrities than any other employee. A short, pert woman—with a flashing wit to match her Irish temper—Anna was renowned for what some staff looked upon as "old-fashioned loyalty" to the Bellevue; any employee who dared to criticize its standards or its guests in her presence could expect a salty dressing-down. She feared nobody and was regarded with awe even by senior management, who long ago had given her a free hand in her domain. Her and Chadwick's relationship was one of mutual respect.

Yet his eyes this Tuesday morning offered the highly observant Anna a clue that all might not be well. She wondered whether the rumor she'd heard earlier was true.

Mary, one of the night elevator women, had picked up the tidbit from the late-shift desk clerk and was bursting with the news when Anna walked into the sixteenth-floor room where the hotel's twenty-six elevator women changed into their blue and white uniforms.

Before Mary imparted her news, Anna had sharply reminded her she was breaking a strict rule. Anna steadfastly insisted all her team took off their skirts as soon as they entered the room to preserve the freshly ironed appearance of their dress. Only when Mary was in her panties was she allowed to continue.

Her news deeply worried Anna. She immediately told all the girls not to discuss the matter further until she obtained clarification.

From the day she started work in the hotel, Anna had been taught never to speak while on duty to any guest or superior unless they first spoke to her. But this morning, ignoring the stricture, she asked Chadwick whether there was any truth in the story that he was about to install automatic elevators, making her and the other women redundant.

Chadwick shook his head, promising that as long as the hotel stood its elevators would be manned.

Anna relaxed—and silently vowed she would give Mary a talking-to for listening to gossip.

As the cage reached the hotel's top floor, Chadwick posed a question for Anna: what did she feel about conventions?

The sprightly elevator operator did not hesitate. Borrowing a line Bob Hope once tossed at her on his way to a fund-raising function, she told Chadwick that as long as guests went up and came down sober, she did not mind who they were.

Still chuckling, Chadwick stepped out onto the roof garden to begin an impromptu tour of the hotel.

The regular daily inspections were carried out by Varr, but once in a while Chadwick liked to conduct his own walk-through. It provided him with the chance to prod and peer into corners, to remind everyone he would tolerate no lowering of standards. He knew it was a matter of pride among employees that he rarely found anything to complain of, even in those recesses where the public never ventured.

Nevertheless, Chadwick also knew some employees were involved in whole-scale thieving. It was no longer only flatware, napery, glassware, or food being pilfered. An expensive television set had gone from a suite, a crate of Bellevue sterling silver flatware had been spotted at the city airport—being air-freighted to Puerto Rico. A hide armchair had mysteriously disappeared overnight from a public room. A couple of paintings had vanished from a bedroom wall.

It was another worry for Chadwick. He wondered how much longer he could put off calling in the police—and the risk of unwelcome publicity that would follow.

Yet as he made his inspection round, pausing for a word with a housekeeper, spot-checking how a recently vacated bedroom was being readied for the next guest, he was heartened by the response to a repeated question: the majority of staff *would* welcome more convention business.

A valet—looking like a hobo with his bundle of dirty linen—a person Chadwick had always thought taciturn, was positively voluble in his enthusiasm, saying he had been much entertained by many of the seventeen hundred amateur magicians who had recently used the hotel as their conference headquarters. A passing steward pointed out that the one hundred candlemakers actually holding their convention now in the Bellevue had caused no trouble at all; some of them had even handed staff souvenirs of their products as presents. An elderly room maid who had prepared the beds of minor royalty was no less enthusiastic: beds, she said, were great levelers; one body was very like another. Her sagacity brought another smile from Chadwick.

Only a room service waiter, a gaunt and aged man stooped from years of wheeling tables along the hotel's corridors, pondered Chadwick's question and then shook his head. Many conventioneers were not only poor tippers but also capricious in their orders, often telephoning for a soft drink and a couple of buckets of free ice to go with the liquor they had brought into the hotel, sending a waiter back to get more coffee, sugar, or butter, and at the end of it all giving a tip of only a few cents. There were also the jokers, the ones who thought it was fun to ring down for a large order in the name of some other guest and wait for the inevitable explosion as a hapless waiter tried to deliver a trolley full of expensive food and drink to somebody who had not ordered it.

Chadwick was confident nothing like this would happen during the very special proceedings due to begin the week after the legionnaires had departed. Then the hotel would be headquarters for the International Eucharistic Congress, when around a million Catholics and other Christians would bring ecumenism—and a welcome boost to bicentennial business—to the city. President Ford, Prince Rainier of Monaco, and his wife, Philadelphia's own elegant Grace Kelly, would convene in the hotel, together with archbishops, cardinals, and Mother Teresa. Then would be the time for Chadwick to argue with considerable truth that the Bellevue was still the Philadelphia hotel of choice for the famous and influential. It would be this sort of occasion he hoped to attract in greater numbers in future.

It was an optimistic view. But all his working life Chadwick had been an optimist.

Optimism, alas, would offer no defense against what was about to happen. Nothing known on earth at this time would afford protection from the assassin lurking invisibly nearby.

By 10 A.M. the air-conditioner repairman was too ill to continue work. He was barely able to make the journey home before falling fitfully into bed.

Late that morning she chose the name she would assume for the next four days—Maria Reeves, after her favorite singer, the late Jim Reeves. That settled, the tall, olive-skinned twenty-four-year-old packed her dresses and suits into an expensive leather suitcase. Next she checked the contents of a smaller case. This was her "work bag." It contained, among other items, a selection of crotchless panties, several false penises, a copious quantity of lubricating gel, a pair of riding boots covered with erotic artwork, and a riding crop.

Her skills in using them had, in the past five years, made their owner a wealthy woman.

She had been fourteen when she performed her first trick, for a dollar, in Memphis, her hometown. Her uncle had paid the money in quarters; for a year she had visited him in his room and performed various acts of fellatio. Then somebody talked; she had been hauled off to court and forced to describe the visits in detail. Her uncle was put away for a year and Maria sentenced to a spell in a correction home. Six weeks later she ran away to New York, fell into the hands of a pimp, got busted a score of times, and was eventually jailed.

After her third stretch in prison, she had, on impulse, taken a train to Philadelphia, where she met a hooker who introduced her to a local call-girl circuit. Maria had soon learned to dress and speak to attract an up-market clientele. Eventually she had enough money to work when and where she liked.

Six months ago she had fallen seriously ill with pneumonia. Recovery had been a slow and painful business. High medical bills and an expensive convalescence in the Rocky Mountains had seriously depleted her savings.

She had decided to start replenishing them by working the American Legion convention. She anticipated that a gathering of "raunchy veterans on the loose" would be eager to pay her price.

Maria had no intention of enticing them off the street; she intended to move in among them. She had already reserved a room in the Bellevue for the purpose. Working carefully from there, she thought she could surpass her previous record of $600 earned during one twenty-four-hour stint. At $50 a trick it would mean hooking thirteen customers a day. Maria did not foresee any problems in meeting that target.

With a flash of the irritation that put a flinty edge on his personality, David Fraser switched off the lunchtime news, cutting in midsentence an update on the wrangling over the swine flu immunization program. Nowadays, he complained to Barbara—the striking brunette he had married when he was still in medical school and who was now seated across the luncheon table coaxing their two small children to eat —the media seemed to have nothing better to do than to criticize the CDC.

Barbara's laughter defused his anger; with the same directness she applied to her law studies, she asked him what he expected: all federal agencies were fair game for the media.

Fraser smiled, his good humor restored.

He treasured these moments when the whole family was together. They helped make up for the periods when work took him away, often for weeks at a time. For Barbara, he suspected his absences in the future would be made that much more bearable by her recently begun law course. It was something she had been planning for years. Now that the children were of school age, she meant to begin pursuing an independent career. They both recognized this was important. Barbara was a strong-willed young woman. The marriage of the well-matched couple was cemented by an uncommon respect and trust, a sharing of experience and a total lack of professional competition between them.

It was rare for either to allow their work to intrude upon family life. But it was equally hard to ignore the question implicit in the newscast that had triggered Fraser's annoyance: was there really a crisis over swine flu?

Fraser knew there was a rift within the CDC probably deeper than even the most perceptive reporter had guessed. Many bureau directors and division heads, as well as the chiefs of specialist units like his own, were privately harboring growing doubts about not only whether swine flu was, in fact, about to sweep the country, but whether it made any sense even to think of a national immunization campaign. Those uncertainties were now beginning to be reflected by a captious press with its questions about the safety and efficacy of the proposed vaccine; there was talk in the media of possibly serious side effects, especially among children. Fraser felt some of the reporting was ill-informed scaremongering, but the very real problem of liability insurance remained. On this July 20 the casualty insurance industry had still not found anyone willing to insure the manufacturers of swine vaccine. The manufacturers refused to bottle it until somebody did.

Barbara was as aware as her husband that the credibility of the CDC was coming increasingly under fire as its director, David Sencer, clung determinedly to his hypothesis about the risk of a potential pandemic.

Sencer had repeatedly argued that once the outbreak began, it would be too late to start vaccinating people; the disease was one that spread rapidly. Sencer was a popular and highly respected director whose judgment in the past, as Fraser well knew, had been frequently put to the test, and not found wanting. Even those who now doubted him had to admit he was not a man to panic or misuse the power his office carried. In a real emergency he could cut through administrative red tape and talk personally to the President; it helped that Ford, like Sencer, had been raised in Grand Rapids, Michigan. And indeed Fraser and his wife had just heard Ford saying on the news that he was "going to find a way either with or without Congress to carry out the program."

That promise, thought Fraser, was definite enough. It seemed to confirm the rumor circulating in Washington that his CDC boss had held a pistol to Ford's head; certainly there could be no question that ever since Sencer had sounded the alarm back in March, a number of others had eagerly snatched at the trigger.

With a dismissive shake of his shaggy head, Fraser said matters wouldn't be helped by the sort of pointless speculation that had followed Ford's remarks and made him switch off the television program.

Fraser finished his meal, kissed Barbara and the children good-bye, and began the four-mile bicycle ride back to work. The athletic doctor did the ride most days. It satisfied his urge for hard physical exercise while giving him an uninterrupted period to think. Speeding along the undulating roads on his racer, he worried again about what he would do with Ted Tsai when the young Chinese joined Special Pathogens; the "good outbreak" he needed seemed as remote as ever.

Pedaling up the steeply inclined Clifton Road—which on his return home he would travel down at forty miles an hour—and nearing the CDC, Fraser was reminded of a further problem he faced: where could he safely keep his prized cycle? His concern that it might be stolen if left outside had led him to take action which had already raised eyebrows. Fraser boldly rode his bike right up to the CDC's impressive main entrance, dismounted, pushed open the glass doors, picked up his cycle, and carried it past the bemused receptionist to the elevator. Then, lifting the bike on end, he squeezed inside between white-coated scientists and fellow doctors and traveled up to the fifth floor. As he began pushing the cycle along the corridor toward his office, he was joined by a uniformed guard.

It was unsafe to bring bicycles into the building, the man said.

There was nowhere safe to store it outside, explained Fraser.

Where was he taking it now?

To his office.

That, the officer stated, would be inappropriate use of governmental space.

Fraser countered: he had himself glimpsed the large collection of tropical plants the man kept in his office; was that not equally inappropriate use of governmental space?

The safety officer promptly dropped that particular attempt at persuasion and finally stated flatly that Fraser was *not permitted* to park his bicycle in his office.

Fraser hesitated. *That* he understood. But the issue remained of *where* he could keep his cycle securely. As there was no prospect of resolving the matter verbally, he said he would send the safety officer a memo. Meantime, until he received an answer, he proposed to continue keeping his bicycle in his office. With that, Fraser wheeled the bike into his already cramped room and managed, with difficulty, to shut the door behind him.

He leaned the cycle against the front of his desk, sidled around it, and sat down at the other side, ready for work.

There would be no time for him to write that memorandum immediately. During his absence another pile of paper work had arrived on his cluttered desk to demand his attention: field reports, scientific papers, confidential internal memos.

A report on VD caught his eye. VD now afflicted more Americans than all other infectious illnesses combined—apart from the collection of illnesses called the common cold. Gonorrhea alone had increased some 120 percent in the past decade, to a million reported cases a year. And now a "super gonorrhea" resistant to penicillin had surfaced in Maryland and California. The implications were frightening: the CDC document stated it had just initiated a nationwide surveillance system for the drug-resistant cases.

A World Health Organization agency—IARC—presented a report on the geography of cancer that posed questions of particular interest to epidemiologists. Why, for instance, did men in Tokyo get cancer of the stomach six times more often than those in New York? Why did the disease strike twice as many Maori males as white men in New Zealand? Why, in California, did twice as many black women as white contract breast cancer? And why was throat cancer thirty times greater in one part of Iran than in another?

Fraser made notes, read on, assessed, made more notes, and continued reading. He could spot nothing suitable for him or his small team to act upon directly. In fact, he could hardly remember a quieter period. Fraser was neither superstitious nor a betting man but, had he been pressed, he would probably have agreed that somewhere a mysterious new outbreak was preparing a challenge to his skills—if only he could find it.

Pending that exciting prospect happening, the chief of Special Pathogens decided to settle back for the moment and write the promised memorandum about his bike.

4

Convention

With fears still prevalent of an attack against the city by some radical group, police vigilance in Philadelphia continued at a high level through the early hours of Wednesday, July 21. A watchful eye was kept on the dingy spaciousness of the railroad station and the airport in case troublemakers debouched from either under cover of darkness and made their way toward the squat skyline of the inner city, dominated for eighty-two years by the bell tower of City Hall.

In the craggy vastness of the downtown business and shopping district—an area running due north and south along Broad Street and east and west along Market Street—the policemen were dwarfed by the tower. Topped by a statue of William Penn, it loomed in the night above the extravagant architecture of City Hall, whose massive shape exerted a solemn heaviness over the all but deserted streets littered with old newspapers and accumulating piles of garbage.

The patrols paid only passing attention to the rats scavenging in refuse that grew more pronounced and odorous the farther they went up or down Broad Street into grim black slums, or east or west out from Market Street into the seedy areas of honky-tonk movie theaters and cut-rate department stores.

Other patrols watched over the main shopping streets—Walnut and Chestnut and select segments of Broad and Market—or cruised through silent side streets filled with the darkened shops of Greeks, Jews, and Italians standing cheek by jowl with an old church, a Friends' meetinghouse, or one of Philadelphia's long-established gentlemen's clubs.

Nothing untoward disturbed the relaxed charm and slovenliness of the sleeping city.

By 3 A.M. the crew of a police patrol car routinely noted that the last of the prostitutes who had hovered near the Bellevue since late afternoon the previous day had departed.

Shortly afterward, inside the hotel, cleaning parties began to move through the recently regilded lobby and public rooms, polishing metalwork, putting a new gleam on wood, vacuuming carpets, and leaving a pleasant aroma of wax in their wake. Around dawn—and well before any of the registered guests had awakened—the cleaners completed their work, disassembled and stored their equipment, and made their way to a cheerless room in the basement for coffee.

Passing through the kitchen area, one of the woman cleaners paused to speak to a man helping to prepare for the early-turn chefs due on duty in an hour to start cooking the first of hundreds of breakfasts. The man was carrying trays of fresh eggs from a storeroom to the bank of gas-fired rings in the center of the kitchen. Without pausing in his work, the man appeared eager to talk; it seemed only natural for the woman to accompany him as he returned to the room to collect more eggs. Still conversing animatedly, the couple stepped into the walk-in larder. In the seconds they were out of sight of anyone in the kitchen, the man pulled a plastic-wrapped package of meat from inside his jacket and handed it to the woman. She hoisted up her skirt and fixed the package to a special hook attached to her girdle for this purpose. She quickly lowered her skirt, leaving the meat invisibly but securely suspended between her legs. Still deep in conversation, the pair returned to the kitchen. Over the years they had stolen hundreds of pounds of prime steak in this way, dividing the spoils between them to help feed their families.

In another part of the kitchen another well-tried trick had been neatly executed. A trainee cook calmly took a fourteen-pound can of ham and slid it into a garbage bin. Shortly afterward the bin was trundled out of the kitchen for disposal. Along the way the ham was retrieved by an accomplice who had a ready market for the item: a sandwich bar in a black suburb.

With over two hours to go before executive chef Castelli arrived, there was ample opportunity to carry out such pilfering. And dodges like these were the bane of the Bellevue's contracted-in security force, whose radio-controlled guards supplemented the hotel's resident detective. While the security men had scored some notable successes against in-house thievery, their vigilance failed to foil all the rackets contained in the hotel. Even so, their very presence was sufficient to keep the filching down to a level where it hardly impinged on the mainly trustworthy Bellevue staff.

Now, all over the hotel, those employees were contributing to the running of an organization which, in some ways, was more complicated to operate than many large businesses.

In the seventeenth-floor telephone room the night shift sorted through requests for wake-up calls. There were over a hundred for between seven-fifteen and seven forty-five. Before then, exactly at six forty-five, an experienced finger depressed a key and the telephone began to ring in a bedroom one floor below.

Maria Reeves groaned. The ringing was an unwelcome interruption: she had managed hardly any sleep the previous night.

After checking in late, the smartly dressed young hooker had been escorted to her room by one of a squad of bellboys on duty in the lobby; "boys," she mused, was rather a misnomer. Most of the uniformed men grouped around the bell captain's desk were middle-aged, and the man who carried her two light bags behaved as though they were filled with bricks. It was an old ruse that almost always guaranteed a guest would give the bellman a generous tip.

Maria also noticed the speculative way the hotel employee had eyed her. As they walked to the elevator she supposed he was wondering why she had requested a room with a double bed. It worried her that he might pass the information along to the house detective.

On the way up to her floor, two hotel guests in the elevator leered at her. She froze both men. It was important that in public she maintain a decorum and distance from any potential customer; it made her all the more desirable and, when the moment came, made it easier for her to get her price.

Maria had tipped the bellman lavishly, and as he turned to leave, she murmured that the hotel held a special memory for her. Then, in a flood of words she had rehearsed coming up in the elevator, she explained that a few years ago she and her husband had honeymooned at the Bellevue. With a catch in her voice that had hooked many a client, Maria added that her husband had just died in the fifth year of their marriage. The rheumy-eyed employee shuffled his feet in embarrassment. Maria couldn't be sure how much he believed, but it might make him hesitate to alert the house detective. She hoped she had confused the bellman sufficiently for him to dismiss her as just another of those lonely, although perfectly respectable, young widows.

After unpacking her clothes and placing her "work bag" inside the larger case—a precaution against any curious maid's snooping—she had retired to bed. Sleep would not come. The street noises kept her awake. Then, when the bell atop City Hall boomed out its funereal chimes for midnight and the traffic finally dissipated, a new and closer sound emerged: the air-conditioning unit mounted in her window began to malfunction. Every few minutes it rattled and whirred. Presuming it was useless at this hour to ask the front desk to send up a serviceman, she switched off the machine. The room quickly became unbearably warm, driving sleep further away. For what seemed like hours, Maria lay on the bed, her skin glistening with perspiration. Finally, when the sonorous chimes of four o'clock drifted across the city, she had switched on the air conditioning, showered, and, close to exhaustion, returned to bed. She had barely fallen asleep when the ringing of the morning call awoke her.

Almost three hundred feet below where Maria Reeves now lay awake, one of the hotel's engineers checked the gauges on the hot water system. Automatically the time-controlled thermostat had stepped up the temperature, ensuring there was enough hot water available for the peak morning period—7 to 9 A.M. when upward of five hundred people might decide to bathe or shower simultaneously.

In another part of the basement, the leaking 800-ton air-conditioning chiller unit hummed smoothly, cooling the eighteen floors above this echoing and strictly functional area. Close to the machine the garbage detail began sifting through the waste before shoveling it into the incinerator. The furnace was still being improperly operated, its afterburner unused. Nobody with knowledge or authority had yet come down to this torrid enclosure to have the situation remedied.

Precisely at seven-thirty William Chadwick was awakened.

Five floors above him, in suite 1301–3, overlooking Walnut Street, Harold Varr was already dressed and telephoning his first orders of the day.

Whatever criticisms might be leveled at the way the Bellevue had slipped from its position as one of the nation's leading hotels, no blame could be laid at Varr's door. During the eight years he had been at its helm, the Bellevue had become his life's work; he frequently gave the hotel up to fourteen hours a day, sometimes seven days a week, sleeping in instead of going home to his wife and children. He loved the Bellevue with a passion few suspected lay beneath his stern and austere exterior. Varr found it hard to accept that the hotel no longer enjoyed the prestige and glamour it once had. He was convinced "a good break" allied to an injection of new capital would restore the establishment to its previous position among America's ranking hostelries.

As he made his calls to departmental heads already at their desks on the executive floor, the hard-driving Varr reminded them of the "guidelines" he had specifically laid down for the legionnaires due to begin registering in just a few hours.

When accepting the convention, the general manager had bluntly spelled out those conditions to the Legion: "We don't permit rowdyism, destruction in rooms, breakages, throwing things out of the window, being obnoxious to other guests, or using electric prodders." Further, the Legion must provide "its own nurse corps, its own military police division, and understand this was a hotel with other guests."

Six hundred and twenty-two legionnaires were due to register during this Wednesday; in all, Varr expected 807 guests, including a number of permanent residents, to be in the hotel by nightfall.

He was determined to stamp hard on any legionnaire who tried to resurrect those times when the veterans had almost run amuck, acting in concert as a "frolicking, rowdy, messy group." At past conventions they had marched behind their bands down through the bedroom floors and poked other guests with electric chargers; and on one memorable occasion a legionnaire had grabbed a brace of turkeys from a buffet table and tossed the lot out of a window over the unsuspecting heads of astonished passersby.

While Varr felt he had done all in his power to suppress a repetition of such antics, he knew the next three days would nevertheless be demanding. And though he himself felt capable of meeting any challenge head on, he did not feel confident about Chadwick. Varr was now certain his immediate superior was carefully guarding a secret from everybody in the hotel. It had taken time for Varr to spot the signs: a sudden shortness of breath, a tiredness that had not been there before, and an occasional flicker of unease in Chadwick's normally alert eyes. To Varr they pointed to one grim conclusion: Chadwick had a serious "heart problem." Any untoward event could precipitate an infarction that could kill him.

By nine o'clock, with the arrival of executive chef Castelli in his kitchen, the day shift of the Bellevue Stratford was present and fully occupied.

On each of the guest floors, maids stripped bedding and towels from just-vacated rooms. In the restaurants, busboys bundled away used linen as waiters prepared to lay the tables for lunch.

The spoiled items were trundled to the hotel's laundry, which occupied a large portion of the subbasement it shared with the wine cellar, incinerator, and air-conditioning engine room. By the end of their day the laundry staff would have processed some fifteen thousand items: bed sheets, pillowcases, washcloths, towels, napkins, tablecloths, greasy coveralls from the engineering staff, and stained whites from the kitchen. In a week the staff ironed more cloth than even the busiest housewife would press in fifty years.

But—and this, too, was seen by some as a sign of the times, a drop in standards that had allowed such people into the hotel in the first place—the laundry staff increasingly had to cope with guests who used ball-point pens to draw on hotel napery. Today, as on any other day, there was a separate pile of linen that had been written upon. It was essential to catch these items before they went into the water, as there was almost no way to remove ball-point ink once it became wet. A member of the laundry staff was steadily working through the stained items, spotting out the offending ink with carbon tetrachloride. It was a slow and laborious process, but one that saved the hotel thousands of dollars.

In service departments throughout the basement and other areas—in the carpenter's shop, printing plant, and plumbing store, in design and decorating, in the television and radio repair shop—men and women went about their daily routine.

Few noticed that the air-conditioner repairman had not reported for work. Those who did wondered briefly whether he had just sneaked a day off. Lots of people did.

None of them knew the young war veteran was still in bed at home, growing sicker by the hour. Or that his two small children would soon develop the same disturbing symptoms as their father had.

The moment Anna Taggart opened the elevator door a great burst of sound almost drove her back into the cage. The racket caromed off the hotel's high-ceilinged lobby and bounced back and forth between its walls. It was the miscellaneous clamor of the Legion convention members registering and getting into their stride.

Some four hours had passed since the conventioneers began checking in, and now, at one o'clock, Anna thought the confusion in the lobby resembled a disorganized cocktail party crossed with a parade ground. Legionnaires, often bellowing greetings and gossip at the tops of their voices, weaved between the cocktail lounges, dining room, and florist and gift shops. A number held tumblers from which they drank before hurling welcomes to new arrivals pouring in past Bellevue doorman Bill Rainer, whose smile seemed to have become glazed by the melee thundering around him.

Anna thought ruefully that if the volume of noise could somehow be harnessed it would provide enough power not only to operate her ten elevators but to "light the entire building."

She didn't mind the noise as such; it was part of any convention. But already Anna was uncomfortably aware that the Legion gathering was going to be altogether different from any convention the hotel had yet hosted this year—perhaps different, even, from previous Legion meetings. It wasn't that there were more hell raisers among the legionnaires than on former occasions; it wasn't that all her elevator operators had already had men brushing suggestively against them or blowing noise-makers in their faces or touching their hands and legs with battery-operated tinglers that gave off mild shocks. It wasn't even the lack of manners of some, the way a few openly belched or scratched their backsides or how once, to the delight of his companions, a particularly ill-mannered member broke wind with a thunderous clap.

It was something else: a faint but unmistakable aroma that lingered in the elevator long after legionnaires got out. It was a blend of cooked meats, bread, garlic, fruits, and vegetables, all of which the conventioneers were transporting up to their rooms in large quantities. In addition to the food, many of the men carried crates of liquor; some of them even waved unlabeled bottles that Anna strongly suspected contained home-brewed hooch. A few of the veterans passed the moonshine among themselves before swaying and staggering to their rooms.

Anna was upset by such goings-on; in all her time at the hotel she had never known guests to bring in their own food and drink so openly. When she questioned Harold Varr about it, he explained that in the case of the legionnaires it was to be tolerated. Anna immediately accepted his decision.

She could see Varr now, standing by the marble-topped front desk, watching the long lines of boisterous conventioneers still waiting to register. Some 4,500 legionnaires, their families, and members of the Legion's Women's Auxiliary were on hand for the three-day convention. Those not among the 622, mainly legionnaires, booked into the Bellevue were dispersed in other downtown hotels.

With Varr was a legionnaire who, increasingly, Anna hoped epitomized the majority of the conventioneers. Ever since he arrived in the hotel, she thought Edward Hoak, the adjutant of the American Legion in Pennsylvania, had behaved "like he was born to the Bellevue." Soberly dressed and mannered, fifty-two-year-old Hoak had conducted himself with decorum and dignity from the moment Anna had taken him up to the sixth floor, where he had a corner suite. Hoak had checked in on Monday and since then had spent most of his time watching the Montreal Olympics on television, sipping Tab, and wishing his heavy cold would disappear. During his infrequent outings to the hotel's executive offices—Hoak was responsible for the convention agenda and for seeing that everything went smoothly—he gave Anna the latest news of some American track or swimming victory. In spite of his cold, his voice had been soft and courteous. Anna was surprised to learn Hoak had been a baton-swinging MP in the Army and that among the state's 260,000 legionnaires he was known as a tough and forthright officer. It was these qualities which many of those milling around the lobby thought would help Hoak realize a cherished dream —being elected as national Legion commander at its all-states convention in Seattle the third week of August.

Now, in the lobby, a trio of legionnaires, the one in the middle crooning tipsily, stumbled toward Anna's elevator. Accompanying them was one of the Bellevue's elderly bellmen, pulling a trolley laden with beer. Entering her cage, the guests eyed Anna openly. One of them asked if she would like to party with them.

Drawing herself up to her full five feet two inches, the fiery operator fixed the man with a stare. In a steely voice that could quell the most amorous of guests, she reminded the veterans that this *was* the Bellevue Stratford, where it was normal for *gentlemen* to have only their *wives* in their rooms. In frozen silence Anna shot the men up to the seventeenth floor.

There the tipsy veteran straightened himself and solemnly apologized to Anna for any offense caused. Then, pointing at the elevator controls, he added, "Lady, we could have used you at Pearl Harbor. I ain't gone up faster since the day I took off after those Japs on December 7, 1941."

Anna laughed appreciatively, her anger gone as quickly as it had come. Perhaps, after all, the legionnaires would pleasantly surprise her.

One floor below, Maria Reeves was also being mildly surprised by the behavior of some of the legionnaires she had brought to her room.

Maria's technique was a throwback to those days in New York when she had worked a number of uptown hotels. She would walk demurely down a corridor, an unlit cigarette in her hand. When she spotted a likely prospect, an obvious out-of-towner, she would shyly ask for a light. From there it was simple: a brief conversation, laced with a cleverly planted innuendo, a carefully timed look of awakening excitement in her eyes, and then, once a positive reaction was received, a sudden mouthful of explicit sexual promises, "a guaranteed turn on" for those who normally got their kicks fantasizing over *Penthouse* or *Playboy*.

At that point Maria linked arms with the man and walked him to her room. To any passing hotel employee, the pair looked like guests who had struck up one of those instant relationships common to all conventions. And even if the hotel's security staff did become suspicious, they were, Maria believed, powerless until they could somehow prove she was soliciting. That would almost certainly require the cooperation of a client—somebody who was prepared to confirm she was a whore and involve himself in a scandal. Without that, she felt there was little the hotel could do. If they canceled her room she could threaten to sue; it would not be difficult to find a lawyer willing to fight the lawsuit for a share of the profits. The Bellevue wouldn't want that. All in all, as long as she was careful, Maria concluded the risks were small—and certainly worth the financial return. Since ten-thirty, when she had accosted her first legionnaire, she had made $250.

Even so, she was surprised by the kinkiness of some of the men. One had produced a banana, peeled it, insisted she use it on herself, and afterward nonchalantly walked off eating it. Another asked for a beating, whimpering like a child as she flogged him with her riding crop. A third had received satisfaction by simply looking at and listening to her as she sat in her crotchless panties on the bed chanting erotic obscenities.

None of the requests were new to Maria, but now as she guided yet another respectable-looking middle-aged legionnaire to her bedroom, she could not help but wonder what further perversions she would encounter before the convention was over.

Early in the afternoon a way miraculously opened through the Bellevue's still jam-packed lobby. Completely oblivious to the hurly-burly around her, an eighty-year-old permanent hotel resident walked majestically out of the Stratford Garden restaurant on the arm of its suave maître d'. She looked neither to left nor to right at the ranks of conventioneers moving respectfully out of her path. The staff affectionately referred to her—behind her back, naturally—as "the great uncrowned royal."

At the elevator she thanked the maître d' for lunch: they both behaved as though she had been his only and very private guest. Then she stepped into the elevator Bill Chadwick was specially holding for her. Not once had she given the slightest indication of being aware of the legionnaires' presence. The space that had opened for her just as quickly closed. The lobby was back to its bustling noisy self, filled by a gathering that seemed to be getting endless pleasure out of just being there.

The crowd was swollen by legionnaires who were staying at other hotels beginning to arrive at the convention's Bellevue headquarters.

Among them was George Chiavetta, a former post commander at a small town near Harrisburg. Chiavetta had come to the Bellevue "to browse around and to watch the other legionnaires checking in."

Unashamedly fascinated by the minutiae of life, Chiavetta found his attention suddenly attracted by a stranger on the sidewalk a few feet from where the veterans were stamping up the Bellevue's entrance steps past doorman Rainer—his smile now more glazed than ever after a legionnaire had blown a particularly loud noisemaker in his ear—and into the lobby.

Something about the man made Chiavetta suspicious. He decided to observe him carefully, which was not always easy as the stranger was walking rapidly about, changing direction for no apparent reason, moving swiftly up to a legionnaire and then just as quickly stepping back into the crowd.

At first Chiavetta thought the man was a harmless street vendor or pimp touting for a girlie bar. Yet there was something about him, a quality Chiavetta couldn't define but found vaguely worrying.

He noted how the man was dressed: in a bright royal-blue single-breasted suit; and how he looked: lank light brown hair, thick lower lip, aged "38 to 45 years," height between five-ten and six feet. He was smoking.

Moving closer, Chiavetta heard the man telling the veterans, "It is too late now, you will not be saved."

Chiavetta was not inclined to dismiss the stranger simply as some religious fanatic, a street zealot. Yet he had to concede that the rolled-up paper the man carried might be a scripture. But if it was, why didn't he consult it instead of keeping it close by his side before pointing the paper in the direction of each of the legionnaires to whom he uttered that strange warning?

Before Chiavetta could himself investigate further, or summon one of the security men posted in the lobby, or even one of Mayor Rizzo's famous mounted policemen standing duty a short distance up Broad Street, the man abruptly turned and vanished into the crowds of bicentennial sightseers walking past the hotel.

Chiavetta was a cautious and careful person. He did not wish to appear foolish. For the moment he decided to keep his observations to himself. Then a disturbing thought struck him: the rolled-up paper would make an ideal container for concealing some sort of noxious substance. He decided to keep a watchful eye open for further sightings of the man in the dazzling blue suit.

By late afternoon this Wednesday, thousands of Legion men and women had established the pattern that would serve them as a matrix for the entire convention. They would attend caucuses, lobby for their candidates for the many offices up for election, vote on dozens of resolutions, and listen to the speeches from the podium at one end of the Bellevue's ballroom. In spite of his cold, Hoak was expected to deliver one of the best—and did; the adjutant had a reputation for catching exactly the patriotic mood of the delegates.

And when convention business ended or momentarily palled, the majority of the delegates went sightseeing, streaming out of the Bellevue in their hundreds, their Legion caps set at angles that would have made a top sergeant wince.

Many of the veterans noticed that the pigeons, long a feature of the sidewalks around the hotel, seemed more numerous, their droppings more evident, than in previous years.

The piles of refuse—blackly sinister in plastic sacks—were proof for many legionnaires of what until now they had only read about or seen on television: Philadelphia, for all its grandeur, its keynote role in the

Bicentennial, was a municipal mess. The refuse strike was a stark reminder of the conflict between Mayor Rizzo and the city's employees.
Rizzo had been scheduled to welcome the delegates officially to Philadelphia, a long-standing tradition of incumbent mayors. Instead, he
sent a deputy to deliver the greeting. Rizzo himself was seldom seen in
public nowadays. A recall petition had been circulated in the city
signed by over 200,000 citizens with the purpose of ousting Rizzo from
office prematurely. Albert Gaudiosi, the mayor's top adviser, had apparently advised Rizzo to keep a low profile during this painful period.
Philadelphia's deputy director of commerce had welcomed the legionnaires. The man reminded the delegates it was in Philadelphia that the
Marine Corps, Army, and Navy had all been founded, "as well as the
Flag and the Nation itself." He had spoken of the need to keep
America strong—a recurring theme among the speakers, who delivered
dire warnings about the Soviets and other potential enemies of the
United States, including the worldwide terrorist movement. As if to re-
inforce that danger, there seemed to be more policemen on duty
around the hotels where the legionnaires were staying.

Nevertheless, for delegates from such far-flung communities as
Clearfield, Lewisburg, Athens, and Republic; for those who had traveled from such pretty-sounding places as Roslyn and McAdoo or had
journeyed across the wide expanse of Pennsylvania from such cloistered
townships as Edinboro and Muse; even for those who had come from
Pittsburgh: for them all, Philadelphia in bicentennial time was the
place to be.

Singly and in groups, the legionnaires surveyed the city at street
level, from the top of the Pennsylvania Mutual Building, from the air-
conditioned comfort of buses that toured them from one local historic
spot to another where they could feel the weight of the past made
heavier by some of the startling new concrete plazas and hotels as
garish as Miami's, or gleaming glass-walled office towers as fearsomely
modern as any to be seen in New York.

For the most part the citizens of Philadelphia paid little attention to
the legionnaires. They were caught up in other events. A slowing in the
nation's economic growth was sharply reflected locally; unemployment
was creeping upward; people spoke of "stagflation." And with each
passing day in the simmering labor dispute between the city and its
workers, the Rizzo administration and the union leaders grew more en-
trenched in their negotiating positions. In some quarters there was
even a suggestion—so far unfounded—that the unrest could spread to
involve public health employees; few people realized how hard-worked
and underpaid those workers were.

But there could hardly be a Philadelphian who did not know that
the mayor was making a determined effort to rid the city's streets of

vendors. For two months his campaign had brought headlines and heated controversy. Wednesday morning's *Inquirer* contained pictures and reports of the latest arrests of peddlers. There was no mention of any attempt to remove the high number of beggars who had infiltrated Philadelphia's downtown area in order to fleece the anniversary crowds congregated there. Even so, most Philadelphians thought the police department would be better employed tracking down the killer of the city's latest murder victim, an elderly woman stabbed to death in her bed; as in many American cities, crime was a growth industry in Philadelphia.

By Thursday the first photos of Mars taken by Viking 1 cameras dominated the front pages. Closer to home, as part of the Bicentennial, the tall sailing ships of the world were arriving at Penn's Landing; inevitably a few overpatriotic folk questioned whether it was "right" for sailors from the communist tall ships to be wandering the streets of Philadelphia at this time of national fervor. They would have been even more critical had they known that some of those sailors were guests at Legion hospitality suites in the Bellevue. Still, the mood of jingoism was satisfied by such films as the local smash-hit success *Midway*, an account of the great United States victory in the Pacific during World War II. Scores of legionnaires joined the lines waiting to see Charlton Heston and Henry Fonda wipe out the Japanese.

As conventions went, the Legion gathering was, by Philadelphia's yardstick, of no great import. Numerically, it was small for a city already gearing itself to welcome a million people for the Eucharistic Congress; compared to that influx, the veterans were making "about as much impact as a platoon does on an army." In the years it had been using the Bellevue as its headquarters—the state convention alternated annually between Philadelphia and Pittsburgh—the Legion had a reputation for careful spending. Its officials drove hard bargains on room rates—it had even forced the Bellevue to give bookings at nine dollars a person—and tried to get discounts for its members wherever possible.

Apart from those street vendors who had so far evaded police arrest and were presently doing a lively trade in noisemakers—each of which was worked by a chemical propellant similar to that still escaping from the Bellevue's air-conditioning unit—Philadelphia's shopkeepers received little extra profit from the convention. In turn, veterans complained that prices had been hiked for the Bicentennial.

Critically comparing costs with those back home, groups of legionnaires wandered through downtown department stores or strolled up quiet side streets reminiscent of a bygone age with their shops devoted exclusively to old coins, stamps, saddles, and leather goods. Some penetrated deeper into a part of the city most visitors were unaware of, passing tiny shops selling fig candies or theatrical costumes or rare books.

Then, suddenly, they were among the old houses, the homes of the perennial Philadelphians. Here the summer sun was shielded by aged trees, the energy-sapping heat shimmering on the midtown sidewalks dissipated by secluded gardens. And beyond these were still more shops filled with curios and antique knickknacks.

It was among them that retired Air Force Captain Ray Brennan hoped he might find another item for his collection of seashells. Brennan, a tall, graying man of sixty-one, was bookkeeper at Legion Post 42 in Towanda. As for so many legionnaires, the high spot of his year was the convention. This time Brennan was cramming more into his four days in Philadelphia than he had ever done before. He told friends it might be the last annual gathering he would attend. His heart trouble was getting worse.

Frank Aveni told those fellow veterans he had not seen since the last convention that he was now in his sixtieth year and never felt fitter. Aveni was from Clearfield and had mapped out his own sightseeing tour of the city. It took him through the old curiosity shops on Pine Street, around the self-imposed gloom of City Hall, down the Benjamin Franklin Parkway—an elegant avenue of trees graced by an occasional fountain—to the tawny stone vastness of the Museum of Art.

Louis Byerly, a sprightly fifty-nine-year-old veteran from Post 344 in Jeannette, had a different itinerary. He had already hit many of the Legion hospitality suites, had eaten at Bookbinders, and was, on Thursday evening, in the process of prowling the late-night bars.

The three men did not know one another. At the various Legion functions they attended, they did not sit close to one another. Often they were not even in the Bellevue Stratford at the same time. It made no difference. They were all to die from the same cause.

It hadn't worked for years, thought Dicko Dolan. J.B. was right: Post 239 should have long ago withdrawn from the Nineteenth District, the largest of all the Legion districts in the state. Geographically, culturally, "in every damned emotional way," Dicko now felt that 239 had little in common with the Nineteenth's other posts. But it was wishful thinking; he knew there was no way he could pull Williamstown out. That realization did not improve Dicko's mood. The lantern-jawed post commander continued to push his way in through the mass of legionnaires and their women who were filling the Bellevue rooftop Rose Garden for an early morning breakfast on Friday, July 23.

Dicko was not a man for parading his post's votes around the convention floor; he preferred to operate clear of the well-lit ballroom, dealing with a few key people at a time. It made him formidable—and feared. And despite its small size, it made Post 239 one of the most respected among the scores of posts at the convention. Everybody knew once Dicko gave his word, there was no more to be said. Some even felt that if he had so chosen, he could have made a successful run for one of the offices up for election. Dicko would hear none of it; he was content to remain as 239's commander.

All around him he could hear the endless politicking—the little deals, the trade-offs, the unwritten agreements, the nod and wink that sealed the fate of a candidate or resolution. Ordinarily he would have loved it—this manipulation and wheeler-dealing, the persuasions and pressures, though none of them would have made him blindly follow the Nineteenth's line and throw 239's votes into the collective district pot. He had made that clear from the opening sessions on Wednesday, when he had spent an hour in the Bellevue going from one hospitality suite to another, taking "soundings."

That night in the Bellevue the Legion had held its most somber ceremony of the week. In the grand ballroom almost one thousand people gathered to look upon a pyramid of rifles stacked upright in the center of the floor, a solitary silver helmet at their base. The names of legionnaires who had died during the year were written on slips of paper and placed in the helmet. As taps was played, the papers were set alight. By this ritual were the souls of the dead men transferred to what was known in the Legion as the Post Everlasting.

Dicko decided to give the memorial service a miss. Instead he had gone gallivanting in Chinatown and returned to his hotel at 3:30 A.M. On Thursday he was back in the Bellevue for a couple of hours, attending the Nineteenth District caucus and "generally acting like a backroom politician." Afterward he called in at a liquor store to replenish his diminishing supply. And now this Friday morning he had come to the Rose Garden to join some seven hundred others for breakfast and to continue the endless process of assessment that preoccupied him during much of the convention.

Jammed among the seething mass, acknowledging greetings, pausing to listen to somebody trying to enlist his votes for a resolution or candidate—and careful, as always, to remain uncommitted—Dicko wondered whether he felt unwell because "the real politicking" had kept him for long periods in 239's hospitality suite in the Holiday Inn, seven blocks away on Market Street.

Like J.B., Dicko had developed a cold since arriving in Philadelphia. Dicko put it down to a faulty air-conditioning unit in the suite; it had leaked so badly that a large patch of carpet was soaked. He had repeatedly raised a ruckus with the Holiday Inn management and the unit, in the end, had been fixed. But nothing had been done about the soggy carpet.

And from what Dicko had seen, things were not much better at the Bellevue. Every time he walked into the hotel he got the definite im-

pression many of its staff were "uppity—they overrated themselves."
He couldn't understand why Anna Taggart's "girls" spoke sharply to
several veterans "who were just horsing about with noisemakers and
having fun"; he thought elevator operators should expect that sort of
behavior at conventions.

If Dicko had his way, this would be the last annual meeting the Legion would stage at the hotel. In his opinion, the Bellevue's basic
amenities left much to be desired. Yesterday the hotel had run out of
ice, forcing legionnaires to buy in supplies from wholesale vendors.
There were no paper cups at several of the drinking fountains. Long
lines formed for the elevators. The lobby was often jammed to capacity. The hotel was simply not able, in every sense, to cope with the legionnaires. Worst of all, Dicko had the overall impression the veterans
were accepted only on sufferance.

Both J.B. and Jimmy, following visits they had made to the hotel
during the previous two days, told Dicko they also got the feeling the
Bellevue did not relish having them as guests. Standing near the front
desk, on Thursday, looking into the Stratford Garden dining room, J.B.
had informed Jimmy that soft lights and snooty waiters were not for
him. The two men had decided to walk across the street and eat at
Horn and Hardart's, where the service and company were likely to be
more convivial.

In the Rose Garden this Friday morning, Dicko could find no fault
with the service. The breakfast was served with speed and civility. It
was the food that made him and many other legionnaires grumble: it
was cold. Some of the men complained that their rolls were not just
cold but still *frozen*, as though they had just been taken out of the
freezer.

Dicko left the breakfast. Feeling out of sorts, he found it an effort to
answer those who continued to question him about how he would cast
239's votes during the morning ballots.

By midday the last of those votes were used and counted, and Dicko
was thankful to be able to escape the stuffy atmosphere of the
Bellevue. He began to walk back to the Holiday Inn. It would give him
time to think.

In many ways, he had to admit, it had so far been for him a disappointing convention.

From the moment he and the others had stood in line waiting to
register at the convention desk in the Bellevue, sensing the hotel's "uppity" staff eyeing them critically, Dicko felt things go flat. Their first
night in Philadelphia, J.B. had insisted on going off alone to the
Phillies ball game; he did not seem his usual self when he came back.
In an effort to liven things up, on Thursday Dicko had taken J.B. and
Jimmy on a tour of the hospitality rooms; in the evening they had gone

to an exotic restaurant where a belly dancer entertained them as they ate. Afterward they had partied in their suite until three-thirty in the morning. Yet somehow—in spite of the jokes, the eyeing of pretty girls, the joshing with old friends, the good food and fellowship, the unlimited booze—in spite of it all, nothing had quite clicked.

J.B. had spent much of the time in his room. He often seemed downcast and lifeless. When he drank he became morose and talked constantly of his two sons. Dicko felt for him; he knew how wretched he would be if he ever lost contact with his children. Both of J.B.'s companions realized that what he missed most was the security of a wife and family. He was the type of man who could not survive alone; he needed not only to give but to receive affection. Without that, Dicko thought J.B. would continue as he had been this convention, totally unconsolable.

Jimmy, too, had been quiet and withdrawn, fending off all Dicko's attempts to find him a "nice Irish girl." There were several at the convention. But when Dicko had invited one to their suite and introduced her to Jimmy, his cousin had talked to the girl only of Doris and her children.

As Dicko continued his walk back to the Holiday Inn, he reluctantly came to the conclusion there was no more he could possibly do to stop Jimmy from marrying Doris.

Another disappointment to Dicko was the absence so far of the expected "radicals." In fact, he couldn't remember a convention passing more peacefully: "no pinkos, crypto-communists, antiwar jerks, or long-haired gurus." Certainly there were unconfirmed reports of a few legionnaires having been threatened. And the story related by George Chiavetta—a man J.B. knew personally and vouched for as being as reliable as they came—was, mused Dicko, at minimum a strange one.

Since first spotting him on Wednesday, Chiavetta had seen the mystery man in the bright blue suit several times lurking around the Bellevue. In the latest sighting, he had noticed that as the man moved purposefully through the hotel lobby, he appeared "glassy-eyed, his face was flushed." Amid the jostling crowd his jacket had come open and Chiavetta had been startled to see at close hand an "odd contraption" that resembled a tobacco pouch partially hanging out of the man's inside coat pocket. Connected to this pouch was a thin plastic tube leading up and around the man's neck and then down inside his sleeve to his right hand, where he still held that rolled-up paper which he constantly pointed at legionnaires. When the man realized Chiavetta was staring at him, he had forced his way out of the lobby and disappeared up Broad Street.

Dicko was still pondering Chiavetta's story when he reached the Holiday Inn. He took the elevator to the eighth floor and walked down a corridor lined with identical plywood doors, passed an ice chest and candy vending machine, and reached 822–24.

He opened the door. On the far wall of the two-roomed suite was a sealed window, hung with drapes of synthetic fiber. Below it was the offending air-conditioner. The carpet was still visibly wet; a dark patch extended several feet from the wall almost to the first of several leatherette barrel chairs scattered around the room. The chairs matched the synthetic-walnut table and TV on a swivel stand, its feet buried in a shaggy synthetic-fiber carpet. On top of a long synthetic-walnut combination of desk and bureau was the last of the beer the Williamstown contingent had brought with them. Plastic buckets of melted ice stood on stationery with the Holiday Inn logo: "Your Host from Coast to Coast." Beside the buckets was a card bearing the words: BE A WATT WATCHER.

Dicko crossed the room, oblivious of the odor of reconditioned air, cigars, and alcohol, walked past the bathroom, and reached the second room of the suite. Its beds had headboards of synthetic walnut and bedspreads of synthetic fiber. Between the beds was a fake-walnut table holding a lamp, ashtray, and telephone with a red light that flashed whenever a call came through or to indicate a message awaiting collection in the lobby.

Here, in this unprepossessing suite, since their arrival on Wednesday, Dicko, Jimmy, and J.B. had entertained and slept.

J.B. and Jimmy were now slumped back on their pillows. Their colds, they complained to Dicko, were getting worse.

He noticed that J.B., in particular, seemed distressed, and wondered whether his friend was having another of his well-known bouts of hypochondria.

Dicko brusquely told them both they would feel better if they showered and then joined him for lunch and a few whiskeys. He firmly believed there was nothing like alcohol to knock out any bug.

By early Friday afternoon a weary Anna Taggart detected a new mood among the legionnaires as they prepared for the climax of their convention—the Legion parade through the city. Men were bursting in and out of elevators, running up and down corridors, banging on bedroom doors, lighting sparklers in the lobby, and generally creating bedlam throughout the hotel.

Anna effectively minimized the legionnaires' misconduct by mentally recalling the contrasting behavior of other Bellevue guests of the past whom she had been so pleased to serve. There had been President Franklin D. Roosevelt: pensive, concerned with the seemingly endless depression, he had apologized to her that his wasted legs were always a problem when riding in elevators. Anna had been twenty-two at the time and too nervous to reply as the great man went on his way to address some meeting in the city.

Almost a decade later, another President, Harry S. Truman, rode with her on his way to make another speech—to mark the end of World War II. He had been ebullient and spoke to Anna of the dawn of a brave new world.

John F. Kennedy, then a baby-faced young senator, astonished her by the nervous way he tried to memorize parts of a speech as he rode down to the Stratford Garden to address local Democrats; it was another stepping-stone in his march to the White House. Years later, in the afterglow of his inauguration, he returned to the hotel as President. Standing proudly in the elevator beside Jackie, Kennedy had reminded Anna of the previous time they had traveled together. She had been a JFK fan ever since.

Lyndon Johnson had towered over her and spoken just like John Wayne. And when Wayne stayed at the hotel, he had acted as he did on screen, slow and courteous, studying the controls Anna used to operate the cage as though they were part of a space station console. The astronauts themselves were well mannered, but without their space suits they looked only like successful industrialists. President Nixon had been friendly, smiling and saying thank you; that was before Watergate. President Ford was relaxed and casual, reminding Anna of Bing Crosby.

How differently all those had behaved from the motley crowd of veterans Anna could see crammed into the lobby this Friday afternoon.

And now a group of them were trying to persuade a shaven-headed giant to take up a drum and lead them around the lobby. Suddenly the dark-suited Bill Chadwick was among them. The noise level made it impossible for Anna to hear what Chadwick was saying, but he was speaking directly to the giant, who began to nod in agreement. He finally lowered the drum.

Shrugging, J.B. walked out of the lobby to join Jimmy and Dicko on the sidewalk.

Watching him go, Anna knew she would remember the man not only for his size and eggshell-smooth head, but also for the sadness in his face.

At least, she thought bitterly, he could walk straight; on several of the upstairs floors she had glimpsed legionnaires sprawled on couches or lurching from one hospitality suite to another. By now she had received complaints from each of her operators about being pawed by some of the men. And one of them reported to Anna she had been astonished when, dropping a group of veterans off on the sixteenth floor, she noticed a smartly dressed young woman clinging lovingly to the arm of a middle-aged legionnaire.

Neither the operator nor Anna knew Maria Reeves had caught another client.

Almost immediately below the lobby, well insulated from its noise, executive chef Castelli continued supervising the centerpiece for the Burgundy Room's cold buffet that night. He ordered cooks not to use aspic to decorate the silver-plated serving dishes on which turkeys, hams, and joints were being positioned. Mayonnaise instead was to be piped around the edges of each plate. The men looked disappointed; they had just finished dicing the aspic into cubes. Castelli explained that mayonnaise would lend a more enticing appearance to the cold cuts. The aspic could be saved for later use.

Satisfied, he went to his office to resume the task he had started before the luncheon rush intervened: there appeared to be a discrepancy between the amount of meat ordered and used this past week. Twenty pounds of prime steak seemed to be missing.

Abruptly one of the junior cooks caught his eye. The man was preparing chickens incorrectly: the legs were being cut too short, the wing tips improperly trimmed.

Castelli hurried to the station. Shaking his head, more annoyed than angry, he told the man to stop. The chef had the ability to criticize without destroying confidence. He was, furthermore, an excellent teacher. He quickly demonstrated to the assistant how the chickens should be prepared, lecturing as he worked. He turned a chicken on to its breast and trimmed the wing tips; next he cut off the feet well below the knee joints so the skin and tendons would not shrink during cooking. He handed the knife back to the cook and watched carefully. The man copied exactly the movements Castelli had made. Pleased, the executive chef returned to his office and finished scrutinizing his books.

There was no doubt about it: the meat had been received but, according to the meticulously kept daily records, not yet used. Nor was it in cold storage. With a sense of shock, Castelli realized there could only be one explanation. Somebody had stolen it.

In the hotel's executive offices a feeling of relief coupled with anticipation grew as the afternoon passed. The Legion convention would soon be over. The Eucharistic Congress was that much closer, when the presence of church leaders and European royalty would be a very necessary balm for all the minor wounds inflicted by the roistering legionnaires.

Although nobody wanted to admit it—least of all Chadwick—the presence of the veterans in the hotel had, on balance, probably provided more headaches than profits. Some of the men *were* abusive;

many of them *did* use their bathtubs as ice chests; at least one *had* urinated in a flowerpot; a pair *had* bowled baseballs at beer bottles in a hallway; several *had* tried to bring in street girls past Mike Smylie's hard-worked security men in the lobby. None of the complaints, by themselves, were serious. But even Chadwick had to admit the legionnaires were not a total success.

Surprisingly, Harold Varr was more charitable. Though there had been flagrant breaches of the conditions he had laid down, he felt in most cases the veterans reacted from nervousness; they were simply out of their depth in the grandeur of the Bellevue, with its impeccable flunkeys, stylized service, and still-pervasive atmosphere of moneyed elegance. While he in no way countenanced the excesses of the veterans, Varr sympathized with those who would have been uncomfortable dining in the Burgundy Room or sipping vintage port after dinner in the Stratford Garden. Such men, he guessed, had probably never before been inside a luxury hotel like the Bellevue.

Varr went down to the lobby in late afternoon to watch the legionnaires troop out of the hotel to form up for their parade. They were as roistering as ever. Having witnessed some of New York's wildest shindigs—when conventioneers could strip a hotel with the speed of a swarm of locusts—Varr was probably one of the few Bellevue employees who was not surprised by the veterans' high-spirited behavior.

A heavy shower of rain preceded the Legion parade, soaking marchers and spectators but doing nothing to dampen the merriment. For a time some of the onlookers were distracted by a fire in a building on Broad Street. Apart from that, the procession passed without incident.

By mid-evening the Bellevue's lobby was again full to overflowing as legionnaires and their women milled around waiting for the convention's Closing Dance to begin. A good many young people, members of bands that had marched in the parade, were also in evidence. They had come to Philadelphia just for the day and would return home by bus after parading again in the Bellevue's balconied Grand Ballroom during the dance.

Almost no one noticed that a number of legionnaires were already absent. They were still in their rooms, feeling listless and unwell. Some felt bad enough to retire to bed.

Their symptoms were similar to those that continued to afflict the Bellevue's air-conditioning repairman. Like him, all the veterans, at one time or another, had been close to one of the many air-conditioning units in the hotel.

Nobody in the Bellevue yet knew of the fear expressed in nearby City Hall: if terrorists were to strike, one of the most feasible ways would be to infiltrate a noxious substance into the air-conditioning system.

At ten o'clock that evening Maria Reeves, as she did at the same time the two previous nights, rode down to the lobby and deposited $700 in the safe-deposit box she had rented. It now held over $2,000, exceeding even her expectations. Returning to the sixteenth floor, she once more went to work.

She had developed a sore throat and felt a headache coming on. She planned to retire early. But first Maria meant to hook one more client.

In a short time she singled out a man. Together they went to her room.

The veteran faced the hooker across the bed and said he was willing to pay a good price if she would satisfy his request.

Maria asked what he had in mind.

The man told her.

She said it would cost him a hundred dollars.

He handed over the money.

Maria told him to undress. She went to the bathroom and drank several glasses of water. Then she slipped out of her clothes and called for the man to join her.

Stark naked, he lay down in the bath. Maria straddled the tub, placing one leg on either rim. Then, at a signal from the man, she started to give him what he had paid his hundred dollars for—the degrading act euphemistically described in Maria's trade as a "golden shower."

Jimmy coughed again and again, deep coughs that seemed to tear upward from the bottom of his lungs before bursting out of his mouth. He had a dull pain in his body that he had never felt before.

J.B. groaned. His head throbbed, his neck ached, his throat was raw, and his body was filled with bone-prickling sensations.

"Good Christ," he said. "We've both got the flu."

Dicko eased the car into the Saturday morning traffic in Philadelphia and began the three-hour drive to Williamstown.

"It's not the flu," he said firmly. "It's just a lousy cold."

A number of veterans he had said farewell to in the Bellevue lobby earlier seemed to have come down with similar colds.

Dicko didn't think it was anything to make a fuss about. After all, his own cold had by now almost gone.

Early Sunday evening, J.B. told Jimmy on the telephone he felt like "death warmed up." Then he stumbled out of the house and walked a hundred yards up Market Street to the Legion post. Jimmy, who lived about the same distance from the post, had told J.B. he was "just too darned tired" to get out of bed. He had wished J.B. "good luck." They were the last words he would speak to his friend.

By the time J.B. reached the post he was sweating profusely.

Dicko privately wondered whether J.B. was merely nervous about what lay ahead. The post was packed with the curious and excited, all of whom had come to see Tommy O'Regan, the world darts champion from Ireland, who had flown in specially to demonstrate his skills. The high spot came late in the evening when O'Regan positioned J.B. before the dart board. In J.B.'s right ear was stuck a lighted cigarette. O'Regan went to his mark. An expectant silence fell over the crowd. Then, with a flick of his wrist, O'Regan sent a dart flying through the air to pluck the cigarette out of J.B.'s ear and pin it to the board. In the thunderous applause, J.B.'s bout of coughing was drowned.

He left the post, intending to collect a jacket from home as protection against the shivering that gripped him.

He would feel too ill to return.

5

Separation

Walking briskly along at about one block a minute, Dr. Robert Sharrar turned into Broad Street, passing the elderly woman huddled in a doorway. Despite the early Monday morning heat—a nearby neon sign blinked out a temperature of 74 degrees—the woman wore a heavy winter topcoat and a black bandanna on her head. She was arranging her shopping bags, sorting out stale bread crusts, moving them from one bag to another. The Pigeon Lady, as she was known in the city, was preparing to begin her day's work of feeding some of the thousands of birds in the area. Sharrar doubted she knew the risk she was running: psittacosis, a disease spread by sick pigeons, could still be a killer.

Farther on, a young man scowled at the passing crowds. To anyone who was interested he explained his expression helped him to see into people's minds with his invisible third eye; a spokesperson for God, he said, had directed him to Broad Street. Sharrar thought the man might have been better directed into psychiatric care.

The thirty-five-year-old doctor paused at a traffic light. Almost automatically, he studied the person beside him. Anemia, he thought to himself. The girl's pallor and breathlessness were clear indications. Probably due to an insufficient intake of iron because of an inadequate diet, a common enough story, Sharrar knew, in this era of junk food.

The light changed and he broke into his stride again. Down a side street he glimpsed a pile of garbage. How long would it be before Mayor Rizzo declared a health emergency? A few more days, a week at the outside? Yet Sharrar believed the garbage looked worse than it really was: it might well attract more rats than usual out of the sewers, but the refuse was some way from becoming a serious threat to the physical well-being of Philadelphians.

In the time he had spent at medical school and then for the past two years working among them—or, more precisely, for them—Sharrar had come to know much about the mentality of the people of his city. Even if the garbage were allowed to rot forever on the streets, it would not faze them. They could cope.

He walked on, instinctively noting and registering. That was second nature, part of his job. People were pouring out of the subway, getting off buses, stepping out of cabs or—a very few—from chauffeured cars, all on their way to work. Some of them looked tired and dejected already. Sharrar was glad of the rewards his work afforded. And every day was for him a new challenge; he never knew what he would be involved in before he retraced this route at the end of the day.

Another block, then the Bellevue. He was pleased to see the hotel was restored to its resolutely old-fashioned self. In place of the legionnaires, well-dressed gentlemen and their ladies strolled past the Bellevue's doorman, himself once more composed and deferential. Sharrar liked the hotel. It was part of the vaguely outmoded charm so much of the city's real estate possessed; the Bellevue represented that almost indefinable quality called "Philadelphia Taste."

A few blocks farther south and Sharrar came into an area where the graces slowly disappeared, where drab and sometimes run-down buildings became the rule. He turned and entered one of them, 500 South Broad Street, the city's Health Center. Hurrying, anxious not to be delayed by any of the scores of other employees entering the warren-like building, he strode quickly to his cramped office on the second floor.

Sharrar, a CDC-trained epidemiologist, was chief of Philadelphia's Acute Communicable Disease Control Program, a post that effectively made him medical consultant to the city's doctors and adviser to the general public on all health matters. His wide-ranging responsibilities currently included preparing a program to vaccinate Philadelphia's citizens against swine flu. For weeks he had been on the alert for symptoms that would strengthen his worst fear—that the flu that left a trail of deaths throughout the city fifty-seven years earlier was about to ravage its inhabitants again.

Of all the United States Public Health Service officers working in city and state posts, Sharrar was one of the most enthusiastic supporters of the CDC commitment to mass immunization. As a result, Philadelphia was now in an advanced state of readiness. The money was there to buy sufficient vaccine to inoculate some 2 million people. Sharrar was determined that, once the vaccine became available, Philadelphians would be among the first to start getting their shots.

The bearded, bespectacled, and mild-mannered doctor possessed a ferocious appetite for work. Early on, it had brought him high scholastic honors and, later, the approbation of his seniors. After graduating from the University of Pennsylvania School of Medicine, he had been an intern at New York City's Bellevue Hospital, then a resident and later a fellow at the prestigious University of Colorado Medical Center in Denver. Following a two-year period with the CDC—like David Fraser, he had used it as an alternative to military service—in 1974 Sharrar returned to Philadelphia with his wife, Karen, also a doctor. The couple were married in 1971. In a few weeks Karen was due to have her first baby. Partly in preparation for this event, the couple had bought a new home, which they planned to move into at the end of the week.

From the moment he stepped into his office, Sharrar was engulfed in the residue of what had already begun as "a difficult year." Philadelphia's schools were hit by a major measles epidemic in February; there had been 1,500 cases, and some 30,000 children and adults were immunized before the end of the school year in June. The outbreak was still being studied, and all of the data collected flowed onto Sharrar's desk for epidemiologic analysis. There were also reports on the latest deaths in the city's fourteen hospitals, an update on the garbage strike, a note from the local medical society, letters from citizens complaining about dirty streets and rats, and a CDC publication about one of the hundred or so epidemics the agency tackled every year in the United States alone.

Sharrar did not entirely agree with the view, common in some Philadelphia medical circles, that the CDC style was to fly in, study an outbreak, and then rush back to Atlanta to write up the results for some prestigious journal. And the time he had himself spent with the CDC taught him tradecraft that had proved invaluable in these first seven hectic months of 1976.

Nevertheless, Sharrar enjoyed his present job even more than working for the big federal agency. Here in Philadelphia the work had more of a grass-roots quality; it was more local, seemed altogether more neighborly—particularly the telephone calls that even now interrupted him. A mother in a suburban slum was anxious to know when and where she could get her children inoculated against swine flu; a man complained he had awakened with diarrhea and vomiting and wondered whether it could be food poisoning; a schoolgirl wanted to know if she could catch measles a second time. Sharrar dealt with each of them gently. He was careful never to diagnose, always referring callers to their own doctor or the nearest clinic or hospital.

He also liked his work because of its variety. At any given moment news could come that would plunge him into the sort of medical drama few doctors experienced. He relished the prospect.

It was a similar outlook in David Fraser that had initially made Sharrar single him out. When Sharrar was already established at the CDC, Fraser was knocking at the door. Sharrar interviewed the confident young doctor and recommended he should go on an EIS course. Fraser, Sharrar recalled, had been an outstanding entrant, displaying an inborn facility for medical detection. With a blend of admiration and pride, Sharrar had watched Fraser climb the CDC tree to his present position, poised at Special Pathogens ready to leap to the more precarious upper branches of the agency.

Locally, Sharrar was perched well down the health department ladder. His small unit was on the same rung as Environmental Health Services, Emergency Medical Services, and the Health Program Analysis Division. They and the city's many other medical services were ultimately responsible to acting health commissioner Dr. Lewis Polk, a one-time pediatrician who wielded similar power to the police and water commissioners. Towering above them all were the city's finance director, solicitor, managing director, and, doubtless the strongest of the group, City Representative Albert Gaudiosi. More than any other employee in this pyramid, Gaudiosi was the one with the swiftest access to—and probably influence over—the man at the top, Mayor Rizzo.

In the event of a major epidemic occurring in Philadelphia, it was with those on the many rungs of this bureaucratic ladder that the indomitable Sharrar would have to contend. From past experience he knew it could be almost as exhausting as having to cope with the actual outbreak itself.

His telephone rang yet again. Commissioner Polk's office wanted to know how the training course was progressing for the teams being prepared to give swine flu shots. Sharrar suspected Polk wanted to have all his answers ready in case the gathering national storm over the entire program burst. Sharrar still hadn't considered that if the immunization scheme collapsed, he could find himself in an awkward position because of his total support for it. In any hunt for a scapegoat, he might be thought an acceptable sacrifice.

Suddenly a cough exploded in J.B.'s chest and then another. He could not stop coughing. The sound drowned the mindless chatter of the game show host on the television at the end of the living room.

His mother rose from the armchair in which she was dozing and hurried across to look anxiously at her son, lying on the living room couch, pale and perspiring. J.B. had hardly stopped coughing since returning home from the post on Sunday night. And since then, apart from staggering to the toilet, he had not moved from the couch. At times his body was racked by bouts of shivering violent enough to make the blankets shake. His mother and sister, Virginia Anne, took it in turns to stay with J.B. and keep him covered and supplied with the jugs of iced drinks that never seemed able to quench his raging thirst.

Mrs. Ralph begged him to let her call a doctor. She had seen a lot of illness in her time and was becoming convinced that her son "was growing sicker by the hour."

J.B. shook his head. It was, he croaked, only a bad summer cold.

He fell back on the couch and drifted into an exhausted and troubled sleep.

Farther up on Market Street, Doris stood at the apartment window watching Arthur Grubb, who had once been Williamstown's milkman and was now its long-serving mayor, talking to Police Chief Robert Seip. She liked both men: they were always friendly, and never by so much as a word had they shown any disapproval of her relationship with Jimmy. And even Dicko had surprised her when he brought Jimmy back from Philadelphia. Dicko had been affable and, sensing her concern, told Doris that Jimmy only had a bad cold.

Now she was not so sure. Apart from his cough, he complained of severely aching joints. She had dosed him with linctus, pouring spoonfuls of the syrup down his throat. It hadn't worked: Jimmy's coughing kept the children awake all night. This morning his temperature was up until she cooled his entire body with a towel filled with ice cubes.

Afterward she tried again to get him to talk about the convention, hoping this would take his mind off his condition. But Jimmy seemed to have only voice enough to ask for more ice water. Doris was surprised by the quantity he swallowed; already she thought he must have drunk a gallon this morning in between lurching to the bathroom from the fold-up bed in the living room he had slept on ever since their vow of celibacy.

She kissed him gently—and was astonished how dry and hot his lips were. She checked his temperature again. It was 102 degrees. She gave him another cooling wash, noting that the heat from his body appeared to melt the ice cubes even quicker than before.

But Doris still did not "rush for the doctor." While it might be more than a summer cold, the chances were, in the end, the doctor would only prescribe the sort of tender loving care she had shown Jimmy these past two days. That, she implicitly believed, was a more powerful medicine than any antibiotic.

Trying to find another way of holding his interest, standing by the window, Doris continued to describe what was happening in the street.

It never occurred to her to telephone and inquire how J.B. was. Nor, in spite of his newfound warmth, did she feel it necessary to alert Dicko that Jimmy was still sick.

Jimmy was her man, her responsibility.

And now, looking out on the normal, everyday ebb and flow of life in Williamstown, Doris was somewhat reassured. Nothing much could happen to Jimmy while life went on so normally. It was irrational—but reassuring.

Doris, of course, did not know that all over Pennsylvania scores of other legionnaires were in bed on this Monday, as sick as J.B. and Jimmy. Some were already at death's door.

Next day, Tuesday, July 27, in Philadelphia, the Bellevue's air-conditioner repairman was again back at work, feeling a little better after being sick for six days with what he thought was a bad cold. But today his two young children became unwell. Whatever it was that he had he seemed to have passed on to them. They had the same debilitating symptoms: headache, body aches, cough, and a fever. And those symptoms were similar to, although not yet as severe as, the ones being displayed by J.B. and Jimmy.

In the hospital at Sayre, Ray Brennan, the Air Force veteran with a passion for collecting seashells, having been increasingly ill with chest aches, breathing difficulties, and a fever, suddenly collapsed and died as his lungs filled with a bloody froth. His cause of death was diagnosed by a doctor as myocardial infarction—a heart attack.

They must dig beneath the surface and never accept a diagnosis at face value, intoned the lecturer in Auditorium B of the CDC: being a disease detective was not like normal doctoring where a physician was able, when baffled by a death, to conceal it, or to refer a dying patient to specialists; an EIS officer *was* the specialist, who, by the nature of his job, often struggled on alone, to be rewarded at the end by being "in at the kill" of one of the dangerous agents threatening a community—or even a nation. And the risks, the speaker reminded them, should never be forgotten: CDC files were filled with stories of scientists who had contracted contagious diseases from patients or had been stricken in the field with severe infections of the nervous system or even become paralyzed; one doctor had been in a coma for three years, another suffered severe mental retardation, a third was bedridden and unable to speak.

Ted Tsai listened attentively, aware that in a few hours' time, when the course ended this Wednesday, he and the other embryo epidemiologists sitting at desks in the auditorium could find themselves facing similar risks.

During breaks between lectures, Tsai had occasionally wondered not only how he would cope with such situations, but also how some of his colleagues would fare. He was not given to histrionics—nor would he have allowed himself to alarm Sherry by repeating some of the gruesome tales lecturers had used to illustrate their points. But the prospect of facing death in this way was a new one to him; doctors normally saved lives with little risk to themselves—he had chosen a medical career where his own life could be endangered. It was a sobering thought. He wondered how many of those seated around him had pondered it.

Throughout their time together in the auditorium, the soft-spoken and perceptive Tsai had observed his fellow students carefully; some of them had already revealed traits that were bound to influence their future careers. Many would probably do no more than the obligatory two-year stint with the CDC after the end of the course. Others would stay on with the agency, but gravitate naturally to less-demanding departments than the EIS.

Tsai felt sure that James Beecham, sitting a few desks away—a young surgeon chosen by the Pennsylvania Health Department to work at its headquarters in Harrisburg—would return to private practice once he had completed his two-year term. Though they were divided by background and mores, Tsai nevertheless recognized that in many ways Jim Beecham was similar to himself: he was independent-minded, liked to be his own boss, wanted the freedom to follow his own interests. But whereas Tsai was serious and quiet, the twenty-eight-year-old Beecham was gregarious and openly good-humored. Tsai liked him. He wondered whether their paths would ever cross again after Beecham went to Harrisburg at the end of the week.

Then there was the athletic Phil Graitcer, one leg extended awkwardly beneath his desk, a legacy of his road race mishap. Born in the same month that Tsai's father had helped launch a major Chinese offensive against the Japanese, the thirty-one-year-old dentist and inveterate diarist was above the average age of his classmates. He had already firmly established himself as the man with an astounding ability to circumvent the thickets of federal and local government red tape. His degrees in psychology from Duke University and tropical medicine from Harvard, his fluency in French, his work as a dentist in Sierra Leone shortly before Lassa fever took David Fraser there, his spell as one of Ralph Nader's Raiders, and his subsequent time in various U.S. government posts: they all helped give Graitcer an easy assurance that allowed him to sail confidently through the EIS course.

Sitting close to Graitcer was his friend the authoritative Robert Craven. At the end of the course the two would be joining the swine flu surveillance setup in Auditorium A. Craven, too, had a varied career before coming to epidemiology; it included working in England and Egypt. He had already spent a year with the CDC in analytical bacteriology before transferring to the EIS. Those twelve months he had spent with the agency had given Craven a polish—a mixture of incisiveness and charm—that many of the others had yet to acquire.

As he looked around the auditorium, Tsai realized he was surrounded by some of the most promising and ambitious new members of America's medical fraternity, all listening attentively as the lecturer ended his talk with a warning: once in the field, they would face danger. But they must never react from fear; they must proceed always with due regard for the safety of themselves and others by moving forward methodically, step by step.

It was good advice. And although Ted Tsai did not yet know it, events were already shaping that would answer his unspoken question much more quickly than expected about how he, Craven, and Graitcer would respond when put to the test.

Doris watched Jimmy's chest rising and falling. He was washed with perspiration and panting from the strain of coughing.

She finally made up her mind.

"Honey," she whispered, "I'm going to get the doctor. You're real sick."

Jimmy was too weak to answer.

The doctor decided to admit Jimmy to the hospital at once. While Doris telephoned her brother to drive them, Jimmy slowly dressed in the brown suit he had worn to the Legion convention. Then, as Doris packed him a bag, they both agreed it would be best for the moment not to tell Dicko he was going into the hospital.

When her brother arrived and had to support Jimmy as he walked to the car, Doris could see Jimmy was having great difficulty with even the slightest physical effort. That, more than anything else so far, made her frightened. During the forty-minute drive she tried to hide her fears by talking brightly of the future but, realizing Jimmy felt too tired to talk, she sat back silently beside him, squeezing his hand.

Pottsville Hospital was neither new nor particularly old. Established in 1895, it had been regularly renovated and extended down the years. Being a teaching hospital for nurses, it was run with anonymous efficiency. Jimmy had been born there.

While Doris attended to the admissions procedure, Jimmy was led away to undress. When she next saw him she was given his clothes to take home. Doris thought that, in his pajamas, Jimmy looked not only ill but apprehensive. A nurse explained to her she could not accompany him to his room, as the doctor wanted to examine him.

Blinking back tears, Doris drifted to the shop in the main lobby to buy some magazines and candy for Jimmy. Her brother returned to the car.

When Doris reached Jimmy's room with her purchases, the doctor was there. He seemed irritated as she placed her gifts on the bedside cabinet; the nurse with him swiftly whispered to Doris to leave. Once more she wandered around the hospital, killing time by orienting herself. The building appeared cheerful enough, but there was a vague aura of impending crisis about the place. At the Admissions Office she had been given a brochure. She sat in the lobby and read it from cover to cover. Then she walked back to Jimmy's room. Another nurse blocked her path. She was older and even more authoritative than the others. She brusquely told Doris not to return before evening.

Her tears now falling freely on her cheeks, Doris walked to where her brother waited in the car. She had no idea what to do next. Her brother suggested the only thing, really, was to go home.

Back in the apartment, completely alone for the first time since Jimmy had returned from Philadelphia, Doris sobbed loudly as she hung his brown suit in the wardrobe beside the blue one Jimmy was saving for their wedding.

On Friday, in Washington, negotiations between the swine flu vaccine manufacturers and the insurance companies finally collapsed. No further meetings between the two sides were envisaged. Without insurance coverage against the possible lawsuits resulting from any side effects caused by administering the vaccine, the manufacturers adamantly refused to release it for use. CDC director David Sencer's worst fear had been realized. The way was now wide open for Americans to be struck by the lethal virus without the prior protection Sencer had so strenuously urged.

The same day, Frank Aveni, the fit-as-a-fiddle legionnaire from Clearfield who had so much enjoyed sightseeing around Philadelphia's historic landmarks, was one of four conventioneers who died. Six more, scattered in towns all around the state, were seriously ill with the same symptoms—headaches, chest aches, high fevers, and lung congestion.

J.B. kept running out of new things to say as he attempted to fill in the silences between his heaving bouts of coughing with repetitious talk, hoping that simply by speaking, his fears would diminish.

His mother sat patiently beside him, inwardly very troubled but determined to remain calm. It was the only way she thought she could help J.B. see sense, to go to the doctor.

Once more he returned to the memory of his marriage. Even now he could not pinpoint where it had started to founder, or what portion of the blame should be laid against him. He was as bewildered as ever, he mumbled to his mother, by Carol's attacks over his fondness for Jimmy and Dicko.

Mrs. Ralph fed him another iced drink, her eyes never leaving him, listening carefully to his hoarse breathing as he forced himself to recall a past that still pained them both. It was Dicko who had first pointed out how Carol always danced especially close to other men—J.B. hated to dance—and it had been Mrs. Ralph who intervened when J.B. remonstrated with his wife, something else he had hated doing. Later he tried to smooth things over by showing an interest in Carol's appearance. J.B. had suggested she restyle her hair.

"Remember how she turned away?"

Mrs. Ralph remembered.

He recalled also how, during one of those increasingly rare passages in their stormy marriage, Carol admitted her tongue was sharp; J.B. had laughed happily, accepting, in turn, that her words were only defensive weapons against his own unpredictable behavior. He promised then to try to mend his ways and said, to mark the occasion, he would like to buy Carol a new dress. She had spoiled everything by suggesting he use the money instead to see a doctor who might be able to sort out what she had called his "crazy moods."

Listening now to that story, Mrs. Ralph thought: *If only she had asked me. I would have told her how much J.B. fears doctors.*

J.B. continued to be gripped by the past, dragging up one hurtful episode after another: the day Carol went to his mother and said she would no longer be his wife; the night she had taunted him about her being with another man; the way she had taken the boys from him, forcing him to feel he had to use drink to dull the pain.

Mrs. Ralph saw an opening.

She told J.B. that, if nothing else, he had a duty to his sons. He must ensure their mother did not change their surname. The best way he could prepare for that was by seeking proper medical help to get well; he would need all his strength for the battle ahead. He should let her drive him to a doctor in Harrisburg.

J.B. began to protest: he was going to no doctor—

His mother cut him off. In Harrisburg they could see the lawyer as well.

J.B. weakened. He would go only if he could see his attorney first.

Mrs. Ralph quickly agreed, rose to her feet, and hurried to Virginia Anne, telling her daughter to pack a bag for J.B. and place it in the car trunk, "just in case." When she returned to her son, he had another stipulation: he would drive the car.

She looked at him steadily. "J.B., you have a temperature of one-oh-two. You could get us both killed driving with a fever like that. And what good would that do?"

"I ain't being driven out of here by you, by any woman."

Mrs. Ralph offered a compromise. "You can drive to the edge of town. Then I'll take over. Okay?"

J.B. agreed. An hour later she helped him into the attorney's office in Harrisburg. His condition had appreciably deteriorated during the fifty-mile drive. Both his headache and his fever had worsened. The lawyer insisted J.B. should go straight to his doctor. J.B. was too ill to protest. Thirty minutes later, after examining J.B., his physician said he would make immediate arrangements to have him admitted as an emergency case of probable acute pneumonia at Holy Spirit Hospital, Camp Hill, one of the finest in the area.

Some three hours later, at about four o'clock in the afternoon of Friday, July 30, a doctor in Bloomsburg, Pennsylvania, called the state health department's regional office in Williamsport. He had three legionnaires in the hospital; tests suggested they had typhoid. They had all been at the convention in Philadelphia. The public health nurse who answered the telephone told him that nothing could be done; any specimens she might collect could not be delivered to the state laboratory before it closed for the weekend.

At almost the same time the infectious-disease-control nurse for Chambersburg Hospital telephoned the health department office in Chambersburg, a town some one hundred twenty miles to the southwest of Bloomsburg. She also had three patients who had just returned from the Legion convention; one of them had already died. In this case the public health nurse who took the call tried to inform others. But by the time her news was passed up and down the ladder—a process slowed, in part, by bureaucratic restrictions on long-distance telephoning—all the public health offices had closed for the weekend.

During that Friday afternoon, reception staff at the Bellevue Stratford began to complain that the air-conditioning vent above their heads seemed to be clogged. They were promised it would be looked at next week. Later, in the basement of the hotel, not far from the malfunctioning air-conditioning unit, the regular biweekly rodent fumigation process was carried out.

Although the hotel was not fully booked, no one was worried; the Eucharistic Congress delegates would be checking in during the weekend. Even the cautious and fastidious Harold Varr was overheard to say that, having removed the last vestiges of the presence of the legionnaires, the hotel and its staff could look forward to a period of rising prosperity.

Doris and her children spent the last part of Friday evening watching television. The children bombarded her with questions.

When was Jimmy coming home?

Soon.

What was the matter with him?

He was sick.

How sick?

Sick enough for the doctors to have to make him better.

Could they go and see him?

Soon.

But wouldn't he be home before that?

She didn't know. Following her second visit to the hospital that evening, Doris still had no idea what was the matter with Jimmy. Nobody at the hospital had approached her and she hadn't dared speak to anyone. The nurses seemed too busy to answer questions; the doctors were far too important to interrupt. Jimmy had dozed all the time she sat with him. Looking at him lying there, his head sunk into the pillows, his eyes closed, his breathing weak, she could only think he looked even more ill than he had in the afternoon. Yet nothing seemed to be happening. In the end Doris had come home and broken the news to Dicko.

He asked even more questions than the children. She tried her best to answer them, sensing an increasing tightness in Dicko's voice. But he remained outwardly calm and offered to drive her to Pottsville the following afternoon. She accepted.

In the Ralph Funeral Home, Mrs. Ralph and Virginia Anne also watched television late into the night. They had both agreed there was nothing to be done except to stay beside the phone. They were certain the hospital would call if there was any important news to impart.

That same Friday night, Edward Hoak, the Legion's adjutant in Pennsylvania, drove to his hometown of Manor, some two hundred miles west of Harrisburg. Early Saturday morning he received a call from a friend who said he had felt ill the night before but hoped to be at the installation ceremony for new officers of Post 472 in Manor later in the day. Hoak, the top paid official of the state Legion, was scheduled to be the main speaker at the ceremony. When he reached the post he learned that a legionnaire who lived in nearby McKeesport was dead and six others from the same area were sick. Among those now in the hospital was Hoak's friend.

Tragic though it was, Hoak did not find the news unduly alarming: "We have a lot of elderly people, so it's not unusual to have a couple of deaths after a convention."

The adjutant had no idea that throughout the state there were now seventy-four people seriously sick, all of whom had attended the convention that he masterminded.

As he drove away from Post 472, he was still blissfully unaware of the crisis that was brewing. Its effect would swiftly sweep across the United States—and then the rest of the world.

6

Valediction

Robert Sharrar and his wife, Karen, returned to their new home late on Saturday morning laden with purchases. She carried curtain rods; her husband, a stack of stools for the kitchen counter where they proposed to eat their meals. Already, after less than a day, the house was beginning to have a definite lived-in look; a couple more weekends—about the only real time they both had free—would see all the boxes unpacked and their home more or less furnished. Like many other working couples, the Sharrars regarded their weekends as sacrosanct, a time when they could temporarily forget the considerable pressures of their professional lives.

Just as Sharrar put down the stools, the telephone rang.

He looked at Karen.

"It's for you. I don't get calls on Saturday."

She shook her head, smiling.

"Bet it's not. I haven't given our number to anybody yet. It must be for you."

Still laughing, he picked up the telephone. The neutral voice of a City Hall operator identified herself.

"Dr. Sharrar?"

"Which one?"

"Dr. Robert Sharrar, the city epidemiologist."

Sharrar covered the mouthpiece and mouthed to Karen she'd won. He removed his hand and briskly confirmed he was the city epidemiologist.

The operator said a doctor was calling from Carlisle about "pneumonia in the city of Philadelphia."

"Put him on."

There was a short delay while the operator linked Sharrar with the caller.

The physician was worried. He had a patient in the hospital with an infection of the right lower lobe which he thought was mycoplasmal pneumonia—a dangerous illness caused by a small organism intermediate in size between a virus and a bacterium. His patient had a dry hacking cough and a fever. The doctor said he had also heard "of other cases in Philadelphia."

Sharrar's mind raced. From what the physician was saying, it seemed his patient might well have mycoplasmal pneumonia. There was really no way for Sharrar to be sure. He suggested the doctor draw some of the patient's blood and have it tested in the state laboratory when it reopened on Monday. In the meantime, if he was reasonably certain it was mycoplasmal pneumonia, the doctor should consider starting treatment with the fast-acting antibiotic erythromycin. It could produce dramatic results in forty-eight hours. But there was that other and more puzzling aspect, the question—

His caller repeated it: Did Sharrar know of any more cases of pneumonia in Philadelphia these past few days?

"No. I'm not aware of any."

The physician then fed Sharrar another tantalizing tidbit. He had just heard of a patient who had died of pneumonia—he wasn't sure whether it was mycoplasmal or viral—in the town of Lewisburg, not far away.

Sharrar jotted down the few details the doctor knew, and ended the conversation by again urging him to begin a course of antibiotic treatment. Sharrar then decided to call the pathologist in Lewisburg. There was no harm in checking.

While Karen waited patiently, her husband questioned the pathologist. He confirmed he had just completed an autopsy on a legionnaire whose lung tissue suggested the cause of death was a viral-type pneumonia; again, there was no way of telling except by laboratory analysis. Sharrar asked the pathologist to arrange that suitable samples be taken and sent to William Parkin, the state epidemiologist in Harrisburg, on Monday. Parkin could then arrange for the specimens to be analyzed at the state laboratory.

Sharrar continued to question the pathologist. It sounded as though influenza could have killed the man. He frowned. Could this legionnaire possibly be the first case of swine flu? He stressed to the pathologist the importance of getting specimens to Parkin to ascertain whether the death was, in fact, caused by an influenza virus.

After the calls, Sharrar realized it didn't make sense to jump to conclusions on what he had heard. The cases sounded not only different but unrelated. And so far as he knew, there were no other reported cases, least of all .in Philadelphia. Even if there were, it would not be unusual to have one or two in a city that size. He shrugged. There didn't seem anything to worry about. It could wait until the laboratory passed judgment on Monday.

On Saturday afternoon, as promised, Dicko drove Doris to Pottsville. They traveled in uncomfortable silence. Neither knew what to say to the other. Jimmy's sickness had, if anything, widened the gap between them again. They did not wish to share their mutual anxieties or hopes, preferring instead to keep them carefully concealed. On arrival at Pottsville Hospital they were told Jimmy had just been transferred to the intensive care unit, the ICU.

Doris was nervously biting her lips as they stepped from an elevator onto the sixth floor, the critical-care area. The afternoon sun filled the corridor with a glow which reminded Doris of that Sunday before Jimmy had left for Philadelphia—when they had sat in "our place," the dell overlooking Williamstown, and spoken of marriage. She wanted to cry.

Dicko stared at a red-painted surgical cart positioned halfway down the corridor.

It was the "crash cart," the ultimate emergency aid in this aseptic world. It contained everything possible to resuscitate a patient. The cart's top shelf was empty, a work space for the mass of materials on the two shelves below. Here were drugs to help make up for the sudden loss of oxygen during cardiac arrest, to help stimulate cardiac output, to bring back a patient from the dead. Here were sponges, tourniquets, solutions, syringes, needles, probes, suction catheters, airways, an aspirator, and a defibrillator, the boxlike instrument capable of giving a powerful electrical shock to start a stopped heart beating again.

To Dicko the cart looked alarming.

A nurse appeared from a side room. Dicko explained who they were. She escorted them in silence down the corridor, Dicko peering through each successive glass door port until they reached Jimmy's cubicle. The nurse told them they could go in. As they opened the door Jimmy began a bout of violent coughing.

Dicko and Doris stood in the doorway, uncertain whether to enter or not. Both were stunned by Jimmy's appearance. Green plastic prongs hung from his nose; the prongs were connected to a rubber pipe plugged into a wall socket from which flowed oxygen to assist his breathing. Wires ran from electrodes positioned on his chest to an ECG cart. A portable heartbeat monitor had been placed by his bed.

Towering over the clutter of equipment was a drip stand; a clear liquid trickled from its suspended bottle down a tube and into a vein in Jimmy's right arm.

The nurse beside the bed turned to them. She asked if they were relatives.

Dicko nodded.

She turned back to study the graph paper coming out of the ECG machine. It was a permanent record of the spiky lines tracing endlessly across the monitor screen. The strip confirmed the serious deterioration in Jimmy's condition. The nurse started to write on a clipboard, ignoring Doris and Dicko as they moved, almost on tiptoe, to stand at the foot of the bed.

Doris began to absorb what she was seeing. Jimmy was clearly very sick, yet all these wires and machines didn't seem to be helping. Great bouts of coughing welled up from his chest and burst through his mouth in a spray of phlegm and mucus.

The nurse continued to write her notes.

Doris moved toward Jimmy, to wipe away the dribble from his jaw.

The nurse sharply motioned her back and herself cleaned Jimmy's face of sputum.

Dicko asked what was the matter with his cousin.

The nurse turned to him briefly. He was very sick. It looked like a severe case of pneumonia.

Dicko asked: How bad?

The nurse replied: Speak to the doctor. She completed her notes and looked again at the heart monitor.

Doris began to plan how she could brighten up this stark room. She would bring flowers, a holy picture or two, perhaps a snap of the children: anything to remind Jimmy of home. Maybe she should bring the collection of dried palm leaves she had kept down the years to remind her of all those Palm Sundays she and Jimmy had sat surreptitiously holding hands in a back pew at Sacred Heart while Father Simpson spoke about the ways of the flesh.

Dicko watched spellbound as Jimmy's chest heaved and fell each time he gasped for breath. He knew the ICU was a place of last resort: only the worst cases, the real emergencies, ended up here. The intent way the nurse watched the graph and dials on the equipment deeply worried him.

Doris sensed Dicko was holding his fear tightly in check. She felt he might be even more frightened than she was. She began to whisper prayers for the sick, improvising passages she had forgotten, repeating those she knew by rote. During a pause between incantations, she tried to convey to Dicko her assurance that all would be well, smiling at him.

He just looked at her blankly.

The crisis came so swiftly not even the nurse was fully prepared. For a fleeting, frightening moment she stared at the heart monitor. The line was skipping beats and faltering. She whirled, running past them, shouting something that made no sense to Dicko. But the barely controlled panic in her voice told him this was no place for an outsider. He left the room.

Doris remained transfixed at the foot of the bed, eyes going from Jimmy to the hesitant green line staggering across the monitor. Firm hands suddenly seized her from behind. White-coated figures rushed into the room, propelling the crash cart before them. Doris found herself pushed out into the corridor, the cubicle door closed firmly behind her. She pressed her nose against the glass port and peered frozen-faced into the room.

The medical team knew they had perhaps four minutes, no more than six, in which to resuscitate the unconscious Jimmy. Through long experience they worked closely together, displaying speed, knowledge, and accuracy of observation. Jimmy's heart was in ventricular fibrillation, beating wildly and ineffectively. He was already as close to death as any person could be. A nurse swiftly disconnected the wires on his chest and plucked out the prongs from his nose; a doctor tilted back his head and began to feel for the pulse in his neck; a third team member smoothly inserted an airway deep down in his throat, fitted a bag-valve mask securely over Jimmy's mouth, and began to squeeze it, providing oxygen to inflate Jimmy's lungs.

Outside in the corridor, Dicko stood a few feet behind Doris, totally stunned by the speed of events.

Doris saw one doctor adjust the dials on a machine. Another was poised over Jimmy's chest, his gloved fist clenched and raised. He delivered a hard blow to Jimmy's breastbone. Doris winced. She had never heard of, let alone witnessed, an attempt to reactivate a patient's heart by a precordial thump.

A third doctor set up a plastic bag on the drip stand; the bag contained a solution similar to Jimmy's own adrenaline. As it began to flow into his body, the sluggish ripples on the monitor screen started to speed up. On a nod from a doctor, a nurse scissored open Jimmy's surgical gown, completely baring his body.

Instinctively, it seemed to Doris, for a brief moment the group around the bed stepped back.

Every one in the room knew time was running out; they would have to use the defibrillator on the crash cart to administer the emergency countershock they hoped would revive Jimmy. Working as quickly as they could, yet without the undue haste that could be fatal, a doctor and nurse coated with paste the defibrillator's two paddle-shaped electrodes and placed them on Jimmy's chest, one just to the left of his left nipple, the other slightly above his right.

The doctor checked the machine was set at maximum voltage. Then, making sure his own body was not in contact with Jimmy's and that everybody else was standing clear of the bed, he pressed down hard on the paddles while at the same time touching a button on each. A measured electrical shock was passed through Jimmy's heart.

Doris was shaking and perspiring. She wanted to look away, but now something else held her glued to the door port: she saw Jimmy's muscles go into spasm, his spine arch, and his powerful legs stiffen as the shock coursed through his body. The electricity even forced his penis erect.

The team around the bed waited nine critical seconds while the defibrillator recharged itself. The monitor continued to flutter unevenly, confirming total cardiac collapse. A nurse increased the drug dose flowing into Jimmy's vein. Another carefully controlled electric shock was administered. Another nine-second pause. Then a third shock galvanized Jimmy's body, almost lifting his 220 pounds clean off the bed. He sank back, limp and lifeless. But suddenly there was a change on the monitor screen, a momentary break in the line. Then, just as quickly, it steadied as Jimmy's heart began to beat normally by itself. The team around the bed waited.

Doris could see some of their faces. They showed no sign of emotion.

Finally one of the doctors nodded and turned. The others followed, saying nothing, pushing the crash cart before them.

Doris backed away from the door port, almost bumping into Dicko. They both retreated as the medical team emerged into the corridor.

Dicko asked one of them how Jimmy was.

The doctor shrugged and added, almost as an afterthought, that they could return to the cubicle.

The team dispersed. An orderly began to prepare the crash cart for the next emergency.

When they went back into the room, the nurse was propping Jimmy up with pillows and covering him from the waist down with a sheet. The monitoring equipment was back in place and his chest once more wired up to the ECG cart.

Doris saw Jimmy's lips move. She went quickly to his side and bent her face close to him, trying to catch his words. He was asking to go home.

Doris straightened, her cheeks wet. She rejoined Dicko. He was plying the nurse with questions. She repeatedly told him to talk to a doctor. Dicko finally left the cubicle in search of a physician.

Doris did not know how long she stood by the bed before she remembered the rosary in her pocket; she had counted the beads several times that day as part of her intercession for Jimmy. She held the rosary up for the nurse to see. Then she passed it to the woman, who placed the beads in Jimmy's hand, closing it firmly. Doris continued to pray. The nurse offered her a chair.

Darkness had fallen when the doctor entered the room. He carefully checked Jimmy's pulse, listened to his heart, and studied the graph printout from the ECG machine. He spoke quietly to the nurse. Then he turned to Doris and asked whether she was Jimmy's wife.

She shook her head, explaining they were getting married soon.

The doctor said he was sorry.

Doris looked blankly at him. She did not understand what he meant.

The doctor asked whether she would like to call a priest. Doris instinctively shook her head; she would not know where to find Father Simpson at this time of night. The doctor persisted. Should he arrange for the hospital chaplain to come?

Doris finally realized: the doctor was saying there was little time left. A priest was needed to administer the Last Sacraments. Jimmy was dying.

The doctor repeated his question.

Doris nodded, too numbed to speak. The doctor left the room and the nurse came to Doris, placing a comforting arm around her shoulder. Supporting Doris, she led her to the head of the bed. The two of them looked down at Jimmy. The nurse picked up a swab and placed it in Doris' hand. She began to wipe away the mucus from his mouth. The nurse handed her another swab; Doris dabbed at Jimmy's cheeks and forehead. She noticed his skin was deeply flushed and damp, his breathing loud and heavy. The nurse said gently that he was not in any pain.

After a while Jimmy's labored breathing eased and he even managed to say he felt a little better. But his voice had thickened and was difficult to understand. He was sweating so much that the bedding was soaked.

Doris asked if they should change the linen.

The nurse shook her head without taking her eyes from the heart monitor. Doris thought the spiky lines were slower and weaker. She held Jimmy's hand, fingering the beads and praying softly.

The chaplain arrived in the final hour of this Saturday and administered the Last Sacraments with professional compassion.

Jimmy's eyes never left Doris.

His ministrations over, the priest joined the nurse; together they both stared at the heart monitor.

Doris felt Jimmy squeeze her hand; he whispered he could not see her properly. She bent down, kissed his cheek, and asked whether he could see her now.

He nodded.

She remained there for a moment, her lips pressed against his skin. Jimmy whispered again he could not see her. She straightened, looking carefully into his face. He was smiling. Doris felt she should smile back, his expression was so relaxed and pleasant. Then she stopped; the way the nurse acted seemed to suggest something was wrong. She checked Jimmy's pulse and listened to his heart. Then she pulled up the sheet until only Jimmy's smiling face was visible.

She turned to Doris and spoke: He's gone.

Doris thought: *She means dead.* The priest came and stood beside her, murmuring prayers.

Doris continued to look at Jimmy's face. The smile seemed more fixed, more difficult to interpret.

The priest squeezed her arm and said it was all over.

Doris looked at him quickly and asked whether he was sure.

The priest nodded.

Doris placed her fingers on Jimmy's lips. They were still warm.

She turned to the nurse and reiterated: Was she sure?

The nurse nodded.

Suddenly Doris began to sob uncontrollably.

The doctor returned and briefly examined Jimmy. He whispered to the nurse, who looked at her watch. She wrote on the clipboard that James Dolan had died at 12:10 A.M. on Sunday, August 1, 1976.

They paid no attention to Doris' suggestion he might not, after all, be dead. With the doctor holding one elbow and the priest the other, she was persuaded to walk out of the room. She was too emotionally exhausted to resist; she showed no reaction when the nurse hurried after them to hand her the rosary. It was only when she was in the elevator that Doris finally accepted that her Jimmy was dead. A line had been drawn, an invisible barrier between a world that had contained somebody who needed her and one where she somehow had to go on alone. Dicko drove her home in silence. The gap between them had widened to a gulf that would never be bridged.

Some time later two orderlies appeared with a wheeled stretcher from an elevator at one end of the intensive care unit corridor. One went ahead and checked the cubicle. He switched on the light. Jimmy's corpse lay on the bed. He motioned for his companion to wheel the stretcher into the cubicle.

For a moment the attendants dispassionately studied the body. It remained abnormally warm despite the cooling onset of algor mortis—the "chill of death." Even though there were fever blisters on the lips, Jimmy's face appeared relaxed. The men checked the body for jewelry. It would be entered on a hospital inventory form. There were no valuables. One man opened Jimmy's mouth; there were no dentures to be

listed. The attendant closed the jaw. The other man placed a name tag
on the right wrist: DOLAN, J. T.

Between them they spread a plastic bag on the stretcher, unzipping
it. Then, one supporting Jimmy under the arms, the other grasping his
legs, they slid the corpse off the bed onto the plastic covering. One of
the men zipped the bag shut; only the vague shape of a body was
outlined.

They quickly wheeled the stretcher back to the elevator, descending
to the basement six floors below. It was the first hour of a new day and
the normally busy area was deserted. Harsh lights cast shadows from
the group emerging from the elevator. Pushing the stretcher along the
concrete floor—past storerooms containing medicaments in sealed
boxes and spare medical equipment—the men reached a locked door.
They opened it and pushed the stretcher into a walk-in cold-storage
chamber. There they removed Jimmy from the plastic bag and left him
naked on the stretcher. Locking the door behind them, they left the
basement. The lock was to stop anybody's interfering with a corpse. No
one at Pottsville Hospital could recall anyone's trying to tamper with
the bodies stored in this cold keep, but several doctors on the staff had
ghoulish tales of colleagues who had turned into necrophiliacs at other
hospitals. Better a lock than a scandal.

During the night the body suggilated—a continuous process in
which the blood settles into the most dependent parts of the vascular
system—leaving the skin pallid. After about five hours the first signs of
rigor mortis also became evident: a stiffening of the muscles in the
face, jaw, and neck.

At eight forty-five on Sunday morning, two other attendants arrived
in the basement. It was busy now, the hospital's rush period, with
nurses and orderlies collecting supplies. Nobody paid attention to the
two men. They unlocked the door and entered the chamber. One of
them checked the name tag. To their trained eyes further indications
of death were apparent: the eyeballs had sunk and flattened, dehydra-
tion was discernible, the skin had lost its elasticity, and rigor mortis
had spread to the arms and trunk.

The men wheeled the corpse out of the chamber. One locked the
morgue, the other unlocked the door of the nearby necropsy room. Together they pushed the stretcher inside, closing the door behind them.

In one corner of the windowless room stood a surgical cart holding
sets of instruments: bone cutters, scalpels, scissors, long-bladed knives,
hammers, and probes. On a worktop stood a wooden box marked SAW.
Close by was a still camera mounted on a stand. Against a tiled wall
was a cart with a couple of small handsaws plugged into outlets. Their
leads were long enough to reach the stainless-steel table in the center of
the room; it had a series of holes in its surface through which liquids

could drain into a grilled opening on the floor. Above the table was a powerful set of lights set in a reflector. One of the men switched on the lights. Along another wall were closets holding surgical trays, pots, and specimen jars, larger jars of formaldehyde, bottles of dyeing agents, culture slides, stainless-steel buckets, and kidney-shaped basins. A powerful pump capable of sucking out all body fluids in minutes was on a cart. A second worktop was covered with neat piles of blank report forms, one for each organ of the body. Taped to a third wall were specific instructions on how to handle a radioactive corpse. In another corner was a large sluice basin where used instruments were cleansed.

Tidy though the room was, perhaps because of its starkness, perhaps because of its function, it had an unkempt appearance. In the well-ordered routine of the hospital it existed for one purpose only, an almost ritualistic process that few members of the staff were permitted to witness.

The men lifted the body onto the table. Next they wheeled into position a stainless-steel table, on the top of which they positioned a set of scales. Then they left, locking the door behind them.

Shortly before nine o'clock the chief of pathology at Pottsville Hospital stepped out of his office with two other doctors.

He locked his door, possibly to prevent the curious from seeing his selection of skulls, poisons, and the unusual collection of antique contraceptive coils that he kept on display in a cabinet.

Slightly built, with quick probing eyes and bristle-bar moustache, the pathologist moved like a ballet dancer, all exact hands and feet. This natural grace enhanced his conservative dress and soft voice: rarely raised, it fitted his precise speech pattern. He never used two words when one sufficed.

The four years he had been at the hospital were time enough to establish him as a careful and thorough pathologist. He had his own marked style. Local morticians claimed they could always tell his touch: his neat incisions and precise stitches made their embalming that much easier. The pathologist's written reports were a faithful reflection of the man: taut, frill-free, totally lacking in hyperbole, and absolutely reliable. Those reports made him a favorite forensic witness in serious crime cases, leaving no room for lawyers to quibble. By the time he became chief of pathology in early 1976, he was respected far beyond the confines of Pottsville.

He was already familiar with Jimmy's clinical collapse. The case notes had been on his desk this morning when he arrived for work. He had studied them, noting the amount of drugs and other treatments administered. After a brief discussion with the attending physician, the pathologist had decided to perform the postmortem at once. As he and his colleagues changed into surgical smocks, trousers, and shoes and donned impervious rubber aprons, he told them he was "fairly certain it was a case of pneumonia."

The trio reached the necropsy room. The pathologist unlocked its door and led the others inside. They pulled on rubber gloves. Although regulations specified they should, none of them put on protective masks. They rarely did.

The pathologist walked over to the corpse and checked the name tag: DOLAN, J. T. Satisfied, he began to gather together his tools. As with any autopsy, what he would do had five separate yet interrelated objectives: to determine the cause of death for the death certificate; to determine the manner of death; to determine the contributory factors; to continue the clinical study of a case; to investigate all problems of a physical, chemical, bacteriological, pathological, and anatomical nature.

The men positioned themselves around the table, the pathologist on one side, his assistants on the other.

He began to run his gloved hands over the torso, arms, and legs, squeezing muscle and fat, confirming that complete cellular and molecular death had occurred. He searched the groin, looked between the toes and under the arms. As he worked he dictated brief observations to one of his assistants. The other helped him turn the body on its stomach. The pathologist continued to palpate and prod. He buried his hands in Jimmy's hair, feeling the scalp. Next he carefully inspected the base of the neck before tracing his hands down the spine. He prodded the rib cage. He moved to the buttocks, spreading the cheeks so he could inspect the anus. He ran his hands over the thighs and then moved to the legs. Finally he examined the soles of the feet. He found nothing untoward.

The pathologist positioned Jimmy's head more to his liking. He snipped off patches of hair and deftly shaved the scalp with a razor, leaving a wide path running from ear to ear.

A cranial autopsy was always the first stage of the postmortem. Incisions into lower areas, the chest or the abdomen, could allow blood to escape from the brain and give a wrong clinical picture of its original condition.

Once more the pathologist paused to study the exposed patch of scalp. It glistened under the powerful overhead light. He picked out a scalpel from the instrument tray and made an incision extending from behind the left ear, up over the middle of the head to behind the right ear. A trickle of blue-black blood followed in the wake of the blade. He began to use a set of retractors to peel the skin flaps away from the incision. He worked quickly, not merely following textbook procedures but relying largely on his own long experience. At last he had fully exposed the skull. When he stepped back from the table, his apron was speckled with blood.

He called for an electric saw. An assistant handed it to him. The pathologist switched it on; its sound changed pitch as he pushed the blade firmly against the bone, beginning to execute one angle of a wide V-shaped cut that would go inward from the back of the head. He paused periodically. The human skull can be anything from one quarter to three quarters of an inch thick; he had no way of knowing the thickness until he completed the cut. Each time he resumed, a shower of fine bone dust sprayed into the air. The room began to fill with an acrid aroma.

It took him some minutes to make the first cut. He made an identical one starting from the forward side of the head. The smell of singed bone increased. He finally switched off the saw and passed it to an assistant. Using elevators, spatulalike instruments specially designed for the task, the pathologist pried loose the segmented bone section from the rest of the head, almost as if removing a skullcap. Below lay the dura, the tough membrane covering the brain.

Once more he paused, this time to inspect the dura. He saw nothing to concern him. He reached for a small scalpel and nicked a corner of the membrane. Then, using pointed scissors, he cut the dura, exposing the brain. All three men carefully studied it. There were no visible signs of malformation.

Using a long-bladed knife, the pathologist snipped the nerves and blood vessels at the base of the skull, steadily loosening the brain from the roots that had linked it since before birth to the spine. He then began to lift out the organ, pausing once in a while to let an assistant cut a remaining vessel or nerve. At last the soft ball of grayish white matter was placed on the scales. It weighed almost three pounds, an average weight. Next he cut a piece of tissue from the brain that would later be microscopically examined; he did not expect the sample to reveal any disorder that could have contributed to death.

The pathologist watched as one of his assistants replaced the bone and skin flaps in their original position. The scalp was then sutured neatly along the line of the original incision.

The three men turned the body on its back. Fluid began slowly to seep through the sutures, dribbling its way to the holes in the table and on down to the drain in the floor.

Once again the pathologist reached for a new knife. He sank it expertly into the skin at the top of the breastbone and, using steady pressure, continued the cut down the entire middle line of the body, ending the incision at the upper edge of the pubic bone. Peeling back the muscle from the chest cavity revealed the rib cage. With a pair of surgical shears, he split the breastbone, neatly segmenting the ribs. His two assistants began stripping away the tough membranous sheath covering the ribs, opening a pathway to the heart and lungs.

That work completed, the membrane coating the surface of the lungs and the one enclosing Jimmy's heart were now visible.

As an assistant put a gloved hand into the chest opening to hold aside a lung, the pathologist carefully severed the ligaments and blood vessels attached to the heart. He then lifted it out of the cavity. It weighed some fifteen ounces, a couple of ounces heavier than normal. He snipped and peeled back the fibrous sac enclosing the heart, so that its surface glistened under the bright light. He examined the aorta; there was nothing alarming there. He turned his attention to the left and right coronary arteries; again there was no sign of any defect. He cut a tissue sample and placed it in a jar. He put Jimmy's heart beside his brain in a pan.

In turn the stomach, kidneys, and liver were removed and examined, and segments taken from each. The pathologist expected that none of the specimens would reveal signs of malignancy or malfunction.

During all this work it was the lungs that continually drew his attention. The large spongelike organs were filled with thick yellowish pus and covered with purplish red patches of pneumonia-like inflammation.

He carefully separated the lungs and weighed them. Each was some four times heavier than normal. To his highly trained eyes, they were "the worst pair I'd seen for a long time."

While he completed the task of taking lung tissue samples, his assistants began to place the organs in no special order in the chest and abdominal openings. Jimmy's brain and heart were put in the pelvis, just above his pubic bone.

The pathologist then rapidly tie-stitched the long frontal incision to hold the organs inside the body. He didn't say anything to his assistants, but privately this experienced doctor now wished that they had all worn protective masks: the condition of the lungs he had found "scary."

That Sunday afternoon, in Williamsport Hospital in north-central Pennsylvania, Dr. Terry Belles, a freckled-faced young resident, was working on a backlog of patients' charts when a nurse interrupted him. Richard Snyder, the commander of the town's Legion post, had arrived at the hospital to see five friends—Maxine McKay, Marjorie Martin, John Sheleman, Arlene Muffley, and William Hartman. All of them, like Snyder, had been to the Legion convention, and all were now sick. Snyder was demanding to see a doctor to find out what it meant.

Belles was already taking care of two of the patients: both were suspected viral pneumonia cases. When Belles found Snyder in Maxine McKay's room on the fourth floor, the post commander was visibly upset. Mrs. McKay, the wife of a veteran, also seemed to have pneumonia. And a nurse had told Snyder that John Sheleman's wife, who had accompanied her husband to the convention, had just been to the hospital complaining of a fever and cough. She had been sent home with a course of antibiotics.

Hoping to calm Snyder, Belles offered to take him to see his other friends. When they reached Arlene Muffley's room, they found the sixty-five-year-old legionnaire's wife being packed in ice to try to reduce her temperature.

Snyder became even more upset.

Growing increasingly perturbed himself, Belles went with the post commander to see his best friend, William Hartman. He, too, was showing signs of pneumonia. Snyder then said he had heard yet another veteran, Frederick Greene, was a patient in nearby Lock Haven Hospital. That, counted off the post commander, made seven conventioneers who had been struck down. What was going on? What was Belles going to do about it? What was *anybody* doing about it?

Belles said he would make further enquiries.

First the young doctor called Lock Haven Hospital; the legionnaire there had pneumonia. Next he telephoned Sheleman's wife at home and asked her to return at once to the hospital for a chest X ray. Then Belles went back to check the charts of Snyder's friends. He noted the fever and respiratory symptoms common to them all.

Belles was confused at the end of his investigation. Only Arlene Muffley had a positive laboratory finding—but it was not for viral pneumonia; it was for pneumonia caused by a rare group of bacteria, *Klebsiella*.

Baffled, the enterprising young doctor telephoned one of the hospital's pulmonary specialists. He told Belles he did not think they faced an epidemic of *Klebsiella* pneumonia since it was not a very communicable disease, but he did think it sounded as though "something's going on because these people were all at the same convention and now they are all showing up with fluid in the lungs."

He asked Belles to keep him informed of developments.

At six o'clock Belles went down to the emergency room to check on Mrs. Sheleman's X rays: the plates showed the same pulmonary infiltrates that her husband's chest film had revealed. She was admitted to the hospital at once.

When the hospital's epidemiologist was told what was happening, she immediately concurred that all the pneumonia patients should be transferred to an isolation ward. Then, at last, the state's local health director, Dr. Harry Buzzard, was informed. He in turn telephoned Pennsylvania's director of communicable diseases, the elderly Dr. William Schrack, at his home in Harrisburg.

The first links had been forged in a chain reaction. But for the moment nothing more was done: Schrack thought it too late on Sunday night to do anything further.

Dr. David Fraser and the members of the swine flu surveillance unit —all of whom, for their own reasons, were still on the lookout for an outbreak—had no idea anything untoward was occurring. The switchboard at the Center for Disease Control in Atlanta, manned twenty-four hours a day to receive emergency calls from anywhere in the world, heard not a word from Pennsylvania.

In Williamstown the wake for Jimmy, a happy-sad affair fueled by endless tots of liquor, continued in Dicko's kitchen late into Sunday evening. All the Dolan family were present, and throughout the day scores of friends had dropped in to pay their respects. Only Doris did not show up, an absence that caused a degree of speculation. Nobody considered she might be at home alone, grieving for Jimmy.

From time to time Dicko called Mrs. Ralph for news of J.B. There was nothing to report: she did not want to keep telephoning the hospital; she knew how busy the staff there were.

Jimmy's death had come as a shock to her, the more so as she had first learned of it when Dale Hoover called to say the Dolans wished the viewing for Jimmy to be at the Ralph Funeral Home, and it would therefore be sensible if Hoover embalmed Jimmy on the premises. Mrs. Ralph had agreed, and the body was due to be delivered the following afternoon.

Mrs. Ralph had considered telephoning her condolences to Doris. But in the end she decided to wait until they met in person. Even then it wouldn't be easy. She had often in the past made plain her disapproval of the relationship between the unmarried couple.

Doris came to a decision. She fetched from a drawer a pair of Jimmy's shorts, a white shirt, and a blue tie. Next she selected a pair of his black shoes and dark blue socks. She placed them in a pile on the table, tears welling in her eyes. She went to his wardrobe and stood for a while, crying openly, undecided. Then, in a fit of resolve, she reached up and pulled out his still-unworn blue suit. She folded it and placed it with the other clothes. Doris parceled them all up. In the morning she would deliver the package to Mrs. Ralph. The clothes were those that Jimmy had intended to wear on their wedding day. Now he would be buried in them.

After dinner Sunday evening, Adjutant Hoak had gone to his office near Harrisburg to work on his campaign for election as national commander. He found a letter from the wife of legionnaire Elmer Hafer saying her husband was in the hospital with pneumonia. A few minutes later, Hoak's secretary called to tell him that Hafer had died. Hoak was upset but not alarmed. He decided to discuss Hafer's death with his assistant, only to learn he was at a viewing for Charles Chamberlain, commander of the St. Thomas post in south-central Pennsylvania. Both Hafer and Chamberlain had been at the convention.

Now Hoak sprang into action. He called Snyder; the Williamsport post commander told him about the seven conventioneers sick there.

With mounting fear, Hoak made a spate of calls. Joseph Adams, who had just been installed as the new state commander, had news of more veterans in the hospital.

It looked very bad.

At 3 A.M. on Monday, the telephone rang in the Ralph Funeral Home. The neutral voice of the man on the line chilled Mrs. Ralph. He was an internist at Holy Spirit Hospital. J.B. had died five minutes before. Would Mrs. Ralph give her permission for an autopsy?

"Why?" She didn't recognize her own voice.

"Because your son seems to have died of a massive bilateral pneumonia whose etiology is unknown. It's important we make a determination."

Mrs. Ralph was unable to speak. She felt somebody beside her. Turning, she saw Virginia Anne, standing wide-eyed, her face a mixture of grief and shock.

"He's gone," whispered Mrs. Ralph.

"Oh, God. Not J.B.," cried Virginia Anne.

"Mrs. Ralph. Are you still there? We need your permission now. I'm going to have to ask you for your permission."

She looked at the telephone, hearing, but not listening to the insistent voice at the other end.

Mrs. Ralph felt her daughter's arms around her, comforting and supportive.

Virginia Anne was composed again. "Mom, give them permission. It doesn't matter now. J.B.'s gone."

Mrs. Ralph nodded, still numbed.

"Mrs. Ralph. Can you hear me? We must have your permission. . . ."

At last Mrs. Ralph spoke. She whispered into the telephone, "You have my permission."

"Thank you, Mrs. Ralph."

The urgent voice was gone. Mrs. Ralph put down the telephone. She looked at Virginia Anne. Then, in a suddenly fierce voice, she said that now, more than ever, they must ensure J.B.'s sons kept the family name of Ralph.

INVESTIGATION

7

Interrogation

Dr. Jim Beecham—fresh from the EIS course in Atlanta and just arrived this Monday morning in Harrisburg for his first day at work—could not quite believe his good fortune. Here, in the beehive of a building housing part of the Pennsylvania Health Department, he would have not only his own office—something the young doctor had never had before—but also a half-share in a secretary. And, she said, smiling, even when she wasn't working for him, she would still be at her desk, right outside his door.

"That makes all the difference," kidded William Parkin. "Where your secretary sits determines your standing in this place. Still, I expect you're used to that after the CDC."

Beecham grinned. He was beginning to like his outspoken new boss, the state epidemiologist. Twice already in their first fifteen minutes together, Parkin had dropped little hints about the CDC's being a hotshot outfit inclined to send in experts for an outbreak who afterward disappeared with the data, leaving behind people like himself to pick up the pieces.

"Nothing personal, you understand," continued Parkin pleasantly. "But they do tend to come in for the really good things and, if you'll pardon the terminology, to steal them!" He grinned at Beecham as he led him on a familiarization tour of the building. "You'll find things a bit different here. We can't, for a start, handpick our epidemics."

Parkin flashed another smile. "The best way for you to make your mark in this outfit is to forget all about your CDC allegiance. You work for me now, and I'll want total loyalty from you in the two years you're here."

Beecham nodded. During the EIS course he had been told about such attitudes; they were to be expected whenever CDC personnel were attached to state health departments.

Yet, instinctively, he knew he was going to get along with Parkin. There was an appealing daredevil quality about the man that belied his age—thirty-three—and his status—happily married, the father of three small children. Parkin had a definite presence. He was tall, muscular, and handsome enough to make many a pretty girl's head turn as they moved from one office to another. And his splendid handlebar moustache and casual clothes gave him the raffish look of an RAF fighter pilot from World War II. When he moved or spoke, Parkin radiated vitality, drive, and unshakable confidence in himself. Beecham had met somebody remarkably similar to Parkin just before leaving Atlanta— David Fraser. But he felt, after Parkin's remarks, he would not mention that.

He's quick to catch on and knows how to listen, decided Parkin; he will be an asset. He relaxed. Choosing somebody to fit into his small team was never easy. He glanced at Beecham. In spite of his boyish look, enhanced by lank white-blond hair, there was keen intelligence in his eyes. He'd need more than that, mused Parkin: he would need stamina and that indefinable instinct which made one epidemiologist superior to another. Parkin thought it no handicap that he, himself, was not a physician. Nor had he passed through the CDC mill which had deposited Beecham shiny-bright into his care. Parkin was a veterinarian who had gone on to major in epidemiology at the University of Pittsburgh. For the past three eventful years he had guided the epidemiologic investigations in a population of 8.5 million. The experience made him as much a specialist in his field, he felt, as any medical doctor. Certainly he would have much to pass on to his new acquisition. But there would be time for that later.

"Jim, you're going to find this a relief from your residency and stint at the CDC. It's going to be like two years of vacation. Basically eight to four, five days a week. Occasionally we'll work into the evening, but that won't be frequent."

It sounded like heaven to Beecham; never since leaving medical school had he had an entire weekend off.

"But better you learn the really important things first," continued Parkin, pointing. "There's the door to the bathroom, and down there is the coffee machine."

They moved inside Beecham's office. "Presumably you know how to operate the FTS?" Parkin nodded toward the phone on the desk.

"I think so," said Beecham.

"You should. You're a Fed, aren't you?" Parkin grinned.

Beecham flushed. It was a term he thought applied only to members of the FBI. He had already almost forgotten about his connection with the federal agency in Atlanta.

"Oh yes, FTS—Federal Telephone System. They taught us about that at the CDC, for calling federal government offices cheaper."

"Right," said Parkin. "But you've gotta learn about the state system. You dial 8 and then these numbers here to get into our health centers."

A frail voice interrupted Parkin.

"Bill. Glad I found you. Got something might be important."

Parkin turned. Dr. William Schrack, the health department's venerable director of communicable diseases, a wily seventy-year-old, bustled into the room.

"Got a call late last night at home," puffed Schrack. "From Harry Buzzard, health director for the Williamsport area."

"That's unusual."

"Buzzard thinks they've got an outbreak of pneumonia. He says it could be typhopneumonia—"

"That's pretty rare," cut in Parkin. "Not been around much since the depression."

"Well, Buzzard called me. Sounded all het up. Says they're legionnaires. They were all down at their shindig in Philadelphia."

"Yeah?" Philadelphia, like Pittsburgh, was normally outside Parkin's jurisdiction. But he knew he could, if necessary, get the authority to enter either city and take control of an investigation. He wouldn't want to do that in Philadelphia—not while the capable Sharrar was epidemiologist there. And certainly not with the Rizzo crowd running the place as though it were their own fief.

"Here's Buzzard's number," pressed Schrack. "I said you'd call him."

Parkin took the paper. He didn't know Buzzard personally. But he did know that even doctors out in the boondocks seldom pressed the panic button without reason. Although they might misdiagnose an illness, their alarm could still be a sign something was seriously wrong. Parkin was about to call Buzzard when the telephone rang in his office next door. He hurried to answer it.

The caller was another district health director. The man sounded excited. "I just got word about a couple of legionnaires in the hospital here in Chambersburg. One of them apparently died from some kind of pneumonia."

"What kind? And are you sure it was pneumonia?"

"I'll check."

Christ, thought Parkin, he should have found out before phoning.

"While you're at it, check whether the surviving legionnaire's got the same thing. It may just be a fluke."

He put down the telephone.

Beecham and Schrack were standing in the doorway.

"More trouble, eh?" asked Schrack.

"Maybe. Hustle over to the Legion headquarters and find out all you can about that convention. Whether they've got any reports of others sick."

"Yes, sir," said Schrack, grinning.

"Jim, you come with me," said Parkin. "We're running late. You might as well get blooded now as far as the administration here goes. It's time for you to experience your first Bachman meeting."

He explained they were going to the regular Monday morning conference of departmental heads in the office of Secretary of Health Leonard Bachman.

"What's he like?"

Parkin smiled equivocally at his new assistant. "He'll eat you alive if you make a mistake. He's a ball of fire. Fifty-one years old and still moves like a wrestler."

They strode out of the building and set off to drive the mile to downtown Harrisburg where Bachman had his office, Parkin all the while sketching a vivid portrait of the most powerful doctor in the state. Bachman had held office for a year. He was an avid nonsmoker and ran a tight ship. He held strong likes and dislikes. He liked anybody who worked hard and didn't ask for more money. Among those he couldn't abide were Philadelphia's Mayor Rizzo and, above all, his high-powered adviser Al Gaudiosi.

"I'll try and remain invisible," said Beecham.

"Hell no. You've got to stand up to him. It's the only way to get his respect."

Beecham grinned. He felt increasingly relaxed sitting beside his ebullient companion. As they parked in front of the health department headquarters, he asked Parkin whether he would be mentioning the news he had just heard.

"No—it could be nothing. Bachman isn't interested in rumors. And he sure wouldn't trust anything Schrack or Buzzard said. He's been pushing for those two to be put out to pasture ever since he took office."

Beecham flinched. "Look, I think I'd better just follow your lead."

Parkin smiled. "You do that and you'll be okay."

Beecham was reassured. Walking into Bachman's meeting, he glanced at his watch. It was eight-fifty. He had been working for the state health department for less than an hour and already things seemed to be humming. He felt certain none of his recent classmates could have got off to a better start after their EIS course.

Two of them, Robert Craven and Philip Graitcer—still walking stiffly after the plaster cast had been removed from his foot—were familiarizing themselves with the mechanics of the impressive War Room at the heart of the National Influenza Immunization Program. It occupied almost the entire area of Auditorium A at the CDC: banks of telephones, teleprinters, and computers, the hardware for an unprecedented monitoring system which, to work, also required a typing pool, photocopy machines, and doctors sitting at rows of desks in the center of the room. Yet on this Monday morning any meaningful action seemed as far away as ever. The main talking point was that the battle between the government, the insurance companies, and the flu vaccine manufacturers was still deadlocked—and there seemed no way out of the impasse.

Craven sensed there was a real danger the occupants of the auditorium could grow stale from the weeks of constant alert that had so far produced no result. Graitcer thought many in the War Room must feel like keyed-up combat troops who were being denied the chance to storm some enemy beachhead. Apart from going to the adjacent cafeteria, there was little for anyone to do—except wait.

The two young EIS officers, having completed a leisurely inspection of the War Room, returned to the section to which they were assigned, Surveillance and Assessment. If anything, it was even more dead than the other areas; some people just sat at their desks and watched the hands on the wall clocks.

Suddenly the telephone on Craven's desk rang.

"Beginner's luck." He winked at Graitcer as he picked up the phone and pulled a pad and pencil toward him.

The caller was a doctor with the Veterans Administration Clinic in Philadelphia. He said he had a problem.

"How can I help?" Craven waited, pencil poised.

Carefully hiding his concern, the man began to explain. "Last Friday I started to treat a patient for bronchitis. This morning his X ray shows pneumonia."

Craven waited. Why was a doctor in Philadelphia phoning from several hundred miles away to tell him this?

"My patient has just informed me he has heard of four other people who have died of pneumonia. The point of interest, I think, is that they all attended the recent Legion convention in this city."

Craven's mind raced. Four deaths more than met the statistical criteria for an outbreak. But what kind? Had swine flu finally broken out?

"Can you tell me more about this convention?"

Craven was aware that people at other desks were looking curiously at him.

"My patient is here. Would you like to talk to him?"

Craven questioned the man. He could offer little new information: there had been "thousands" of legionnaires at the convention, the majority of them elderly; they had all had a good time, "a lot of drinking and late nights, that sort of thing."

Craven relaxed. It didn't, after all, seem so unusual; he would have expected a number of deaths as a matter of course among such a large gathering of elderly people, many of whom were probably suffering from some respiratory complaint. Four deaths was high, but not alarming.

"Have you notified your state epidemiologist?" asked Craven.

"I can't get through. The lines seem jammed."

"I'll give Jim Beecham a call," whispered Graitcer, who was bending over Craven's desk listening intently to the conversation. "See if he knows what's going on." Graitcer returned to his desk and began to dial Harrisburg. Craven spoke again to the doctor in Philadelphia.

"It's strange, but we've heard absolutely nothing about these deaths until now. What I need is more information about those dead legionnaires. Their ages. Who their doctors were. Where and when they died. Who were the pathologists who did the autopsies. Anything you can get."

The doctor promised to do what he could.

Craven put down the telephone and continued making notes on the call while Graitcer tried to reach Beecham in Harrisburg; the line rang constantly busy.

As Craven looked up, he saw his division director walk into the room. He immediately read to him what he had written on his pad.

His superior listened carefully to what Craven said. Then he cautiously told Craven that whatever was happening in Philadelphia, he doubted this was the first sign of the long-expected swine flu.

Nobody could be that lucky on his first day at work.

Secretary of Health Bachman wound up the staff meeting faster than usual. No one had to ask why: the normally conservatively attired health chief was dressed for vacation in nautical jacket and trousers.

With a final warning to his aides that he expected no foul-ups while he was away on his boat, he waved them out of his office.

Parkin was the last to leave, taking Beecham in tow. Bachman had stared briefly at the baby-faced EIS officer and growled his standard benediction: if Beecham worked hard, he would do well; if he slacked, he would have the devil incarnate on his tail.

Bachman had liked the way the young surgeon responded: polite but not subservient. He couldn't stand a yes-man; he tried to surround himself with men and women who knew their own minds—and were not afraid to speak them. That was one of the reasons he liked Parkin— that and the man's incredible capacity for work.

Watching the slim Beecham close his office door, the feisty director of the state's medical services could not help but think: They get younger all the time. Still, that was no bad thing.

He slumped back in his swivel chair. As of now he was on vacation. His car was packed, his boat and trailer attached ready to go. In a few minutes he would walk out of this office and for the next few weeks shed all the cares and petty medicopolitics that bedeviled his working life. It had been a grueling year. Uppermost in his mind were his continuing staff problems, in addition to which he had so far been unsuccessful in ridding the health department of its more aged physicians who he thought had been "marvelous men back in the thirties but were now doddering and not up to it."

He toyed with one of the brass fittings he had bought for his boat on the way in to the office. By tomorrow morning he would have the English-designed GP-14 racing through the waters off the Maine shore.

Life, after all, mused Bachman, had many compensations. He was friendly with the governor, had a powerful voice in state affairs, was virtually his own boss, and had an adoring wife and family. In addition he had his health, a decent income, money in the bank, a life-style the newspapers called "comfortable." They also called him peppery, tough, and a grappler, an allusion to those days when he had been a champion bantamweight wrestler. Bachman understood media shorthand; that had helped make him, on the whole, one of their favorites.

He rose to his feet, tossing the brass fitting from one hand to the other. He was moving toward the door when the intercom buzzed. Bachman frowned. His secretary knew he was on vacation; all calls should have been diverted to his deputy. Slightly irritated, he depressed the intercom key.

"What is it?"

"The Associated Press wants to speak to you."

Bachman groaned.

"Tell them to talk to the press officer."

"He insists on speaking to you. Says it's important."

Bachman looked at his watch. Just after ten o'clock; he could still deal with the reporter, get home, and be on the road by noon.

"Okay, put him on."

The reporter's voice was flat as he began to recite.

"Dr. Bachman, Edward Hoak, adjutant of the American Legion in this state, has just issued a statement expressing grave concern that some thirty of his legionnaires who attended their convention in Philadelphia a little over a week ago are now seriously ill with what Mr. Hoak is calling 'mysterious symptoms.' And he says at least eight of his men, and probably more, are dead. What comment do you have at this time . . . ?"

Bachman dropped the brass fitting onto his desk. He knew he

wouldn't be needing it. His vacation had ended before it began. He sat down in his chair and asked the reporter to repeat Hoak's figures.

Dr. Sharrar looked again at the X ray. It showed nothing. Yet he could see that his usually robust assistant, Mitch Yanak, was sick. Yanak was pale and drawn and had a headache and dry hacking cough. But after giving him a thorough checkup in the examination room at 500 South Broad Street, Sharrar could still find nothing that would explain Yanak's condition. He told his ailing assistant to get dressed and go home.

Yanak began to protest; he hated to miss work.

Sharrar shook his head: now was a quiet time. Yanak should be in bed. He would need Yanak to be fit and well for the next flu season—expected to begin in about six weeks—when Yanak would again supervise epidemic investigators in the field.

Reluctantly Yanak agreed.

Still pondering what could be the matter with his assistant, Sharrar strode back to his office. He came through the door to find his telephone console "lit like a Christmas tree."

He pressed a button at random. It was Parkin bringing Sharrar into the gravest epidemiological crisis America had faced for a long time.

In every public health office in Pennsylvania, telephones were now ringing. The switchboards in Harrisburg, Pittsburgh, and Philadelphia were soon completely blocked by the calls.

Jim Beecham thrived under the pressure. During his EIS course he had been taught that an essential part of any investigation was the early gathering of information by phone. The trick, Beecham knew, was to work at top speed without being slipshod; nobody should be cut off before the basic information had been given, allowing for lengthier follow-up calls later.

"Would you repeat that, please. There's a lot of noise here."

Beecham pressed the receiver tight against his ear. He could still hear Parkin's voice booming out from the adjoining office. In other offices people seemed to be talking and shouting all at once.

". . . Who did the autopsy?"

A nurse ran down the corridor calling for Dr. Schrack.

". . . Let me check the spelling of his name. D-o-l-a-n. Initial J. And the pathologist . . . do you have a number for him?"

Beecham continued to scribble on his pad, ignoring the temptation to press the other buttons insistently winking on his telephone.

Next door, Parkin was switching deftly from one caller to another, placing and removing them from "Hold" with an unerring touch.

"You're being wise after the event," he rasped at a local TV station reporter. "We only heard about this an hour ago and we are doing all we can to get to the facts. You want to ask any questions about delay —talk to Bachman. The only delay I'm having is dealing with the press!"

He cut off the reporter and pressed another button.

"Listen"—this to a regional health director—"time is a key factor here. You and I know in our business important evidence can disappear fast. We've gotta get specimens to the lab in Philly immediately. This thing may spread. What? Hell, I don't know. It could be Lassa fever, maybe pneumonic plague. Killers. No, I'm not kidding. Just get those samples in fast. Okay?"

Another button. It was Bachman.

"Parkin, I've got to give the press something quickly. Hoak's gone off on his own and talked to them already. We've got a panic in the making and I want to put this thing in perspective."

"Too early, too early. I'll call you as soon as the picture clears."

"I can't wait. We're already behind because of the problems with our Williamsport office. And there's maybe ten dead already."

"I know. I know. We're trying to get a fix. Once we do, I'll let you know," promised Parkin.

"You listen to me, young man. I want you here for a meeting at noon, I want you here for a press conference at two o'clock, and I want you to bring along that new CDC guy to make things look good. Understand?"

"But we've got our hands full here—"

"You heard what I said. I'll see you at noon."

Parkin thought the health secretary sounded more jittery than he could ever remember. No doubt he was under growing pressure: Governor Shapp's office would be calling him, the media would be laying siege to his telephone. So would a lot of other people. Parkin shrugged. Bachman was a seasoned performer—he would know how to deal with the callers. The annoying thing was having to return to Bachman's office with Beecham. He'd certainly have to prepare the EIS officer for that.

The epidemiologist pressed another button. It was the chief of pathology at Holy Spirit Hospital, Camp Hill. He had news that made Parkin sit bolt upright and reach for pen and paper.

"When?"

Parkin scribbled a note.

"How long?"

Another scribble.

"Doctor, I want those samples as fast as possible."

Parkin's secretary poked her head around the door.

"It's UPI."

Parkin covered his mouthpiece. "Dammit, put them on to Bachman's press officer. I'm too busy for public relations."

He turned back to the pathologist.

"Sorry. We've got a lot of interruptions here. What's his name
again?"

Checking every letter after he heard it, Parkin wrote on his pad:
RALPH, JOHN BRYANT. He circled it and wrote underneath that J.B. had
died at 2:55 in the morning and that his autopsy was now in progress
at Holy Spirit Hospital.

It was going to be close. If it was a flu virus that had caused Ralph's
death—and was responsible for all the other deaths—there was every
chance it had invaded his body, triggered a series of adverse physiologi-
cal and biochemical events, and then disappeared before any symptoms
were evident. If it was something else—perhaps another kind of virus—
it might have persisted in the body for the first few days of the illness
and then disappeared before the peak of the disease was reached.

Only laboratory analysis could determine the situation one way or
the other.

Parkin informed the pathologist he would be sending a state nurse
to collect the samples from J.B.'s body the moment they were available.

J.B.'s body—waxy, cold, and hardening—lay on a stainless-steel table
in the center of the necropsy room in the basement of Holy Spirit Hospital. In size and furnishings it was almost identical to the one in
which the autopsy on Jimmy had been performed. But the doctors at
Holy Spirit wore protective masks and had taken special care to surgically gown themselves. The pathologist had ordered these precautions
after learning that Jimmy and J.B. had both been at the Legion convention.

The pathologist was in no hurry to begin work until he knew everything he could about the sequence of events that had finally deposited
J.B.'s corpse in this chilly and cheerless room.

"The case notes say his main complaint on admission was cough and
fever," said an assistant.

"Look at his HPI," said the pathologist. "That tells us a lot."

The doctor began to read, his voice echoing off the tiled walls and
floor.

"A known diabetic. A known alcoholic who drinks sporadically but
excessively. An ADA diet. Regular Librium, Beminal, insulin—what a
life."

He glanced toward J.B., staring sightlessly at the ceiling, hands rigid
at his sides, toes pointing stiffly upward.

"Drank heavily, beer and whiskey, during Legion convention July

21–24; fell sick afterward. Developed fever, shaking chills, headache. Became somewhat delirious. Temperature reached 105. Admission X rays showed a bilateral pneumonia, left greater than right. Seemed to be patchy and rather diffuse."

He studied the FH—the family history. Nothing much there: J.B.'s father had died from a heart attack at sixty-three; his mother was a fit seventy-five-year-old; there was no history of cancer, diabetes, epilepsy, or hypertension.

"The SR shows a gall bladder operation in 1968; during recent years, since his divorce, he had become short of breath, mainly on exertion. Has had liver problems, but no hepatitis or jaundice. No VD. No varicose veins or phlebitis."

The pathologist nodded, then began to run his gloved hands over J.B.'s body, dictating as he worked: "Bald shaven head, numerous pits over skin."

He prized open J.B.'s mouth. "Has lower teeth, edentulous in the upper, and this was compensated." He felt J.B.'s neck, chest, and abdomen, noting the gall bladder scar. "Normal genitalia. Small external hemorrhoids. Pigmented skin over the shins and around both ankles."

He straightened up from his examination.

"Let's go to work."

Some thirty minutes later, the pathologist had removed J.B.'s brain from his skull. It was weighed and a sample removed.

He picked up a scalpel, pierced the skin above J.B.'s pubic bone, and drew the knife straight up to the breastbone. Then he made an incision toward the right armpit and another toward the left. He had executed a large blood-rimmed Y. He called for an electric saw and traced it back down each arm of the Y. He then raised the sternum, revealing the internal organs. Working as a team, the doctors cut away the tissues attached to the diaphragm and started to remove the heart, kidneys, and liver, still enclosed in slippery silvery membrane. The pathologist lifted out a final tangle of entrails and dipped into the shell of J.B.'s body to take out the lungs.

There was little conversation now, except the pathologist's voice reminding his companions of what the M.D.'s lung report had noted: bilateral inspiratory rales most marked in the right base. That hardly prepared him for what he now saw. J.B.'s lungs "looked like Brillo pads."

He carefully sliced a section from each lung and weighed the specimens—over 300 grams (10½ ounces). Samples were then taken from J.B.'s liver and kidneys. A portion of his fat deposits was also weighed and placed in Formalin.

The pathologist labeled the containers while his assistants replaced the organs in J.B.'s cavity and loosely sewed together the Y.

J.B.'s corpse was now ready for his friend, Dale Hoover, to collect
and take to the Hoover Funeral Home. There, in his embalming chamber, he would prepare J.B. for his last public appearance on this earth.
Once Hoover finished his handiwork, nobody would ever see that parts
of J.B. had been removed, which, even now, were beginning a journey
that would take them from Holy Spirit Hospital to Harrisburg, to Philadelphia, and finally to the CDC laboratories in Atlanta. There J.B.'s
specimens would prove of more value than anyone at this stage could
conceivably guess.

At the CDC, in Auditorium A, Phil Graitcer eventually got through
to Jim Beecham in Harrisburg. Beecham told him a system of collecting specimens had already been set up. Even so, said Graitcer, the EIS
would want to augment that and become involved in the field investigation. Conditions made it ideal, he argued.

If the outbreak had merely struck a random group of people who
just happened to have been together for a time, the chances were when
later some of them started getting sick and dying there would be little
prospect of their friends or families knowing others were in the same
position. With the legionnaires it was different: they were a closely
knit and identifiable group. From what Beecham told Graitcer, it was
clear the Legion had the facilities to check rapidly on the medical status of all the members in the state. It was just the sort of developing
situation the swine flu surveillance unit needed.

"We don't know yet if it is swine flu," said Beecham.

"You don't know that it's not," countered Graitcer.

He hunched himself forward over his desk so the others around him
in the War Room wouldn't overhear.

"Look, Jim, we're going to want to come up there, and you've got to
help get us an invitation."

"Phil, I've only been here a couple of hours. I hardly know where the
bathroom is. But I can tell you one thing. Parkin, who runs the setup,
is not actually enamored of the CDC."

"Listen. We both know the federal government doesn't go into a
state without an invitation. So how do we get it?"

"I guess it must come from either Bachman or Parkin."

Graitcer grunted. "Okay. There are guys here who'll be in touch
with them. But we *are* going to want in. When the time comes, will
you give your support?"

"Sure, Phil—for what it's worth."

Graitcer sat back, satisfied.

Close by, Bob Craven picked up his phone. It was the doctor from
Philadelphia calling again. This time his voice was not calm.

"How does eleven grab you?" he almost yelled down the line. "There are eleven dead now."

The doctor made no attempt to conceal his concern, heightened by his continuing inability to get through by telephone to the public health offices in Harrisburg and Philadelphia.

Craven called across to Graitcer, asking whether Beecham was still on the line. Graitcer shook his head.

Craven urged the doctor to telephone again with any further news. Then to the astonishment of those in the War Room, the normally controlled Craven shouted out loud enough for almost everyone to hear, "This is it. This is the beginning of swine flu. We're in business!"

At the Bellevue Stratford, Harold Varr and Bill Chadwick were also pleased with the way their business was going. It was midmorning, Monday, and the hotel's two senior executives stood at the top of the marble staircase watching the orderly and spectacular scene unfolding below. Throngs of soberly dressed clergymen—the standard grayness of their garb enlivened by the splash of a monsignor's purple or cardinal's red—moved about in the lobby, delegates to the first International Eucharistic Congress to be held in the United States for fifty years. The area was filled with the voices of priests from Asia, missionaries from Africa, nuns from Ireland, as well as many of the religious leaders of Europe. A group from the Vatican conferred in one corner of the lobby; in another a bishop and his retinue conversed; at the gift stand, still others were buying postcards.

"How civilized they all are," murmured Varr.

"And how different from the last lot," added Chadwick.

"The staff certainly think so. I haven't seen so many real smiles for a long time."

They watched approvingly as the front desk clerks dealt smoothly with the delegates, as the bell captain directed his men with the minimum of fuss, as Anna Taggart greeted each arrival with a deferential smile.

Satisfied all was well, Varr and Chadwick walked to their offices on the mezzanine floor. They both still basked in the dazzling smiles Princess Grace and Prince Rainier had bestowed on them when they earlier escorted the royal couple and their three children to their suite; they had left before the princess turned off the air-conditioning unit—something she always did in any hotel suite she stayed in.

Varr had barely settled down to study a beverage consumption report before his secretary announced there were two reporters demanding to see him.

Varr settled back in his chair; he didn't normally deal with the media, but a little publicity was always welcome.

"Show them in and bring some coffee."

"They say they haven't time for coffee."

"Perhaps a drink—"

"Mr. Varr?" The taller of the two men in the doorway had an aggressive voice. "You in charge here?"

"I'm the general manager, yes."

"Then you'd better listen to this." The second man began to read. "At least twelve American legionnaires are dead and another forty hospitalized in Pennsylvania following their convention in Philadelphia—"

"They stayed here, right?" asked the aggressive reporter.

Varr felt his hackles rising.

"This was the headquarters for their convention, yes. You would be correct in saying that."

"And would we also be correct in saying you have been killing them off with the food you served them?"

Varr rose to his feet, fighting to control his anger.

"You boys got any proof for what you're saying? You'd better have. If you print anything like that you'll get sued to the wire."

The second reporter looked at the sheet of Teletype in his hand and smiled deprecatingly, trying to defuse Varr's anger.

"No need to get sore, Mr. Varr. Like you, we've got a job to do." He tapped the paper. "It says here all these people are dead or sick with the same illness. This was their headquarters—"

Varr cut him off. "The Legion was spread through a lot of hotels. Why pick on the Bellevue?"

The reporter looked solemn. He said he was not picking on the Bellevue, merely trying to establish the truth.

Varr was not mollified. "This is a hell of a way to go about it. Barging in here, making accusations." He spread his hands on his desk, fighting down his fury. "We didn't have any complaints about our food. If there had been anything wrong, we'd have the Health Department on top of us in a minute—"

"You still might," snapped the first reporter.

Varr had had enough. He told the reporters he was taking them to see Chadwick. After listening to their story, Chadwick moved to divert it from the Bellevue.

"Gentlemen. There is nothing you have told us which can remotely connect this hotel with this tragedy. We did have some six hundred members of the Legion. But there is nothing in that Teletype to suggest any of those now sick or dead stayed here."

The reporters looked at each other, uncertain.

"At the very minimum you need to establish where the legionnaires stayed. I'm sure you will realize the damage any inaccurate reporting could cause."

Chadwick looked carefully at the reporters. Inwardly, Varr admired the way his superior was handling them. He began to relax.

"Gentlemen, you strike me as responsible members of the media. I'm sure you will wish to check further before involving us in this matter."

The first reporter's tone changed. His voice had lost its aggression but somehow, thought Varr, he now sounded more menacing.

"Mr. Chadwick, we will check. And we will be back. You yourself said this was the convention headquarters. If it wasn't the food in this place which killed them, then how can you say something else here isn't responsible?"

"Pure speculation," said Chadwick pleasantly.

Only Varr noticed the sudden tightness around Chadwick's lips. Varr's own well-attuned antenna was also signaling: "Trouble. Big trouble."

In silence the hoteliers watched the reporters leave.

All morning Doris had been formulating her thoughts. Death was so terribly final. Never again would she hear the voice that for so long had been part of her life. What, she thought, was she going to do now?

Throughout the weekend relatives and friends had gathered around and were of great help. Life, however, seemed to be unreal. Something of her own self, as it were, had gone; she wondered how life could be worth living without Jimmy.

Gradually she came to realize that death was part of life. It had to be accepted. She knew there was no way she could escape the sorrow of bereavement. Jimmy's death *had* broken up her life, and only the passage of time would help her to accept and understand what had happened. She began to see death as a human reality of which she must take account in the midst of continuing to live.

Father Simpson had only this morning, when discussing the funeral arrangements, pointed out the burial service itself would encourage Doris to share her loss with others. He urged her to see it as a healing and creative experience.

Now, as part of that process, Doris gently explained to the children over lunch that Jimmy would never again play with them—but that they must all retain his memory forever. She began to remind them of all the happy times they had shared with him. Soon the children were laughing at those memories, vying with each other to tell stories about Jimmy.

Doris drifted into a reverie, remembering, among other things, how she had once sat with Jimmy in their dell when he read her a quotation of Hemingway's he had noted in a magazine article: *If two people love each other there can be no happy end to it.*

Instead of making her cry, the words somehow gave her inner peace and strength.

Shortly before two o'clock, reporters and radio and television crews assembled in the press room of the state capitol, not far from Leonard Bachman's office. Bachman had a healthy respect for the media; he worked on the basis that, given the facts, reporters would generally report responsibly. This open policy—only recently injected by Bachman into the stygian bureaucracy of Pennsylvania's health department—had further established him as a popular figure with the media.

Many of those setting up their lights, cameras, and microphones glanced curiously toward the health secretary. Usually he had a dry aside or a joke for them. None were forthcoming today.

Seated stiffly beside Bachman on a dais at one end of the room were Parkin and Beecham; on his other side were two other anxious aides.

Beecham was particularly nervous. Following the midday meeting that Bachman had insisted he and Parkin attend, Beecham witnessed a heated argument between the two men. Parkin felt it was far more important he and Beecham got back to their offices and continued to oversee developments there; Bachman instead insisted they stay with him and attend this press conference. Parkin continued to argue that he was leaving his office virtually unmanned at a crucial time, that if he did not return immediately there was a real danger he would lose control of the investigation, that there was now no one implementing the important decisions taken at the midday meeting. But Bachman was adamant: "Dammit, Parkin, can't you understand the press is important? Our first duty is to inform everyone what is happening. And you and your CDC man are going to help me do just that."

Still protesting, Parkin was finally forced to give in. He tried to reassure Beecham, explaining that the health secretary's volatile personality made it inevitable they would be working in a hothouse atmosphere during the days to come. Beecham must get used to it and learn to play Bachman's political games and turn them to his advantage.

Just before entering the press room, the three men met to compare notes in a small antechamber. Beecham was shocked to see that Bachman's "hands were visibly shaking. It was scary. How were we going to explain to a group of reporters what we ourselves didn't understand?"

But what frightened Beecham most of all was the thought that if the disease was communicable, person to person, the cases could escalate stratospherically, creating a pandemic to equal that of 1918. He felt at the press conference he was "witnessing history in the making."

Bachman had decided he would hold nothing back. He was banking on his reputation for honesty and forthrightness to defuse a potentially explosive situation. Yet as he glanced around the rapidly filling room, he was not so certain he would succeed. The press conference had attracted a number of journalists who in the past had sensationalized his statements. Still, he knew he had the governor's backing for what he was doing. He had spoken to Shapp before calling the conference. The governor had wished him good luck and told him to "do whatever you think is necessary."

Parkin, too, had been busy on the telephone, opening up contact with the CDC, talking to a number of departmental heads in Atlanta. He had also suggested that Bachman discuss the situation directly with Sencer. And finally, putting aside his own well-entrenched attitude toward the CDC, Parkin had swallowed his pride and admitted to Bachman that the agency would have to be brought in: there was simply no way the state's epidemiologic service could cope with the burgeoning crisis.

"We're all set, Dr. Bachman," yelled a TV reporter.

Arc lights suddenly bathed the dais in a harsh glare. A silence settled over the room.

Bachman straightened in his seat, adjusted his spectacles, and read a short prepared statement describing the illness and its symptoms. He then began to review the events of the weekend.

A reporter cut in: "The first deaths occurred last Friday, maybe before. Today's Monday. Why did it take so long for you to get into the action?"

It was one of the many questions that had exercised Bachman all morning. His own inquiries suggested there had been a breakdown in the reporting system he had been struggling to improve throughout the department. Even now his staff was trying to establish what exactly had gone wrong at, among other places, Williamsport. But until he had all the facts Bachman was not prepared to throw his staff, or himself, into the jaws of the media.

"We acted as fast as the information came in," he answered. Moving back to his notes, he announced there were now six confirmed deaths and some fifty cases from what looked like an outbreak of an infectious respiratory disease. Once more he was interrupted.

"Dr. Bachman, those numbers don't tally at all with what the Legion's put out. They say there's at least *sixteen* dead as of last night and another sixty-six in the hospital."

Bachman nodded to Parkin to reply.

"We've only been able to confirm six deaths so far. As we don't at this moment know exactly what the disease is, it's impossible to say exactly how many have died from it."

"But we've no reason to doubt that the Legion's figure is accurate," added Bachman quickly. "I can assure you we are on top of this situation and there is no cause for panic."

"Is this swine flu?"

The questioner identified himself as a Philadelphia *Daily News* man. Bachman smiled: only a journalist from that free-wheeling newspaper would have tried to nail him so quickly. He had mixed feelings about the *News*. It was a hard-hitting tabloid that often exposed social injustice, yet in his view it too often also looked for the easy option—a headline-grabbing story that would set its staider rivals in anxious pursuit. Bachman was determined that neither the *News* nor any other newspaper was going to use him to float a swine flu scare story. There was enough alarm in the air already without a newspaper blazing a trail that could trigger off God-knows-what.

He fixed the reporter. "Swine flu is only one possibility."

The *News* man was not satisfied. "How'd you rate it on a scale of ten?"

"We don't rate possibilities like that," responded Bachman patiently. It was a loaded question; to flatly deny any possibility of swine flu would be digging a pit for himself. He explained that until the labs came up with a definite finding, which would take about three days, swine flu must be considered; *everything* must be considered.

"How do you rate your department's efforts so far?"

Having baited the line, the reporter had unwittingly let Bachman off the hook.

Nodding vigorously, the health secretary said it was a good question and proceeded to answer it fully, carefully explaining how all morning Parkin had been mobilizing the entire resources of the department to deal with the outbreak: Bachman preferred the word "outbreak" to the more emotive "epidemic" and was careful to avoid any suggestion of mystery or danger. It was a masterful exposition of playing down; while fully recognizing the gravity of what had occurred, Bachman somehow contrived to give the impression that the search for a solution was well in hand. He explained how public health nurses from the eight regional departments and over sixty county offices were visiting every hospital in the state to check on all suspected patients. Top priority was being given to collecting specimens for immediate analysis in the state laboratories in Philadelphia. The specimens were being taken there by state police helicopters.

"Are you working closely with the Rizzo administration?" asked a writer from the Philadelphia *Inquirer*.

Bachman studied the reporter. Was he trying to draw into the open the barely civil relationship that nowadays existed between the health secretary and Mayor Rizzo's people? Was this one of Al Gaudiosi's devious ploys? Bachman decided to choose his words carefully in reply to the questioner.

"We shall be working with everybody—and that, of course, includes especially our colleagues in the Philadelphia Health Department."

"Will you be sending anybody to Philadelphia?" asked another reporter.

"I'm advised the city has a perfectly capable epidemiologist, Dr. Robert Sharrar. Dr. Parkin is in close contact with him."

"Are you aware Mr. Gaudiosi is also holding a press conference this afternoon?"

It was the *Daily News* man again.

Bachman flinched. "No, I was not aware of that. But it doesn't surprise me."

The reporter smiled. He sensed he had caught Bachman off guard. He pressed his advantage.

"Will you be calling in the CDC to help you?"

Bachman grinned. "You've anticipated me. After consultation with Dr. Parkin, I have spoken to Dr. Sencer, the director of the CDC, and he has agreed to assist us."

An excited murmur swept the room. Cameras focused on Parkin as reporters questioned him.

Parkin explained that the sheer physical diversity of the outbreak—people were now reporting sick all over the state—had influenced their decision to bring in the CDC. The agency had skilled physicians and other specialists specifically trained for such emergencies. Indeed, one had joined him this very morning—Beecham beamed beside Parkin but said nothing—and other EIS officers would be arriving later in the day.

A newsman asked who would be in charge of the investigation.

Bachman quickly interjected that the CDC would be working with Parkin.

The reporter persisted. "With Parkin—or for Parkin?"

The health secretary's patience snapped. He had an outbreak to deal with, not time to waste debating semantics.

A TV reporter addressed Parkin. If this was not swine flu, could it be something equally lethal?

"Like what?"

"Like Lassa fever."

Parkin did not hesitate. "We have nothing to support that."

"How about pneumonic plague?" continued the reporter. "Could this outbreak fit into that category?"

Parkin hesitated. Plague was a disease that did worry him. Every epidemiologist knew that since 1970 the number of reported cases was on the increase. One possible reason was that more people were venturing into remote areas of the United States where the disease still flourished in the rodent population. In medical circles there was a genuine fear that eventually some nature-loving person would contract the plague—a fleabite would be enough—and return to city or urban living to spread the deadly disease. Parkin knew that even to suggest such a dire possibility at this stage could produce a panic that would overwhelm every health department office in the state. He told the reporter it was most unlikely to be plague of any kind: "In the households we have contacted, we have found no secondary spread to family members."

A radio reporter asked Parkin to say simply what he thought the outbreak was.

The epidemiologist shook his head. He was not going to be drawn into speculation.

Bachman said the closest he could call it was a viral pneumonia.

Another reporter shouted a question. "Has anybody considered the possibility the legionnaires may have been killed?"

Bachman and Parkin looked at one another, bemused.

"I don't follow your question," said Bachman.

"Could they have been poisoned? Murdered by a maniac?"

"We have not considered that," began Bachman.

"Will you now be doing so?"

"If we find any evidence we will notify the police—"

"You planning to call in the FBI?"

"No."

"Why not?"

"Because we have no evidence—"

"If you get evidence?"

"I'm not speculating."

"Are you keeping an open mind on this, Dr. Bachman?"

"I am keeping an open mind on everything. You have my word this will be an aggressive investigation."

"Then you will consider every possibility?"

"Yes."

"Even murder?"

"My God, you'll do anything for a headline—"

"Correction! Anything to get the facts. Remember what Mayor Rizzo said about terrorists? Don't you find it strange that all the victims so far are either legionnaires or their friends?"

Bachman shook his head. He repeated he would not endorse such speculation.

A reporter who had arrived late hurried forward. "I've just heard that Rizzo has called in fifty of Philadelphia's homicide detectives to help with the investigation there. Have you any comment on that?"

A babble of voices filled the room, drowning Bachman's answer that he had no comment to make on the mayor's action. As he led his team from the platform, he wondered whether this was just another Rizzo stunt—or was there, after all, something more sinister behind the wave of mysterious sickness and deaths?

During the afternoon, Ted Tsai, Bob Craven, and Phil Graitcer caught flights from Atlanta to Pennsylvania. Tsai was bound for Harrisburg, Craven to Pittsburgh, and Graitcer—against Parkin's wishes—to Philadelphia. All three carried suitcases with clothes for a few days, and kits that they had specially prepared for the collection of samples. The size of Tsai's amused the other two EIS officers: it was far and away the biggest box.

Earlier the independent-minded Graitcer, off his own bat, had spoken to the director of the state labs in Philadelphia and got his agreement to split all the specimens being helicoptered there, sending half of them immediately to the much more extensive CDC laboratories in Atlanta. And after a brief consultation, Craven and Graitcer had also come up with a questionnaire they intended to use when talking to patients. As the two set off they felt they were indeed "in business."

Tsai was still slightly dazed at the speed of events. One moment he had been quietly assimilating himself into Special Pathogens, the next he was swept along by a series of deft moves by Fraser to get him on the team to Pennsylvania.

Fraser knew it was a gamble. Even so, from what he had heard he believed there was every chance he had found for Tsai just what was needed: "a good outbreak, not one founded on rumors but a real event."

Tsai himself had still to work out how, having been assigned to Special Pathogens, he now seemed attached to the swine flu team.

Yet, he reasoned, the very fact he was heading toward Harrisburg could also only mean this outbreak might not, after all, be swine flu. If that was the case, concluded the prescient Tsai, Fraser himself would even now be making discreet moves behind the scenes to get himself involved in the action.

Early on Monday evening, Dale Hoover drove into Williamstown and carefully parked his car outside the Ralph Funeral Home. Like his hearses, the auto gleamed from polishing. Carrying his bag, the undertaker hurried into the professional side of the house.

Mrs. Ralph met him outside the preparation room.

"They brought Jimmy in an hour ago."

"Thank you. I'll go straight in."

She nodded and turned away.

Hoover closed the door of the preparation room behind him and began to unpack his bag, laying out his instruments with the care of a surgeon. Indeed, the room had the tiled and sterile look of an operating theater and Hoover's equipment was crudely imitative of a surgeon's: scalpels, scissors, needles, and hooks were placed in orderly rows alongside injectors, forceps, separators, and tubes. In addition to these basic tools, Hoover had a wide range of ingenious aids to prop and keep a corpse in place. There was the Throop foot positioner, an adjustable device that resembled old-fashioned stocks; the repose block, designed to hold the head and shoulders at just the right height; the Edwards arm and hand positioner, able to maintain both at any desired angle. And there was a selection of mouth forms and lip supports for enhancing the natural living look that allowed Hoover to regard himself both as an embalmer–restorative artist and a dermasurgeon: he disliked the way some trade journals corrupted the word to "demisurgeon."

Most of Hoover's equipment for dealing with the dead was made by the Slaughter Corporation.

His tools would have been of little use without his astonishing array of chemicals, conditioners, cosmetics, creams, jellies, pastes, oils, powders, and waxes, each of which served to harden or soften tissue, to shrink or distend it, to make it dry or moist. There was Claf, a compound that gave flexibility to joints and helped create a good skin texture; Instant, a fast-acting firming agent; Hardening, a preparation for solidifying a body cavity. There were solutions of dyed and perfumed formaldehyde, glycerin, borax, phenol, and alcohol. These aids were all neatly stacked on shelves in handy reach of Hoover. They were standard to any preparation room.

But just as a surgeon often preferred his own set of instruments, so Hoover carried his own cosmetic kit, a small, inconspicuous box the contents of which in his dexterous hands turned the dead back into a semblance of the living. The box contained face creams and finely mixed powders milled to make the skin look velvety smooth. There were jars of Restoration Wax, Lip Wax, Lip Tint, and an aerosol of Leakproof Skin, a remarkable substance that dried in just forty-five seconds. There was also Flax for removing frown marks and It, a chemical to clean nostrils. Weldit Lip and Eye Sealer was an adhesive to permanently close lips and eyes—the product could also be used to bond glass and wood, though the makers warned it must not be used on plastics. The kit was completed with a wide range of cosmetics. They were manufactured by Avon.

When all was positioned to his liking, Hoover donned his modish operating coat, rubber apron, and gloves.

Then he turned to begin a careful inspection of Jimmy, lying face up and naked on a stainless-steel table very similar to the one in a necropsy room.

Hoover set to work.

First he shampooed Jimmy's hair, drying it briskly with a towel. He would set it later.

Next he snipped the tie-stitches holding the pathologist's long incision in place and lifted out Jimmy's brain, heart, lungs, and guts, dropping them into large steel pails. He poured a powerful chemical over the organs. He then washed the body with warm water and soap. Hoover worked quickly, aware that with every hour that elapsed between death and embalming, the risk of complications grew. He had soon completed the first stage of his work, draining the blood from the veins, leaving the corpse looking pale and waxy. Hoover covered Jimmy's face with a thick cream to protect the skin from burns arising from any leakage of the powerful embalming fluid that he now pumped in through the arteries, replacing the drained blood. Almost miraculously, the body began to approach the pinkish appearance of living tissue.

Jimmy was embalmed, but he had yet to be restored. That could only begin when his chemicalized tissues became firm and dry.

Hoover was examining his work when Virginia Anne came into the preparation room carrying the clothes Doris wanted Jimmy buried in. J.B.'s sister was agitated. The early evening TV news reported a spate of deaths identical to those of Jimmy and J.B.; there were also over a hundred persons sick with the same mysterious symptoms that had struck down her brother and his friend. All of the victims were thought to have been at the convention.

"Dale. You mark my words. This is no accident. This is deliberate. J.B. and Jimmy, all of them, I tell you, were murdered."

Hoover stared at Virginia Anne. "How's anybody able to murder them all?" He began to comb Jimmy's hair free of tangles.

Virginia Anne stepped closer to him. "Only one way, Dale. That's by poisoning them. That's why they did autopsies on J.B. and Jimmy. To search for traces."

Hoover looked doubtful. "It would have to be a pretty powerful poison." He stopped, realization dawning. He looked at the pinkish corpse on the table. "Jeez, I'd better be careful. The stuff could still be in his body."

There was every chance, argued a doctor at the far end of the long table, that whatever was causing the Pennsylvania outbreak might well have disappeared by the time the CDC was fully operational in the state.

The score of other specialists in Room 207, a conference room on the second floor of the CDC's Atlanta headquarters, agreed this was a possibility. The meeting had been going on for over two hours and now, near midnight, they continued to debate the meaning of the scant facts before them. From time to time aides hurried into the room bringing news telephoned by Bachman, Parkin, or Craven. It was often contradictory and in the end amounted to very little.

Once more director David Sencer returned to the nub of the problem. Was this swine flu?

Sencer's carefully controlled voice reminded his staff of a terrifying possibility. "If this is swine flu, we are probably in for a massive outbreak in this country and perhaps the world. Our first requirement is to determine whether this is swine flu or not. If it isn't, we can put our energies toward making other diagnoses."

A doctor across the table from David Fraser raised another point. "Whatever this is, it is simply too big for three first-year EIS officers to handle. We need a staff person there. Somebody senior enough to cope with some tricky situations."

There was silence in the room. Then Sencer made his decision. He looked down the table.

"Dave, I'd like you to take charge in the field."

Fraser nodded.

8

Correlation

With the sun just rising over the starboard wing, Delta Flight 209 from Atlanta reached cruising altitude and headed north at nine miles a minute carrying Fraser to Baltimore to catch a connection to Harrisburg. It was the first and quickest route Delta was able to book him on: airline staff had spent part of their night working out the logistics; they were accustomed to sudden requests from the CDC to get one of its staff moving fast.

Fraser had gone to bed at 2 A.M. Three hours later he was awake, showering and dressing quickly to catch this flight. Yet he did not feel tired. He could almost feel the adrenaline pumping through his veins, stimulating further his sheer excitement over what lay ahead. The pleasure of anticipation was made all the greater because he had not expected to be back in the field so soon. He knew it was not every day the head of a unit was dispatched to investigate; it was a mark of the importance and gravity of what was happening in Pennsylvania that he was being sent. And it was also unusual that he, the head of Special Pathogens, whose basic concern was with epidemics of totally unknown cause, had been asked to handle an outbreak Sencer still strongly feared was swine flu. Might it be that, in spite of what he had said, deep down Sencer sensed this was something else—a lethal something that needed all the well-developed and well-honed skills of Fraser to trap it? Fraser simply did not know. But it added another dimension to the sense of euphoria and controlled tension he was feeling.

He glanced out of the window at the receding lights of Atlanta. Somewhere in the darkened city below, Barbara and the boys were still

sleeping. Fraser had told his wife he expected to be back in three or
four days, quickly kissed her good-bye, and taken a cab to the airport,
using to do so most of the ten dollars he had managed to find in the
house. The balance of the money was in a pocket of the green three-
piece summer-weight suit he liked to wear when traveling. The few
other clothes he was taking filled a small battered suitcase that he had
checked through to Harrisburg. He hadn't packed his famous desert
boots; he didn't think he would be doing much walking. That would
be for others. He was going to be the master strategist, the one who
plotted the moves in the investigation, who called the shots that
would, he hoped, lead it to a successful conclusion.

Only then could he happily return home to his family. It needed, he
knew, a very special kind of wife to put up with the unpredictability of
his work. That was one reason he was glad Barbara was developing her
own law career; it provided her with a challenge which, in turn, reduced her emotional dependence on him. This was important for them
both, and for their marriage. They each recognized that while he was a
devoted husband and father, he was almost obsessional about his work.
An inner compulsion few people except Barbara understood drove him
on. It was not merely ambition, though he possessed a goodly share of
that; nor was it just ego or a seeking after power that motivated him.
There was something else even he found hard to put into words. It was
partly to do with his strict Quaker upbringing, partly to do with satisfying the hopes his parents had for him, partly to realize his own dreams,
and partly to do with his well-developed social conscience. The thirty-
two-year-old doctor knew he really cared about some things: poverty in
the Third World, injustice everywhere. Money, as such, did not interest him; he saved very little from his $39,000-a-year salary. Clothes,
finding a niche in society, and playing the local cocktail circuit bored
him. In the end, if he dared admit it to himself, probably his sense of
adventure, his desire to venture into the unknown, the subtle stimula-
tion of facing danger, and finally the knowledge he was doing something that could possibly mean the difference between life and death
for millions were the compulsions that most turned him on. That was
why, while the world below him slept, he was wide awake and raring to
go.

It was, he guessed, going to be "a hard haul." Already he had
gleaned enough to realize something of the parameters of the outbreak
—as well as some of the key personnel already involved.

The CDC was being "invited" in. Bachman had made that much
clear. He's asking for help, Sencer had said, smiling wryly, not for the
agency to take over. There was nothing new in that; Fraser had long
come to terms with the machinations of local medicopolitics. Bachman, he suspected, had a political end to keep up. Well, the health

secretary could be the front man, could talk to the press, appear on television. All Fraser wanted was a free hand to actually run things in the field. How he would get that, he decided, was something he would work out later. There were now more immediate things to consider.

He turned to his pad and wrote: Swine flu?

Sencer had himself set the tone by insisting that, no matter what the hour, Fraser call the moment he established with certainty whether or not it was swine flu. The director had been unusually keyed up and almost emotional, and Fraser sensed the situation was a particularly critical one for him. If it was swine flu, the country was not prepared for it: the trail of devastation that would follow might well be laid at Sencer's door for not succeeding in pushing the mass immunization program through in time; if it was not swine flu, the CDC director was faced with an outbreak that might have equally grave consequences unless its cause was quickly ascertained. Although the responsibility for that fell largely on Fraser, he felt a stab of compassion for Sencer: he was under an intolerable strain and by his own admission was "deathly scared." Fraser suspected the director had gotten little rest this night: he was right. Even as Delta 209 now sped over Georgia, Sencer was sitting wide awake at home, the first time in his life he had been totally unable to sleep.

Fraser momentarily put Sencer out of his thoughts, concentrating instead on a methodical review of everything he had heard during telephone calls with Parkin and Craven in the early hours of this Tuesday, August 3.

A few of the victims, they reported, were not legionnaires at all but women. Even so, the one thing that seemed clear was that all the victims had been in Philadelphia at the time of the convention. The rest was pure speculation. Fraser virtually ignored the press reports he had been read over the phone. Short on facts, the media was long on hypothesis. And even though some of the reporting was undoubtedly accurate, Fraser was resolved to start the investigation from scratch, proving everything to his own satisfaction, step by step. He knew there would be pressure for the media reports to be checked out; he would consider every suggestion made—from *whatever* source—and then decide which should have the highest priority.

He made a note. The cooperation of the Legion would be crucial: its detailed membership list and communications network would act as a starting point for serious fieldwork. Another note. There would have to be a standard questionnaire prepared, to be used by interviewers in the field.

He put aside his pad to eat breakfast, recalling the last challenging words said to him by his immediate CDC superior some seven hours before: You're going to solve with this outbreak an unsolved outbreak of mine. He was referring to the deaths of fourteen people in Washington, D.C., eleven years before. They appeared to have contracted pneumonia while in the hospital, but the cause at the time could not be determined. The knowledge of what was expected of him by his CDC bosses did not worry Fraser unduly.

He cleared everything on his tray, knowing it could be hours before he had the chance to eat again. He turned back to his pad.

He wrote a key word: staff. Before leaving the meeting last night he had overheard others making plans to call in additional backup support; these further EIS officers would help forge a human chain that ran from patients' bedsides back to the laboratories in Atlanta. Those in the field would all have to work long hours in often trying conditions. And there would no doubt be the additional drawback of having reporters dogging their steps. Conducting an investigation in the full glare of the media was something even Fraser had not done before. He made a note to devise a way of handling the press, to work out a means of giving the media the all-important facts without allowing them to trample over the clues.

He glanced at an earlier note. Tsai and Beecham were in Harrisburg. Another newly qualified EIS officer, Stephen Thacker, would arrive today to join them. Fraser didn't know Thacker at all, but one of Thacker's instructors on the EIS course had indicated that the fledgling epidemiologist was resilient and knew how to work under pressure.

He'd soon see the truth of that, thought Fraser; there was going to be plenty of pressure.

There was another name on the pad: Mark Goldberger, a portly, bespectacled epidemiologist whose wit had made him the clown prince of the EIS course. Fraser knew of him only by reputation. Like the dentist Graitcer, Goldberger was said to be strongly individualistic. He was being drafted from his post with the Maryland Health Department in Baltimore to work with Graitcer in Philadelphia. They would doubtless make a formidable pair.

But Fraser knew many more epidemiologists were being called in. He had agreed to that before leaving Atlanta, although he had no control over who would be sent. He made a note to telephone the CDC soon after arrival in Harrisburg to find out who else was coming. Afterward he would have the difficult personnel management job of getting the group of disparate doctors to work as a team.

Their first objective must be to ascertain just where and when people had become ill, and then to establish what they had done that was different from what others in the group who stayed well had done. Knowing the number of sick and dead would also determine the disease's attack rate—the percentage of people it made ill. But to do that he would have to get agreement on a definition of the parameters of the disease, so patients could be included or excluded from the outbreak on the basis of consistent criteria. He began to write rapidly, trying to lay down a rough basis for a case definition.

Again, from past knowledge, Fraser knew that a particularly vexing problem could arise with the media over the case definition question. It was always difficult to explain that the criteria were a basic epidemiological tool used mainly as a means of pinpointing a manageable number of known cases to be looked at, and that they were not an all-embracing formula meant to include everyone who might have the disease.

He'd have to get Parkin to agree to any such definition. Over the telephone the state epidemiologist had sounded bullish and confident, quickly vetoing any idea of Fraser's basing himself and the CDC team in Philadelphia. Parkin maintained that as the patients were spread throughout Pennsylvania, it was sensible for the investigation to be headquartered where he was, in the state capital. It had all been very relaxed and pleasant, but Fraser had sensed Parkin was trying to establish his authority.

Fraser had not argued. He had met this problem before. Although it was seldom put into words, the result was the same: a struggle for ultimate control of an investigation. Dealing with that problem successfully called for toughness and fine judgment. It didn't always make him popular—but then, he was not in a popularity contest. He was confident he could handle things this time.

He continued to review and make notes. He would have Beecham and Tsai prepare line lists—a chart containing pieces of information about each patient: name, age, address, medical and pathologic data. The chart would be updated and added to throughout the investigation. It was a slogging task—so much epidemiologic work was—but essential for the reconstruction process that would follow.

He wrote on a fresh page. Is it lethal? Yes. Is it transmitted person to person? Don't know. Quickly? Incubation period? The eventual answers to these questions could help identify the pathogen, the disease-carrying agent.

The jet was now over Maryland as Fraser continued to write.

The victims seemed to be sited mainly in the central and western part of the state. Wherever they were, it would take time for the data on them to be funneled back to Harrisburg. Nine days had passed since the end of the convention. If the disease was contagious, a secondary wave of cases should be surfacing—especially if it was swine flu. And there was another alarming possibility. Whatever the disease was, many of the conventioneers might be now sick at home, infecting their families and friends. They, in turn, would then infect others. That was the quickest way to spread an epidemic. An urgent check must be made on that possibility.

The plane began to descend into Baltimore as Fraser scribbled on, trying to formulate a set of questions that would allow the EIS officers to obtain a flow of coherent information that could be compared from one patient to another. This was the only way to determine whether there was anything common to all the victims. Had they all eaten the same food? Drunk the same liquid? Been to the same ball game? Stayed at the same hotel or visited the Bellevue Stratford at the same time?

The Bellevue bothered him. As it was the convention headquarters, it was bound to come under early suspicion. He could well imagine how the hotel's management would react to a team of epidemiologists combing its building.

On the short leg to Harrisburg, Fraser continued the process of organization. It would be essential, he knew, to bring order to chaos, "to sort things into neat little packages that can be called knowledge and understanding."

At Harrisburg airport a harassed health department official greeted him.

"It's really hitting the fan," said the man. "Parkin's got his hands full running the show."

Fraser made no reply. His mind was evaluating the shocking figures the official gave him. There were now said to be nineteen deaths among some one hundred suspected cases, suggesting a mortality rate approaching 20 percent. Fraser knew few diseases that deadly.

His escort drove Fraser to Parkin's office, where Tsai and Beecham greeted him. Both men looked tired. They, too, had slept little the previous night and since early this morning had already been preparing a line list. Now, around eleven o'clock, they had begun to collate information under sixty-nine headings for each known victim. The list included a column for the Bellevue hotel rooms the conventioneers had visited, another for the food they had eaten, a third to cover what they had drunk. The chart was mounted on a wall of Beecham's office.

For several minutes Fraser studied the columns of information. They still contained mostly gaps. Even so, a potentially key factor was emerging: the number of new cases was on the decline; no deaths at all had yet been reported today.

"Where's Parkin?" he asked.

"With Bachman, getting pounded by the press," said Beecham.

Fraser looked surprised. "Then who's in charge here now?"

"Me, I guess," said Beecham. "Until Parkin gets back."

Fraser shook his head. This was no way to run an investigation. He would have to act faster than intended.

Neither Bachman nor Parkin seemed to be in any hurry to meet him. Fraser's highly attuned antennae signaled a delicate situation. Part of his success in handling such ticklish situations was a rare ability to see the other person's viewpoint. Applying that skill now, he saw that neither Bachman nor Parkin would wish to appear unable to cope; to neglect or cut short a press conference in order to welcome him could be seen in some quarters—especially by the local media—as an admission of their inability to solve the crisis. On that basis, it was perfectly natural for the health secretary and the state epidemiologist to keep him waiting for a spell. They were busy people, decision-makers, leaders. In due course they would see him. But they were not going to rush. The rules had been laid down. He would play by them, waiting for the moment to make his move.

In the meantime he listened while Beecham explained the mechanics of Parkin's department, who was who, who did what, how far they had gone with their inquiries. Then Fraser gave his first orders.

"Jim, get a schedule of events for the convention. As complete and detailed as you can. We'll base a questionnaire on that. And I want a complete list of people at the convention."

Beecham looked doubtful. "That'll take time. From what I've heard, the Legion people keep good records but there's no master list of who went to Philly."

"Make them see it's important to get one," said Fraser firmly. "Make them see it can save lives."

Beecham turned to his telephone console, its lights blinking with calls.

In the chaotic open office area outside—windowless, cluttered with old desks and filing cabinets, and lit by fluorescent lights—amid bustling nurses and frantic health officials, Ted Tsai sat by a phone not far from Beecham's pretty half-secretary. His specimen collection box was by his side. Fraser liked the way Tsai was coping, displaying to callers the sort of courteous calm he had first spotted in him. Fraser began to think he could trust Tsai's judgments. He led him away from his desk to a quiet corner to talk.

Keeping his voice low, Fraser began to question Tsai.

"Have you met Bachman yet?"

Tsai grinned. "Only by reputation. Everybody says he's a fire-eater."

"What about Parkin?"

"Capable. This is his first big one. He's determined to make the most of it."

Fraser sighed. He hoped it was not going to be difficult. He really did not want a fight.

"What about Beecham?"

Tsai hesitated. "He's good."

Fraser squinted at him. "Anything else?"

"He's Parkin's man now."

"You sure?"

"Positive. I heard Parkin saying to Beecham just after I arrived they must be careful not to let the CDC tramp all over their turf."

"What do they think this is? Their own private outbreak?" Fraser shook his head. He wasn't angry, just resigned.

"I think they're worried you're going to run the show."

"I am."

It had been like this in so many places, thought Fraser, a fixation that the CDC were medical carpetbaggers, ready to grab the evidence and rush to judgment in print. He had really hoped it would be different this time. He shrugged. He would do what he would have to do. If there had to be a fight he would keep it short.

"How do you feel about all this?"

This time Tsai didn't hesitate. "I'm a CDC man like you."

Fraser grinned. Tsai was going to be okay.

"Fill me in on what's happened so far, what everybody is doing, and what they are planning to do."

He listened without interruption as Tsai outlined the initial steps taken in the search to establish whether the outbreak was caused by one of the viruses, bacteria, fungi, or even bizarre toxins.

Tsai marveled at the way Fraser could concentrate his mind, blotting out the noise and chaos all around, which continued unabated. Everywhere there were telephones ringing and being answered, people shouting to be heard, information and advice being passed from one person to another.

Fraser listened to Tsai's exposition with no change in his easygoing expression. The first samples were being processed through the state laboratories; more were on the way. County epidemiologists were starting to supervise autopsies. Records were being completed. Nurses were visiting patients and their relatives. The first steps were being taken to determine whether there was a pattern, a rhythm, to the catastrophe.

"Any firm theories yet?"

Tsai shook his head. "No. But plenty of rumors. Some of them are really way out."

"They'll all need checking. You never know."

Beecham interrupted, shouting from his office doorway. "It's Bachman. He wants you."

Fraser nodded. "I'm on my way."

He walked purposefully out of the room, oblivious of the speculative stares he attracted.

Ten minutes later he was ushered into Bachman's office.

The health secretary and Parkin advanced on him, pumped his hand, smiled, asked about his flight, said how glad they were the CDC was helping. As they still made small talk, Fraser was guided to a chair beside Bachman's desk. The health secretary settled himself in his padded swivel chair. Parkin lounged opposite Fraser.

"Glad to have you with us," repeated Bachman.

Fraser concentrated for the moment on him. He had already sensed that Bachman had managed to reach his post—one of the most important in the public health establishment of America—by doing things his way. Bachman's face was alert and watchful. Fraser had the eerie feeling he was being judged.

"We're going to have to work together, Dr. Fraser."

"That's what I'm here for. You'll get all the cooperation you'll need from the CDC."

"Fine. Fine. Let's get down to specifics." Bachman turned to Parkin. "Bill, let Dr. Fraser know where we're at."

Parkin did, explaining how the public health nurses were the key to his operation in the field, collecting data and specimens, and that he had pulled in extra clerical help from other divisions: "I've even had to rape the VD program for people."

Fraser smiled momentarily. "Good. But what have you actually found out?"

"There's about nineteen dead and upwards of a hundred in the hospital."

"Of course." Fraser's voice was cool. "Not yet much to go on. And if it's not swine flu, the chances are some of the specimens you've collected may not tell us too much."

"Why not?" barked Bachman.

Fraser looked at him steadily. "It's a matter of timing. Ideally they should have gone to the labs much sooner."

"We're getting them in as fast as we can," said Parkin aggressively. "The cases are scattered. It takes time."

"I understand." Fraser turned to Bachman. "If this is swine flu, we should have expected secondary cases by now—"

"Do you think it is?"

"We don't have enough facts to make a judgment," said Fraser. "But if you want my opinion, I'd say this isn't swine flu."

Bachman slumped back in his chair. "And if it isn't, then we don't know what it is."

"That's right." Fraser was in no hurry. "Any idea what's happening in Philadelphia?"

"Sharrar's in charge down there. Probably got his people looking at the Bellevue. It was the Legion's headquarters."

"I know, but that doesn't prove anything. Do we know for sure all the victims stayed there? That big a convention would have used several hotels. They'll each have to be checked. Plus restaurants where they ate. All sorts of places."

"That'll drive Rizzo crazy," said Bachman. "It could wreck his Bicentennial."

"I hope not. But it may have to be done. I'm only concerned to establish the facts," said Fraser levelly.

There was silence in the office.

Bachman finally broke it. "Whatever, we'll have to keep the media informed. That's what we've been doing so far."

"Is that working?" asked Fraser mildly.

"We're staying public on this one," said Bachman. "It's the best way to cut back on the rumors. From now on I'm calling two press conferences a day."

"We had a reporter this morning asking if the CIA could be involved," continued Parkin. "You know, a crazy spook using one of those handy little cans of germs the CIA are supposed to have."

Fraser grinned. "Some reporters will try anything for a story."

"Yeah. And we've got a few hard-nosed ones here," said Bachman. "You gotta watch for the *News*. Some of their men are sharp as a tack. And now the *Times* and the networks are on the way."

"They all want to watch us at work," said Parkin.

"Do you think that's wise?" bristled Fraser.

The three men looked at each other. Nothing was said. But all knew a turning point had been reached.

"How are we going to run this thing?" Bachman finally asked.

Fraser smiled. "No problem. This is a state health department investigation. Bill's the state epidemiologist."

Parkin looked relieved.

"The CDC's here to help. The best way we can do that is if the EIS officers report directly to me and I keep Bill fully informed."

Parkin looked doubtful.

"He'll have his team. We'll coordinate closely between us. I'll just orchestrate my people and handle the CDC end of things."

Fraser sat back and waited. There was really no way Bachman or Parkin could object to his proposal. But in retaining total control over the EIS team, he would, in fact, be effectively controlling the investigation.

"I've only got a few trained personnel . . ." began Parkin.

"That's okay. My people can work closely with them. No problem," said Fraser, heading off further discussion.

There was silence in the room.

"We'll handle the media." It was Bachman, seeming almost relieved. "I'll need Parkin as liaison, to advise me."

Fraser nodded. "I think that's sensible."

Fraser turned to Parkin."Do you have time to brief me so we can decide how best we can go forward?"

It was a polite question. But both men knew it would also be the last briefing Parkin would give before control of the investigation slipped from his hands into Fraser's.

The man on the phone was insistent. "Listen, Doctor. I know what it is. It's contaminated soda. *I know!* I drank a bottle with viral pneumonia in it. It nearly killed me. But I'm okay now. And I still got the empty bottle."

Sharrar sighed. It was getting worse. The lunatic fringe was out of the woodwork. For the past twenty-four hours—apart from a brief respite for sleep—his efforts to lead the epidemiologic investigation in Philadelphia had been hampered by people offering the most extraordinary of theories. There was the Diseased Prostitute Theory, the Bad Booze Theory, the Toilet Paper Theory, the Poisoned Onion Theory, the False Teeth Theory—as well as theories that went from one end of the alimentary canal to the other. But this was the first he had heard of the Contaminated Soda Theory.

"Bring in the bottle," said Sharrar patiently.

"No way!" The man's voice grew indignant. "What you trying to do to me? That bottle's lethal. It could kill people! I could have one of those homicide detectives you got working for you pin murder on me—"

"The police are only helping us answer the phone," began Sharrar. "This is not a crime inquiry—"

"You can't say that," shouted the caller. "That pneumonia came from my soda bottle."

"Bring the bottle in—"

"I already told you. It's too dangerous." The man's voice began to rise. "You're crazy. That's the trouble with you health people. Crazy!"

He hung up.

Sharrar glanced at Graitcer. "A soda nut." He didn't smile. The man should never have been put through to him.

Graitcer was standing by a wall map of Pennsylvania. It was speckled with nineteen red pins signifying the dead and seventy yellow pins for those who were sick. There were more than seventy sick, but there were no more yellow pins available.

"You could ring Polk's office and request some," kidded Graitcer.

"And get my head kicked in." Sharrar grinned. "Then who'd be left to solve this case?"

Such moments of badinage relieved the tension that continued to course through the warrenlike building. It was created through a mixture of fatigue, fear, excitement, and the experience of being involved in something "big"—the realization that, as one employee put it, "the eyes of the world are upon us."

Sharrar was driving himself hard, though it had nothing to do with any feeling of guilt over the way he had acted following the phone call from the physician on Saturday. He had subsequently reviewed his decision-making and not found it wanting. He had, after all, suggested an appropriate antibiotic for the doctor to prescribe, and had also made that follow-up call to the pathologist in Lewisburg requesting he send autopsy specimens to the state health department in Harrisburg. There was no basis for Sharrar to blame himself—just as his subsequent actions were executed with the nearest thing to textbook precision an epidemiological investigation allowed.

Even so, they had so far borne little fruit. Sharrar based everything he did on the fundamental assumption—which every epidemiologist shared—that "infectious diseases do not occur by magic or by chance, and they are not distributed randomly in the population." There had to be a certain something, an agent, that caused the sickness. But as yet there was not even an agreed definition of the disease, let alone what it was or what caused it. As a result, medical practitioners of all sorts were calling in constantly with what in the end could only be informed guesses: typhoid, plague, Lassa fever, psittacosis, and, of course, the front-runner, swine flu.

And the Bloomsburg physician who attempted first to raise the alarm last Friday afternoon had surfaced again. He now thought the disease was caused by contaminated food or water containing a pathogenic species of the salmonella organism. Sharrar knew *Salmonella typhosa* caused typhoid fever, but he didn't think whatever they were dealing with was that. Few, if any, of those ill complained of vomiting or diarrhea, symptoms usually associated with salmonella poisoning. But Sharrar had to agree it was a suggestion that could not be ignored.

All around him, others were taking similar calls and making notes: listening was as important as asking questions at this stage. Some of his staff were combing the obituary columns of local newspapers for recent deaths of legionnaires; so far three suspected cases had been found in this way. Others were visiting Philadelphia's hospitals, searching the records for yet more possible cases, posing to patients identical questions: *When did you become sick? Did you go to the convention? Where did you stay? What did you eat? Whom did you associate with?*

It was still very basic, and there was a long way to go. But already the small triumphs and setbacks were emerging. A police helicopter had flown in samples at record speed: a ghoulish lab technician had joked that the victim's blood was still warm. A number of standard autopsies had been performed. But some relatives were refusing to allow

postmortems—later they would be overruled—thus for the moment re-
stricting access to clues. This delay was somewhat balanced by the samples of blood, urine, feces, sputum, and spinal fluid taken from survivors and placed in a nutrient broth ready for laboratory analysis. Yet
Sharrar knew there was a distinct possibility that tens of thousands of
men and women could by now be exposed to the disease, whatever it
was. The potential, on this Tuesday afternoon, for a widespread and
deadly epidemic was staggering.

He was increasingly grateful to have Graitcer and Goldberger—who
had arrived a few hours ago—close at hand. Within minutes of Goldberger's walking into the health department building, Sharrar had
given him a list of numbers to call, saying they belonged to patients
who had left telephone messages indicating they had symptoms that
sounded suspicious. The jovial epidemiologist had a smooth telephone
manner, sometimes gently chiding and even joking with patients as he
wrote down their answers on a photocopied questionnaire. Inwardly,
though, he was anything but happy. To Goldberger, the situation in
the health department was "simply chaotic, there was no adequate organization structure, and Bob, as city epidemiologist, was literally
swamped dealing with the politicians at City Hall."

Phil Graitcer, on the other hand, felt in his element. He was back in
his hometown much before he had ever expected to be and, as he
would wish, at the very center of the action. As if to reinforce that feeling, his eyes were frequently drawn to the open doorway of a nearby
conference room where Rizzo's homicide detectives had set up their
temporary headquarters. The men were in sports clothes, and to
Graitcer it looked as though some smoke-filled bookie's joint had somehow materialized in the midst of the health department—except that
when those in the room took off their jackets, he could clearly see they
were wearing shoulder holsters, the gleaming pistol barrels protruding
menacingly from them. The incongruous sight added yet another dimension to the already unreal atmosphere pervading the building.

When not watching the detectives or adding information to the city
line list of patients and victims, Graitcer, too, was on the telephone.
From time to time he called his swine flu surveillance unit superior in
Atlanta; the energetic dentist believed it his duty to report to the person he still considered his boss. If the disease proved, as expected, to be
swine flu, Graitcer would be working in the precise area the CDC had
assigned to him and his colleague Bob Craven, now in Pittsburgh.
Since Fraser knew nothing about that disease, Graitcer could well
imagine how uncomfortable the present position was for the senior
epidemiologist. Additionally, Fraser, for Graitcer, was far away in
Harrisburg, nowhere near Philadelphia, where all the most important
decisions about the investigation were being made. And like Gold-

berger, Graitcer thought it also impossible in the circumstances for
Sharrar to show effective leadership. There were just too many demands on his attention from outsiders.

But at least Sharrar was free from badgering reporters. Their calls
were being diverted by City Hall switchboard operators. While Sharrar
deprecated some of the more sensational aspects of the media coverage,
in general he welcomed the publicity; guests at the convention who
had gone home to other states—New Jersey, New York, and even California, almost three thousand miles away—were hearing about the outbreak and beginning to call in.

In the main their messages were being taken by others. Apart from
politicians, Sharrar was having to deal with local businessmen and
hoteliers seeking reassurance and advice; where appropriate, he provided both. But those seeking policy decisions—whether it was, for instance, safe to continue with the Eucharistic Congress—he referred to
City Hall.

While swine flu continued as a strong possibility, the medical data so
far assembled suggested to Sharrar a number of other tentative hypotheses. The incubation period seemed around seven or eight days; most of
the victims—although not all—had visited the Bellevue Stratford hotel
at one time or another during the convention. The thought that "the
grand old lady of Broad Street" might be involved filled him with
foreboding. Some health department staff had already visited the hotel,
making discreet inquiries, anxious not to alert religious leaders or the
media to their interest. Sharrar shuddered at the thought of what some
newspapers would do if the city's most prestigious hostelry were to be
needlessly dragged into the investigation.

The repercussions could be widespread: they would cast an immediate shadow over the Bellevue and blight the city's bicentennial celebrations. Further, he had heard something of the influence Bill Chadwick
wielded locally. He was certain the hotelier would fight tooth and nail
to protect his hotel. Nor would Sharrar blame him; he would do the
same in Chadwick's position. All in all, while he would keep an open
mind, he would consider most carefully before embroiling the Bellevue
in the unfolding drama.

He put aside the question of the hotel's involvement and concentrated on what Goldberger was saying.

The EIS officer was standing by the line list chart. "I'm willing to
bet this is a common-source outbreak." Goldberger pointed to one of
the columns. "Look at the dates of onset. Don't they suggest a common source?"

Sharrar studied the line list. Goldberger was right. It was possible to
deduce from the chart that the victims had probably been exposed to a
disease-carrying agent that came from only one source. Yet the epi-

demic curve seemed to be leveling off, even declining. If that was the true situation—and it was much too soon to be sure—then somehow, for whatever reason, the agent must no longer be in the environment.

Had it gone away for ever? And, just as important, where and how did people contract the illness in the first place?

"Could it be sexually transmitted?" asked Goldberger. "I know Phil is anxious to check the hotels for prostitutes."

"Doubtful," said Sharrar. "Sexual diseases don't normally cause this type of syndrome. And I doubt it's insect-borne either. We'd have heard if there had been a large colony of ticks, fleas, or mosquitoes in the downtown area."

"That seems to leave us with an airborne agent or one borne by food or water," suggested Goldberger.

Sharrar looked thoughtful. He had thought initially that the vector was airborne because of the pulmonary symptoms common to so many of the reported cases. But, again, that did not fit all the facts. If the disease was airborne, an even higher attack rate would have been expected. And if something was in the air at, say, the Bellevue, why hadn't the staff there succumbed?

"Maybe some of them have," said Goldberger. "I want to survey the employees, but the manager isn't being very cooperative."

"Keep trying," said Sharrar, ending the conversation as Graitcer walked toward him.

The dentist had just learned that at least three of the stricken legionnaires lived within ten miles of the probable carrier of the swine flu virus that had killed a soldier at Fort Dix, New Jersey, in February. It was the death of that soldier which had sparked off the entire debate about whether the disease was likely to sweep the United States.

This new information sounded ominous. The symptoms the dead and ill legionnaires showed mirrored closely those of swine flu. Sharrar was acutely conscious of what this could mean: vaccine had not been released for the immunization program and in any case would now be too late—the entire state, the whole country, perhaps even the whole world might get it. The prospect was terrifying.

Sharrar could ignore his incessantly ringing telephone no longer. He told Graitcer to call the state labs to see whether they had any news.

All the labs' numbers were busy. Every division of Commissioner Polk's large city health department was being inundated with calls, as were hospitals and clinics and doctor's offices—most from very frightened people desperately seeking information to calm them.

Graitcer kept dialing until he was through and speaking to the microbiologist responsible for receiving the specimens as they were brought in to the state labs in western Philadelphia. The first had arrived by helicopter at 5 P.M. the previous evening, throat washings from a legionnaire, which had been labeled specimen number E-76-1, indicating it was the first sample of the epidemic. In the intervening period specimens from a further thirty-four suspected cases had been logged—among them J. B. Ralph's, whose were numbered E-76-21.

The microbiologist confirmed that all the specimens she received were split, as agreed with Graitcer before he had departed from Atlanta, and half were then flown, hand-carried by special courier, to the CDC for similar analysis by its labs. The system, she said, was working well in the circumstances. She hoped to improve it to the point where samples would arrive in Atlanta within twelve hours of her receiving them. But at the moment everything was somewhat disrupted by the pressure of the media—press, radio, and even TV crews were actually inside the laboratory building. Their numbers were now being reduced, as some refused to sign the laboratory's liability release form and were therefore escorted from the premises. Those who stayed were being rounded up, confined to a special room, and promised a press conference to be held there later in the afternoon.

Graitcer sympathized. He could hear the strain in the young woman's voice; he could well imagine the pandemonium surrounding her. Normally the state lab was a quiet place, its staff occupied with their regular routine of checking blood for, among other things, venereal disease or measles, and sometimes testing the minced-up brains of bats for rabies. Now they had just been warned, in the chilling words of the Virology Division director, "You are working with something which might kill you—so prepare yourself."

The most stringent safety precautions had been adopted. Only two persons at a time were allowed into the high-risk laboratory; surgical gowns, masks, caps, and gloves were discarded inside the room before leaving. Afterward they were sterilized in an autoclave. Mouth pipetting was banned; rather than follow the usual practice of sucking samples partway up a glass tube, technicians were using a hand-held device to transfer small amounts of fluid from one container to another.

Listening to the microbiologist describing the laboratory procedures, Graitcer could not help but wonder whether even such elaborate precautions offered sufficient protection against the disease-ridden material the scientists were handling.

He knew that well into the previous night and from very early morning this Tuesday—staff had slept on cots in the building to reduce the time away from their work—lab personnel had been engaged almost simultaneously on three different kinds of viral analysis.

The first and quickest way to confirm the presence or absence of a specific virus was the serum test. Red blood cells from victims were mixed with a saline solution. Into this various viruses were added, among them the A/Victoria influenza strain of 1975, the B/Hong

Kong that had been prevalent in recent months, and of course the
swine flu virus. If any one of these was already present in the serum,
the antibodies in the blood would join forces against the new invader,
as it had against those already there. The first evidence of this having
occurred would become apparent later in the day. But the serum test
by itself could not be conclusive, for the microbe might have first invaded the body during a previous illness.

"What about the eggs?" asked Graitcer.

"Not before late tomorrow night. More likely early Thursday morning."

Since Monday evening the microbiologist's colleagues had been involved in the slower—though far more accurate—procedure of trying to
grow colonies of viruses in specially prepared chicken eggs. Unlike most
bacteria, which can grow on almost anything, viruses tend to multiply
only in living cells. Fertilized eggs provided just those and were ideal
for use in the laboratory. But, depending on the virus, it could take up
to seventy-two hours, or longer, for a crop to be harvested and
identified.

"Can't they harvest before?" Graitcer knew he was pushing. Yet
even a day was a long time to wait when people were dying.

"You'll know as soon as we do," she promised.

Even as she spoke, a fellow microbiologist was continuing to inoculate eggs with material from specimens containing what their division
director described as "quite likely the most virulent organism known to
mankind." The woman was perched on a stool in front of a biological
safety cabinet, which was open across the front and covered with a
steel biohazard hood. Air and germs were constantly being sucked up
through ducts in the hood so that no disease-carrying agents could escape into the room. Inside the open-fronted cabinet were cartons of
eggs and racks of test tubes. The scientist was masked, capped, gowned,
and rubber-gloved. She lifted an egg and pricked a tiny hole in its top.
Then, with infinite care, she used an eyedropper to draw off from a test
tube a minuscule portion of a legionnaire's respiratory tissue. She injected it into the egg. If, for instance, the swine flu virus was present in
the tissue, it would be secreted into the egg's fluid, begin to multiply
rapidly, and be available for harvesting from the egg in a little over two
days. Those she had inoculated Monday evening should be ready from
late tomorrow. She numbered the egg to correspond with the number
on the test tube. Then she again precisely repeated the procedure,
selecting another egg to inject.

From a refrigerator in a different area of the laboratory, scientists
were carefully removing live, specially treated human and primate cells.
They were stored in sealed tubes and would provide the basic growing
medium on which tissue cultures could be started. The method was an-

other means of coaxing into the open a virus that would not grow in
eggs. But here again, in spite of the most exacting application of
scientific standards, guesswork came into play. Different viruses had
different needs, and choosing the right medium on which they would
grow contained a large element of chance. Since the bug that was
killing the legionnaires was not yet known, there was no way to be sure
which growing medium to choose; in addition to the swine flu virus
there were many others that could be causing the deaths.

And there was always the possibility that the epidemic was not even
caused by a virus at all. To this end, in the animal section, yet more
scientists were injecting suckling mice with minute amounts of lung
specimens from deceased legionnaires in the hope that whatever was
causing the deaths—whether a virus or something else—would soon
make the mice sick.

The uncertainty surrounding all the tests helped heighten the anxiety permeating the entire state laboratory building.

A feeling of anxiety was also filling the large blue-carpeted office in a
new skyscraper across the street from City Hall. Acting Health Commissioner Lewis Polk fervently hoped that soon the multitude of steps
he had taken, or approved, would bring an end to the newspaper headlines, the radio and television interviews, the media calls from as far
away as Sydney, Tokyo, London, and Paris. Some of the callers made
him wince with their talk of "plague" and the "phantom Philly killer."
Polk had tried to dampen their search for sensationalism. But it was
not easy, especially when the usually sober local morning paper, the
Inquirer, had splashed MYSTERIOUS DISEASE KILLS, and the afternoon *News* screamed BUG THAT KILLED 19.

Yet, Polk had to admit, the *News* had also given considerable space
to the steps he had implemented. Every available health department
doctor and nurse was on the case, often traveling far beyond the city
limits to interview people. An emergency telephone number was now
manned twenty-four hours a day. So far its operators had received 3,600
calls, and they were still pouring in. The slips of paper on which the
operators wrote brief details of the calls were collected each hour by
one of the homicide detectives and taken to Sharrar for scrutiny. Some
of the messages were followed up by personal visits by plainclothesmen
whose interviewing techniques were already beginning to cause comment.

Many of the calls were long-distance and collect; the city was picking
up the tab.

Callers complaining of suspicious symptoms were urged to go to
their doctors or nearest hospital. All the city's hospitals were on
standby, and special isolation wards had been set aside for cases. Polk
had publicly welcomed the presence of the CDC, while at the same

time reiterating his total confidence in his own staff. Nobody, he was certain, could accuse anyone of unreliability.

Scanning the latest edition of the *News*, he was relieved to see he had been accurately quoted. It was true: there was no evidence yet to implicate either swine flu or—the other media front-runner—typhoid fever.

Polk knew his comment would be approved of by Al Gaudiosi. Before holding their first press conference this afternoon, Gaudiosi had told him, "Don't lie, don't hide, and don't fudge the facts."

The city's chief doctor had been asked by a reporter about the possibility of foul play. Polk had ruled it out, unless it involved "a very sophisticated type of bacterial warfare."

Unknown to Polk, Gaudiosi's reaction to that possibility was rather more positive.

From the moment he had learned of the outbreak, the mercurial mind of Gaudiosi had been working to minimize its impact. Well ahead of anyone else he foresaw a situation in which "Philadelphia was a terminal city." As a consequence, some of his actions had been almost brutal: he had been appalled to hear that people such as Chadwick were talking to the media; in no time the hotelier was told to stop speaking to the press. From now on, all statements relating to the epidemic were to come only from Gaudiosi and Polk or their appointed subordinates. Mayor Rizzo, still under threat of recall, reportedly wished to maintain his present low public profile. Although in frequent contact with the city representative—he had given his wholehearted support to Gaudiosi's suggestion that the homicide detectives be brought in—Rizzo seemingly wanted to keep out of the press. The situation suited Gaudiosi. And he would ensure that the voices of those at laboratories and hospitals would soon also be silenced unless their remarks were previously approved. In this way he clamped an iron control over what the media were being told in Philadelphia.

What bugged Gaudiosi was his inability to curb what state secretary of health Leonard Bachman was saying. Up in Harrisburg, in Gaudiosi's view, Bachman had "jumped in with both feet and was running with the ball." It seemed to Gaudiosi that, "as Philly was the focus," Bachman might find more useful ways to expend his energy than by staging twice-daily press conferences.

Gaudiosi's outspoken attitude inevitably made him a target of the editorial pages and columnists. He ignored the sniping. He knew he was right.

Even his allies in the media—and there were never enough—did not always understand him. They sometimes found it hard to defend his public image as a figure of fun, a lampoon for cartoonists, yet behind his euphonious voice and warm Italian embrace was a rattrap of a mind. Gaudiosi, as many knew to their cost, was not a man to be trifled with. And he was at his most brilliant best during a crisis.

After appointing himself the city's main spokesman for the duration of the epidemic, Gaudiosi set about considering whether something more sinister lay behind it than appeared to most people. Perhaps his many years as a newspaperman raised the specter in his mind, perhaps one of his many "connections" first floated the idea, perhaps it was so obvious it simply could not be disregarded. But for whatever reason, within a very short time Gaudiosi was asking himself, and then his most trusted aides, a chilling question: Could all these deaths have been deliberately induced by that most fearful of all modern weapons —an agent of chemical-biological warfare?

A surprising amount of information on CBW was immediately available to the industrious Gaudiosi and his quick-working staff. It was all there in the literature, just waiting to be read.

Biological agents included not only bacteria, but also rickettsiae, viruses, fungi, protozoa, and microbial toxins. All told, there were at least one hundred and fifty serious diseases that could be caused by biological agents. Those agents were classified as either lethal or incapacitating. Bubonic plague, anthrax, botulism, and the various kinds of encephalitis were all lethal. Brucellosis, Q fever, and staphylococcal poisoning were included in the incapacitating category. Two of the most effective ways of disseminating CBW were aerosols and infected insect vectors. The Army and CIA had jointly developed a capability of spreading the medieval Black Death in modern form by using infected fleas; it was also possible to induce various kinds of pneumonia through aerosolized secretions. This method was believed to be a particular favorite among CBW experts; pneumonic plague had the added attraction of complicating a preliminary diagnosis.

For almost three decades countless unsuspecting Americans had been caught in the CIA's covert operations—especially its behavioral studies. The CIA had become obsessed with developing techniques for mass drugging, mass hypnosis, and creating chemically induced disease that would confuse even experienced doctors: CIA drugs could cause illnesses whose symptoms mirrored those presented by, among others, food poisoning and viral pneumonia.

Had the CIA used such a substance in some outlandish experiment in Philadelphia—choosing the Legion convention as the perfect cover? If things went wrong, it would be easy to blame the drug-crazed counterculture. Perhaps the Agency had utilized one of the highly narcotic fungi it had requested be grown secretly at Toughkenamon, a comfortable drive from Philadelphia; in 1953 certain farmers in this largest mushroom-producing area in the world agreed to grow any kind of fungus the government desired, including deadly mushrooms for the

CIA's chemists to use as the basis for mind-blowing hallucinogens. Had somebody, somehow, got hold of a phial of the processed fungi?

Only recently a shocked nation had learned something of the Agency's ruthless attitude toward even its own members. One of them, Frank Olson, surreptitiously pumped full of drugs by CIA colleagues he thought he could trust—the Agency had been covertly experimenting with LSD in the United States in the fifties and sixties—jumped out of a window in a New York hotel. The CIA hushed up his death, but eventually the news leaked. Now President Ford had personally apologized to Olson's family, and Congress was to authorize that they receive $750,000 compensation.

On April 3, 1953, the CIA had formally embarked on its intensive programs for "the covert use of biological and chemical materials." The Agency quickly developed the capability to afflict every man, woman, and child in the United States by drugs so powerful the amount needed could be carried in an overnight bag.

It would have required only a few grams to cause the present mass sickness and death of the legionnaires. Could it have been anthrax that killed them? Anthrax has a number of presenting symptoms closely resembling pneumonia.

The use of biological weapons, Gaudiosi well knew, was old. The Tatars had catapulted plague-ridden corpses into the Crimean city of Caffa. Caffa had fallen—and within a year most of Europe was gripped by the Black Death spreading outward from Caffa. Centuries later, in the 1930s, the Japanese introduced plague-infected fleas in their war against China. And in the sixties the United States had experimented with planting plague among rodents in guerrilla-occupied areas of Vietnam, Laos, and Cambodia. Those operations had been conducted not only in great secrecy but with great care.

Gaudiosi pondered. Could it just be that a dissatisfied Vietnam veteran had managed to get his hands on a plague-carrying agent? A single canister would be quite sufficient to have caused what had happened. He already knew both the Philadelphia police and the local FBI office had, as a result of Rizzo's well-publicized fears of a terrorist attack, ordered increased surveillance of possible suspects. They included a number of Puerto Ricans working at the Bellevue Stratford. But was that enough? How simple it would have been, for instance, to have surreptitiously sprayed plague germs into a pile of festering garbage. Scavenging rats would have soon become infected and could still be spreading the disease. Gaudiosi believed that "whatever was causing the deaths was out there somewhere, as if waiting to slip under your threshold and consume you or the city—even while we all slept."

He would not let that happen. It was time for action.

Gaudiosi reached for the telephone and asked the startled operator on the City Hall switchboard to connect him to Fort Detrick in Maryland.

Within minutes he was speaking to a senior duty officer.

Thick shoulders hunched forward, one hand tightly clutching the receiver, the other riffling through notes on his desk, Gaudiosi began to speak.

Had the officer seen the papers?

He had: the outbreak was front-page news everywhere. But why was Gaudiosi calling Fort Detrick?

Because the disease was so weird.

Weird? The officer became guarded.

Weird, repeated Gaudiosi. Weird enough for him to wonder whether the victims might not have been infected by some CBW substance.

Impossible, insisted the officer. The United States had stopped its germ warfare program in 1969 when President Nixon announced a ban on CBW research.

All his working life Gaudiosi had played the role of a hard-boiled newspaperman. He could not change that role now.

People who had been in Philadelphia were dying mysteriously; Fort Detrick was not far from Philadelphia. Everyone knew it had been America's CBW headquarters. Lab technicians at the base and even their relatives had become contaminated with such diseases as typhoid fever, anthrax, and pneumonic plague.

Surely no one was suggesting plague was responsible for the epidemic?

Gaudiosi sprang to the attack. He wasn't suggesting anything. He was asking for help. He wanted the Army's top CBW expert to be sent to the city at once.

But why? How could the Army help?

The duty officer must certainly know about that incident when, in a joint CIA-Army CBW test, technicians secretly seeded a stimulant throughout three major lines of the New York subway system. Maybe this time Philadelphia had been chosen for another test.

That was almost ten years ago—

And only last year, Congress discovered that specific CBW substances existed for the sole purpose of assassinating people. Is that what happened here? And what about the CIA-Army experiment in which unsuspecting civilians in bars around the country had their drinks spiked with LSD and similar drugs?

None of this had anything to do with what was happening—

Gaudiosi knew that. But the presence of a CBW expert was insurance. Only he would know the sort of bizarre new toxins and mutated killer organisms that had been created, where they were stored and deployed around the country—and if any of them had been lost.

But the germ warfare program does not exist—

"Look," said Gaudiosi. "We don't know if there's any CBW involvement, but if you know of some poison or agent that would cause the kind of reaction the legionnaires have, we would appreciate the information. And if there are problems communicating this kind of information to us, I recommend you pursue it with the CDC."

The duty officer promised to refer the request to higher authority.

Gaudiosi was satisfied. Nobody would be able to say he had left a stone unturned.

Covered from head to toe in protective clothing, the doctor at the state laboratory carefully wrapped each vial in cotton batting. Then he gingerly placed the vials inside an unbreakable jar. He sealed the gasket and lowered the jar inside a collar of dry ice. The ice was inside a core of shock-absorbent Styrofoam that lined the inside of a heavy cardboard box.

The box was clearly labeled in bright red:

ETIOLOGIC AGENTS
BIOMEDICAL MATERIAL
In Case of Damage or Leakage Notify
DIRECTOR, CDC, ATLANTA, Georgia

Beside the words was a warning symbol of red interlocking crescents within a red circle.

Both the method of packing and the label were required by law.

When the box was securely sealed, the doctor handed it to a CDC courier, who carried it to a waiting police patrol car. Its siren wailing, the car was driven to Philadelphia Airport, carrying on the first stage of their journey to Atlanta portions of the bodily samples of J.B. Ralph.

From time to time, undertaker Dale Hoover looked nervously at his right forefinger. It was covered with a Band-Aid.

Hoover could remember the precise moment the mishap occurred. He had been using a curved needle to replace neatly the rough stitches put in by the pathologist following his cranial autopsy of Jimmy when the needle had slipped and its point pricked his finger. Leaving needle and thread hanging from a skin fold behind Jimmy's left ear, Hoover had peeled off his gloves and thoroughly washed his hands with antibacterial soap. The prick had bled only a drop or so.

Virginia Anne suggested he pour formaldehyde on the nick, but he decided not to in case the chemical temporarily reduced the feeling in his hand. Hoover could not risk that: sensitivity was important for the delicate task that had followed—the making up of Jimmy's face.

That restorative process had taken an hour. Then Virginia Anne helped the mortician dress Jimmy in his blue suit. Now they placed him in a coffin.

Hoover had given a good deal of thought to the proper arrangement of the corpse in the casket. First he turned the body a little to the right, depressing that shoulder slightly and raising the other so Jimmy no longer seemed to be lying flat on his back; in some irreverent sections of the trade this elevated posture was known as the "Resurrection Pose," a suggestion the body was poised ready to jump from the coffin on the Day of Judgment. To hold Jimmy in place for that moment, Hoover used special rubber positioning blocks.

Once Jimmy was satisfactorily placed in the casket, Hoover concentrated on his hands. The mortician was justifiably proud that he was renowned throughout the Williams Valley for the unusually lifelike appearance he gave to dead hands.

In Jimmy's case he had already removed all traces of grime from the fingers and manicured the nails. Now he took the right hand and carefully positioned it so the fingers, cupped slightly for a more lifelike and relaxed look, rested on the inside of Jimmy's thigh, while the left lay draped across his chest.

Accompanied by Virginia Anne, Hoover wheeled Jimmy into the adjoining viewing room, overlooking Williamstown's Market Street. Here, until his funeral tomorrow, open house would be held for Jimmy, his lips ever so slightly parted suggesting the faintest of smiles, the upper one protruding a mere trace to give him an even more youthful appearance, his head supported high in the coffin, yet not so high that the lid, when lowered, would hit his nose, which was stuffed, like his ears and other orifices, with cotton wadding to avoid leakage from a body resting at the carefully predetermined angle that reduced the impression of decomposing flesh placed in a very expensive box.

Confident he had done everything possible for Jimmy, Hoover left the Ralph Funeral Home to drive the few miles to his own palatial funeral parlor, where J.B. was awaiting his attention.

Earlier in the day he had collected J.B. from Holy Spirit Hospital and been perturbed when the pathologist told him to take "the greatest care" when embalming the body. As a precaution, Hoover had worn a mask, gown, and gloves while maneuvering J.B. into a vinyl pouch.

Now, driving home, Hoover's mind returned to what the pathologist had said: J.B. had died of something "mysterious" that could be contagious.

Hoover looked again at his finger.

Anxious to take his mind off such troubling thoughts, he switched on the car radio. An announcer said the death toll was rising, the victims dying horribly—foaming, bloody fluid filling the spaces between the air sacs in their lungs, preventing oxygen from reaching the bloodstream before they succumbed with breathless gasps and a pulsating fever.

"Whatever it is," a Philadelphia virologist predicted, "it could be the most dangerous thing in the world."

Hoover switched off the radio. This was disturbing. When he reached home he showed his wife his finger. She said he should go to a doctor at once.

He shook his head. First he must embalm J.B.

J.B. could wait, said his wife; J.B. was not going anywhere.

Her husband remembered something else he had been told earlier that day. Both Jimmy and J.B.'s funerals were going to attract national —and perhaps even international—media attention. All three U.S. networks were planning to send production crews.

Hoover had, he believed, a duty to J.B., to Mrs. Ralph and Virginia Anne, to Williamstown's Post 239, to all J.B.'s friends, to the funeral industry of America, and not least to himself, to let nothing interfere with his professional duties. He would need every spare moment between now and the funeral on Thursday to get J.B. ready for a viewing that might eventually end up in living color on NBC.

He told his wife he would seek medical attention for his pricked finger only after he had prepared J.B. J.B.'s bald head, which had caused so much comment in the last week of his life, could well present the dedicated mortician with problems. It would require all Hoover's great skills to avoid the troublesome "gnomish syndrome"— an unnatural wrinkling of the pate.

Late in the afternoon, the state lab microbiologist whom Graitcer had previously telephoned was ready to read the first of the serum tests set up the evening before. She knew it might be difficult to interpret whatever she found. The tests had been started under far from ideal conditions. Usually such tests involved a comparison between the antibody level in serum drawn from a victim during the earliest stages of an illness and the level found subsequently in serum taken some days after the initial extraction. In the latter stages, antibodies against the specific illness suspected usually started to multiply. But in the present epidemic the victims had been ill for five or six days before the first serum was taken. Without comparisons with earlier results, it was possible to miss altogether any rise in antibody levels.

She carefully arranged her samples before her. She adjusted her microscope and peered at the first specimen.

It showed titers—evidence of antibodies. And swine flu had come up positive.

She was still continuing her examination when Graitcer called again.

"It doesn't mean we've cracked the case," she told him. "It simply means some of the victims could at some time have been exposed to swine flu."

Graitcer scanned a wall chart beside his desk.

"All the victims, apart from a couple of guys, Ralph and Dolan, seem to be over fifty. You could be looking at a residue of antibodies from the epidemic in the twenties. I'll check with the CDC and get their figures for the prevalence of antibodies to swine flu in the general community."

He dialed Atlanta and had the answer in minutes: approximately 90 percent of those over the age of fifty would have antibodies against swine flu.

He turned to Sharrar. "We can't base anything on the serum test."

"Let's wait for the eggs," said the city epidemiologist.

Graitcer grinned. "Better not count your viruses before they're harvested."

Sharrar smiled. The irrepressible EIS officer was a godsend—more so than ever, considering the latest news Sharrar had just been given. Evidence now pointed to the epidemic spreading.

9

Interpolation

Fraser was furious. He was continually forced to make critical decisions in the full glare of the media as he set in motion the largest epidemiological investigation in history. All told, almost four hundred persons were already involved at some level throughout the state and at the CDC in Atlanta; soon scientists in half a dozen countries would be caught up in the ramifications of the hunt he was attempting to direct in a dazzle of flashguns, blinding arc lights, and microphones thrust at him from all angles.

Struggling to ignore reporters from the Philadelphia *Inquirer* and its brash rival, the *Daily News*, perched on either side of his desk, the Washington *Post* and New York *Times* breathing over his shoulder, and the *National Enquirer* and Los Angeles *Times* squatting on the floor beside his chair, Fraser answered his telephone for the twentieth time in about as many minutes.

It was Bob Craven in Pittsburgh. In the past twenty-four hours—during which he had snatched only a couple of hour's sleep and wolfed the odd hamburger washed down with coffee—Craven had firmly established himself in the local health department office. Working closely with the city's resident epidemiologist, Craven had improved the questionnaire he and Graitcer drew up before leaving Atlanta and had used it for collecting information on all known victims in the area. His line list showed a cluster of thirty-seven cases, running from Upper St. Clair toward the Ohio border to Republic, forty miles south of Pittsburgh, and spreading across western Pennsylvania as far as Tipton. Inside this sprawl of industrial muck and rural charm, Craven had

spoken to sick legionnaires, their relatives, doctors, Legion commanders, police officers—anybody who could provide information. He
had supervised several autopsies, specifying which organs should be dis-
sected for specimens, and how.

One of the postmortems was conducted by a pathologist on the staff
of Dr. Cyril Wecht, the coroner of Allegheny County. Ever since he
learned of the epidemic, the enterprising Wecht had been trying to get
control of every legionnaire corpse in his territory. He had sent an "Urgent Memorandum" to hospitals saying they must report at once to his
office all deaths of those who attended the convention; further, he issued a battery of instructions, suggestions, and advice on procedures for
the collection and submission of samples. Wecht's renowned temper
had been aroused when he could not reach Bachman by phone; the
health secretary's lines were jammed with calls from the media. That
was probably the moment Wecht's first doubts emerged about the way
the investigation was being run; those doubts would grow, fester, and
simmer, making the coroner a thorn in the side of Bachman, creating
yet another irritation. For the moment, though, Wecht had contented
himself with firing off a peremptory telegram to Bachman "requesting
clinical and postmortem findings in American legionnaire deaths."
Bachman would choose not to reply to the communication.

Craven had noted Wecht's guidelines on how samples were to be
taken and where they should go. Now he sought reassurance from
Fraser.

"Dave, Wecht's a roughhouse when it comes to getting what he
wants. I've sent off a second lot of samples today. We got to the patient just after he died and the specimens look ideal. But I hope it
won't cause a problem with Wecht."

"You did right, Bob. Tell him to call me if you have any trouble."

Craven was still concerned. "He's a helluva tough guy. And he
knows how to get things going his way. He's got the press up here eating out of his hand on this one—"

"He should be here! Anyway, I want you to continue to collect samples. You work for the CDC—not Wecht."

The *News* reporter pushed closer to Fraser as the other journalists
pricked up their ears.

"Sounds like you gotta problem," said the *News* man. "Wecht's not
a man to cross."

Fraser glowered at him.

"You got any new names?" demanded the *Inquirer* reporter. "I need
names. We're running a list of dead and sick." He leaned across the
desk, scattering Fraser's papers.

"Dammit, get off my desk." Fraser checked the fury boiling inside him. A row with the media was the last thing he wanted. He turned back to the telephone.

"Everyone here's running scared," said Craven. "In fact, it's worse than that. There's a feeling of absolute naked *terror* in the people."

Throughout the day he had repeatedly encountered panic on a wide-spread scale. Most relatives of the dead expected to be struck down any moment; legionnaires and their families were already being shunned by their neighbors. Even doctors and nurses feared that the death-dealing disease could be contagious. Several drugstores in the area reported being overwhelmed by requests for medicines that might ward off the illness. And Craven himself had answered his share of frantic calls from citizens desperately seeking reassurance.

"There's no way we can stop these calls. People here are petrified—"

"Okay. I know you're doing your best." Fraser hurried to cut off Craven; he could sense the reporters crowding in around him. "What was the name of that bus driver you took samples from?"

"Hornack. He drove a bunch of kids to the convention. Several of them are pretty sick as well."

Fraser put a checkmark against Hornack's name on a lengthening list of the dead. "Better find out what they all did in Philly."

"Who are you talking to?" asked the Washington *Post*.

Fraser covered the mouthpiece. "One of my EIS officers in Pittsburgh."

"Let me speak to him," said the *National Enquirer* reporter, rising from the floor. "I want to know if he's talked to the FBI."

"The FBI?" Fraser was astonished.

"Yeah. They're in on this. They've talked to Adams, the new Legion state commander." The reporter looked at a slip of paper. "They've also spoken to some doctor—I'm not sure where—about a letter he received a few days ago. It looks like there could be a paranoid killer on the loose." The reporter reached for the telephone. "Let me talk to your guy—"

"Hold it," snapped Fraser. He spoke into the telephone. "Bob, have you had the FBI around?"

"No."

"Okay. If you do, let me know."

He turned back to the reporter. "He knows nothing about this. Nor do I. It sounds pretty wild to me."

It wasn't. On July 28 Dr. F. William Sunderman, Jr.—who, with his father, was a world authority on nickel carbonyl and its toxic effect —had received an anonymous letter stating the legionnaires had been murdered with a manufactured poison. Sunderman did not at first take the letter seriously, but when news about the epidemic broke, he handed it over to his local FBI office. The Bureau, and later the Secret Service, would become involved in an investigation to trace the letter writer. He was yet another missing piece for the puzzle Fraser was putting together.

"Do you know about the truck?" asked a reporter.

"No, I don't know about the truck," said Fraser tightly. "What truck?"

"It was reported parked near the route of the Legion parade."

"So?"

"It was a military-looking truck. And the number plates are supposed to have *FD* on them."

"What's *that* supposed to mean?"

The reporter shrugged. "*FD*—Fort Detrick or Fort Dix. That must mean something to you."

Fraser was well aware Fort Dix was where, earlier in the year, the first case of fatal swine flu had been detected; he also knew Fort Detrick was where the nation's CBW agents had once been stored—and where many still believed they still were.

The reporter's story sounded a highly improbable one to Fraser. Yet, in the weeks to come, the Truck Theory would continue to engage responsible sections of the media and the police. Out of their inquiries grew a chilling scenario. The truck was en route from Fort Detrick to Fort Dix with a cargo of lethal germs; it was known that noxious substances were sometimes transported between the two sites. The crew of the truck had illegally driven into Philadelphia and left the vehicle in the downtown area for several hours; various eyewitnesses reported seeing it parked for up to five hours near the Bellevue Stratford Hotel. Some viewers had seen it on television during the Legion parade. A popular supposition was that the truck's crew had gone off for a meal, to a movie, or to a girlie bar. Because of its military number plates, the truck had not attracted the interest of the city's otherwise vigilant traffic department, so no official record existed of its being parked for so long. Unknown to the military, one of the containers of germs was leaking—or, went another version, had been left deliberately unsealed. The deadly agents had emerged into the atmosphere. The story was puzzling: Why had only legionnaires been afflicted? But the Department of the Army would prove uncooperative, and even obstructive, in all attempts to establish the identity of the truck and its contents. The theory of a cover-up would take root. Were the facts buried in some restricted Defense Department file? Or at Langley, Virginia, home of the Central Intelligence Agency? These and other questions would remain largely unanswered—just as on this Tuesday evening David Fraser, for quite different reasons, felt unable to answer many of the reporters' continuing questions.

"Dammit, can't you guys lay off?"

"Take it easy, Doctor. People are dying out there. Our readers have a right to know. It's our job to tell them," reasoned the New York *Times*.

Out of the corner of one eye, Fraser saw a TV crew tracking toward him; out of the other, he spotted a radio reporter pushing a microphone closer to his telephone.

"Okay," gritted Fraser. "Everybody in this room has a job to do." He looked at the *Times* man. "You're right. People are dying out there. I'm trying to ensure no more die. So if you'll just let me finish my call, I'll try and answer your questions. Okay?"

The reporters nodded. For a moment Fraser had a respite. He continued to brief Craven.

"Sorry, Bob, it's a bit difficult here. Those kids in the school bands, the drum and bugle corps. I think they're worth following up. . . ."

His words were barely audible in the tumult. All around, people were shouting orders and requests; photographers were jostling each other for better positions. *Newsweek* had gotten hold of a ladder and was perched on the top rung. *Time* had two legmen snapping everybody in sight. A team from NBC news had joined the other film crews in the room. A researcher from "Good Morning America" was compiling notes, a producer from the "Today" show was talking to New York. The wire service reporters were filing updates from whatever telephones they could grab. And every phone not in use was ringing off the hook in this lackluster room—the makeshift focal point of the entire investigation.

Jim Beecham somehow managed to ignore the bedlam and continue his struggle to convince the car rental company he was being serious.

"I need half a dozen cars at seven tomorrow morning. The drivers all have credit cards." Beecham groaned; the girl on the line seemed unusually obtuse. "It doesn't matter what sort of cars or whether they're automatic or not." He paused briefly to look at a TV sound recordist taking atmos. "We need them for a couple of days and they'll be brought back to Harrisburg."

The girl asked why six cars were required.

"Because we have an epidemic. We're sending doctors to check on it. There's not enough government cars for all of them."

Was this something to do with the mysterious outbreak she had been reading about and hearing about on the radio all day?

"Yes, it is."

The girl told Beecham to stay on the line. An agitated manager took over the call. If the disease was contagious there was no way he was going to rent out the cars.

"As far as we know, it is not contagious." Beecham began to use all his power of persuasion. "We have a full-scale emergency here. We need your support. This place is full of reporters. You wouldn't want them to get the idea you're refusing to cooperate . . . ?"

Beecham got his way. The cars would be available next morning.

Ted Tsai was conducting for a group of newsmen what amounted to a basic seminar in epidemiology while at the same time fielding a stream of phone calls. Like everybody else, he had slept only a few hours in the past twenty-four; now he had his second wind and felt he could handle anything. Tsai accepted the presence of the reporters as an essential part of the American way of doing things and thought himself obliged to accommodate them. Partly because he was Chinese and partly because he seemed to possess endless patience, he attracted attention.

Explaining as he worked, he led the reporters through the ramifications of the line list, showing how a wide scattering of information was helping to build a picture of events surrounding the epidemic. Regularly he added to the list information he received from others in the room, by telephone, or from Steve Thacker, another young EIS officer, who had just arrived from Washington, D.C. Thacker had been on the course with Tsai, but until now they barely knew each other.

Within hours of arriving, Thacker had distinguished himself by helping Fraser formulate the critically important preliminary case definition —the criteria by which it was decided whether a person should be included on the list of "official" cases.

To meet the criteria, a patient had to have a fever of at least 102 degrees and a cough, or a lesser fever plus chest X-ray evidence of pneumonia. Because such symptoms appeared frequently in the general public, an epidemiological constraint—some association with the Legion convention—was generally required. In practice, only persons who were or had been hospitalized were placed on Harrisburg's "official" list. The definition was loose but highly useful. It screened out most people with "ordinary" illnesses while keeping in those most likely to have the disease—whatever it was—or to have died from it.

Tsai told his journalist audience that the case definition was a particularly necessary tool for Fraser, helping him decide, among other things, which leads he should order *not* to be pursued. Now, surrounded by a couple of TV crews and a gaggle of newspaper and radio reporters, Tsai felt relieved he was at least dressed for the occasion. He was wearing a tie Sherry had given him and his best suit, a hard-wearing worsted. Even so, he was not prepared for the questions the *National Enquirer* reporter, who had drifted over from Fraser's desk, now directed at him.

"Dr. Tsai, do you think this is murder?"

"No."

"How can you be certain? The FBI are involved."

"I'm sure many people will become involved—"

"Like the CIA? The Secret Service? They're already involved. The CIA is running checks on any missing CBW agents. The Secret Service is deciding whether it's safe for President Ford to go to Philadelphia next Sunday to address the Eucharistic Congress. And I hear the whole congress is in danger. What do you make of all that?"

Tsai became his inscrutable best. Nothing could draw him into speculating.

Another reporter switched tack. "How do you hope to catch this thing before it wipes out more people?"

"Perhaps you should ask Dr. Bachman," said Tsai gravely. "If anyone has a timetable, he does. I certainly don't."

"I just wish Bachman was here. He knows how to answer our questions."

"Then you're in luck." Tsai pointed. The health secretary, flanked by Parkin, had marched into the room.

Bachman was still in a towering rage after talking to Polk in Philadelphia. He considered Polk "a good friend" and had anticipated he would meet with no problems "keeping the investigation on a professional health-related level." Instead he found Polk surprisingly evasive —and Bachman suspected he knew why.

"Polk's probably been persuaded by Rizzo," he growled at Parkin. "And no doubt Gaudiosi sees this epidemic as a publicity coup." Bachman shook his head in disgust. "They're small-timers down there trying to be big shots. That's definitely what motivates them."

He looked around the room. What he saw did not improve his temper. To the aggressive health secretary it seemed as though "some of those EIS guys from the CDC were acting like secretaries, taking phone calls, writing things on boards—physicians shouldn't have to do that!"

The reporters began to gravitate toward him.

"Who let these guys in here?" he snarled at Parkin.

"You did. When you said we should be open with the media, this became inevitable."

"Well, it's not going to stay inevitable," snapped Bachman. "The place is a madhouse. I don't want everybody in the building giving interviews. That's not the way to get a cohesive and factual account into print of what's happening." He made a decision. "I think it would be good if the lot of you were moved out of reach of the media. But I'll need you, Parkin, to be on hand for my press briefings."

"Dr. Bachman! I've got more important things to do—"

"Parkin. You'll damn well do what I say. And that's not a request."

"You better ask Fraser about moving. He seems to be running things—"

"*I'm* running things. And so are *you*. Don't you forget that."

Bachman turned to meet the advancing reporters, once more his composed public self.

He handled questions coolly and quickly. Those he could not, or would not, answer, he neatly sidestepped: the investigation was progressing satisfactorily; the public had no cause for alarm—

"What about the FBI—"

"Ask them. The CIA. Any agency you like," said Bachman, cutting off the *National Enquirer* newsman. "I'm only concerned with what my department is doing."

For the moment no more would be heard about the involvement of law enforcement agencies in the investigation.

"We want to follow your people around. See how they work. It'll make good background pieces," said the Associated Press reporter to Parkin.

"No way. They're up to their eyes. They'll just get bogged down if I let you guys tail them."

A clamor of protest came from the reporters.

"Why don't you ask Dr. Fraser about his people?" said Bachman, winking at Parkin. "Maybe he'll let you follow his epidemiologists."

Parkin thought: *Bachman's at his foxy best. He's showing me I still have a say while at the same time testing Fraser.*

A melee of newsmen swept Bachman and Parkin to Fraser's desk.

He was on the phone, talking to Atlanta.

"That means I've got sixteen EIS officers in the state so far, and another nineteen coming tomorrow. Good. . . . No, I'm not at all sure I want a computer," said Fraser tersely.

He looked up. The reporters were recording this conversation as well. He turned back to the phone.

"You may well hear what I've just said on your late-night news." Fraser hardly masked his anger.

He put down the telephone and looked steadily at Bachman.

"Dr. Fraser, do you have any objection to letting us follow around your EIS officers?" asked a TV reporter. "It'll make a good mini-feature."

Fraser ignored the reporter. "Dr. Bachman, I'd like to talk to you— alone."

For a brief moment the two men stared at each other. Then Bachman nodded and told Parkin they would use his office.

Closing the door behind him, Fraser faced Bachman. He spoke quietly, choosing his words carefully.

"Dr. Bachman, this is an absurd way to run an investigation. I expected it to be chaotic, but the press have made it into a circus. I can't think for twelve seconds in this setup."

"Dr. Fraser—"

"*No one* can work under these conditions. You must put an end to it now. And I mean *now*."

There was silence in the room. From outside, they could both hear the shouts as reporters bombarded Parkin with questions.

"I've already decided. You're moving up with me. I've plenty of space."

Fraser's face froze. "I don't think that's a good idea. Why not just bar the press from this place?"

"Dr. Fraser, when I came into office, I made it a point to keep the media informed. I don't want to bar anyone from anything. Why not move?"

Fraser felt he had a valid reason for not moving: having to work virtually under Bachman's eye would draw his EIS officers even uncomfortably closer to the multifaceted machinations Fraser had already detected in Pennsylvania politics. That could be equally disruptive for them. But to explain that to the explosive health secretary would be impossible; in many ways Bachman was the epitome of the doctor turned part-time politician. Yet Fraser sensed that to back down now would totally undermine his future position.

"Dr. Bachman. To move will take time. We don't have time. There are people dying—"

"I know that. We all know that. I can arrange for the whole thing to be done quickly."

Bachman looked at Fraser carefully. *He's young but tough,* thought the crusty middle-aged health secretary; *he's also determined, bright, and certain of himself. Even his rumpled clothes and shaggy hair denote a man with boundless confidence; that and the fact he's pure Ivy League.*

"Let's put off any decision about moving. Let's just get the press out of our hair so we can work," said Fraser.

"I know how you feel about the media. But we have to live with them on this one. They're not going to go away." He gestured toward the babble of voices from the other room. "You heard them. The FBI, CIA, the whole damn lot is being dragged in. It's a big story." He spread his hands in supplication. "We've got to give them something."

"Like what?"

"Well, how about following your EIS officers—"

Fraser sighed. "Dr. Bachman. The country pays a small fortune to train an EIS officer. I don't think it's the most sensible use of that money to have them fooling around with the media."

"Easy, young fellow. I wouldn't want anybody to think I was

suggesting we squander public money. I simply think we should, if you agree, let them follow your men around for a short spell, take a few pictures, that sort of thing. I can use it as a trade for getting them off your back. What do you say?"

Fraser considered. Bachman had a point. And what he said made a certain amount of sense. He made up his mind.

"*One* EIS officer, for *one* day. Agreed?"

"Agreed."

"Okay. I'll sacrifice Thacker. He's articulate, affable, and one of the most presentable guys I've got. But in return I want that mob out of here."

"Right."

Together they walked back into the chaos of the next room. Both men realized their relationship had undergone a significant change. While the question of moving offices was still in the air, Fraser had won the battle about the media. Free from now on of intruding reporters, he would be left to lead the assault against what one of them was already calling "the disease of the legionnaires," and which would soon be shortened in reports around the world to "legionnaires' disease."

Doris thought Jimmy looked fantastic. He was so lifelike that it seemed at any moment he would open his eyes, sit up, uncup his hands, and crush her to him. What was so incredible—"so beautiful"—was that Jimmy's lips had been permanently fixed in the smile she would always remember him for. Part of her mind told her Dale Hoover must have spent considerable time and effort to avoid what she knew embalmers described as lip drift; the other part clung to the fantasy that Jimmy was alive and just sleeping between the whitest of white linen.

She glanced to her left. Seated there, ramrod straight, eyes fixed on the coffin, was Dicko, with his wife and family. They had totally ignored her when entering the slumber room in the Ralph Funeral Home to participate in a private family viewing and prayers.

Doris clutched her oldest son to her protectively. She had not wanted to bring the boy. Now she was pleased he was there: he had been a special favorite of Jimmy's, and the sight of Jimmy's rosy-cheeked body, "glowing with life," would be a fitting memory for her son and herself.

She was also glad she had gone against Jimmy's specific wish and held the viewing. Yet, sitting in the front pew of the softly lit room—with a single ethereal spotlight cunningly placed to illuminate Jimmy's face—Doris could think of no suitable prayers. Instead she remembered how Jimmy had often said he would not wish her to see him in a coffin. But then, she thought, Jimmy could have had no idea how "well and wonderful" he would actually look when he was dead. Dale Hoover, she decided, was as great an artist as the legendary Mr. Ralph, J.B.'s father. It was he who had replaced her sister's head after it was knocked off by a train speeding through the valley; hard as she had looked, Doris had been unable to see how the head had been joined to the body.

The door of the viewing room suddenly opened and Father Simpson entered. The portly priest moved, as if on well-oiled wheels, in a rustle of vestments.

He beckoned to Doris and the Dolans. In silence they rose and moved to stand on opposite sides of the coffin. Then, as Father Simpson bowed his head, the mourners knelt.

Doris was only inches from Jimmy's face. She had never seen his skin so smooth.

Father Simpson recited the traditional prayers for the dead.

As the final rosary was said Doris glanced across the coffin.

Dicko was staring fixedly at Jimmy. From Dicko's eyes the first tears emerged. They rolled down his cheeks. Doris hoped none would fall on Jimmy's face. She wanted nothing to spoil his perfect look of serenity.

Father Simpson moved to stand behind her. He whispered that she should now say a final prayer for Jimmy.

Doris felt a moment of panic. She had not expected this. She thought: *What do I say? What are the last words I want Jimmy to hear from me?*

Then she remembered. In the kitchen where she and Jimmy spent so many hours planning their future hung a wall plate from Dublin. Painted on the plate was a prayer. She knew it by heart and offered it now: *May you be in heaven half an hour before the Devil knows you are dead.*

Doris rose and stepped back from the casket, oblivious of the Dolans, still praying across the bier. She had two more things she wanted to do. Ever since leaving Pottsville Hospital Doris had carried the rosary the nurse had taken from Jimmy. She fingered it for the last time. Then she stepped forward and placed it in his cupped right hand. Now there was only one last gesture to make. She stared at Jimmy's face for a long moment, then bent over, kissed him on the cheek, rose, and walked slowly from the room.

At the door Doris looked back. Dicko was placing another rosary in Jimmy's other hand. Doris thought: *When Jimmy gets to heaven, God is sure going to know he was a very good Catholic.*

She opened the door and, with her son, walked out into the street—disregarding the small group of waiting photographers and reporters.

They were the vanguard of a media invasion unprecedented in the long history of Williamstown.

Seated in their underwear in their staff room, the elevator operators of the Bellevue Stratford listened carefully as Anna Taggart reminded them of the strict management edict: there was to be no talking to the press.

"Really that means you don't answer questions from anybody. Reporters are people who are smarter than most. They'll try anything to get information. Like posing as guests. Riding with you in the elevators. *Anything*. So be wary."

All over the hotel other departmental heads were briefing their staff along similar lines. Varr and Chadwick imposed the ban following a spate of calls and visits from reporters. In spite of this, no newspaper had so far actually directly linked the hotel with the cause of the outbreak. Varr wondered how long that situation would last.

Throughout the day he and Chadwick conducted a thorough investigation into every conceivable source of infection in the hotel that could be responsible for the sickness and deaths.

Castelli was the first to be summoned to Varr's office. The executive chef, usually one of the most cheerful of employees, was close to tears over the suggestion that his kitchens were in any way responsible. Varr and Chadwick listened carefully as Castelli explained the numerous checks and balances he regularly ran to ensure his kitchens were as free as possible from contamination. Afterward he led them on a tour of the kitchens, pointing out all the health and safety measures in force. Varr and Chadwick were reassured. They had to agree "even a hospital kitchen wasn't cleaner" than the vast areas in the basement which Castelli controlled. Like him, they believed his kitchens were blameless.

Next the hotel's chief engineer was called to the executive floor. He guided them through his work log, detailing, among other things, the present state of efficiency of the air-conditioning plant and mentioning in passing the leaking larger unit.

Varr pounced: Could that be responsible?

The engineer emphatically shook his head. It could not possibly be the cause of the outbreak.

Varr was not satisfied. He started to question the engineer about the air-conditioning repairman. Might his illness be due to the faulty machine?

Again the engineer rejected the possibility. The man had reported that his doctor diagnosed him as having had only a severe summer cold. The leaking machine could hardly be responsible for that. And his children were said to be totally recovered.

What the air-conditioner man had not yet told anyone was that his wife was now in bed feeling seriously sick.

The engineer was sent back to work while the two executives continued to interview the hotel's departmental heads. None of them was able to offer a clue. Despite the reporters' suspicions, the hotel seemed to be in no way responsible for the tragedy.

Anna Taggart arrived in the office and was asked to tell them everything she could about the Legion convention.

Varr and Chadwick listened with barely concealed smiles as Anna revealed something of the wilder shenanigans of some of the legionnaires.

"Did you notice anything else?" asked Varr.

Anna screwed up her face. "I think we all did, didn't we? Those people were bringing in food from outside; they were cooking it and keeping it in their rooms for hours without refrigeration. . . ."

The two men looked at each other.

". . . They had ice cubes in the bath, in dirty garbage pails. They snitched ice from wherever they could. No wonder they fell ill. . . ."

Varr wondered: Might this be the root of the problem? Had the hotel's desire to satisfy the legionnaires' demands led to their deaths?

"Thank you, Anna. You have been most helpful," said Chadwick.

After she left, discreet checks were made with other hotels where the legionnaires stayed. Each reported a similar situation to the one Anna described.

Varr thought it "made sense" and could be the reason no Bellevue staff—apart from the air-conditioner man—had recently been ill. The legionnaires had poisoned themselves by their own unwitting hands.

Or, mused Chadwick, been poisoned. He, too, had heard the reports of possible foul play.

Perhaps that was what decided him. The suspicion that the cause of the outbreak would be traced to the food, drink, or ice the legionnaires brought in would not be passed on to the media. It could only involve the hotel in unwelcome publicity; if nothing else, attention would be drawn to the fact that the once imperious Bellevue had reached such a state of impecuniousness it was willing to meet almost any request to get business.

The self-defensive decision to remain silent was very soon to be called into question.

Dale Hoover was in no hurry. At this stage of his work on J.B. he saw himself as the creator of illusions, of pleasant images that banished all traces of death and suffering and presented J.B. in an attitude of normal, restful sleep. This illusion was known as a "memory picture," one Mrs. Ralph, Virginia Anne, and J.B.'s friends "could recall at will during the succeeding years."

Hoover believed he had a "heavy responsibility"; on his skill would "largely depend the degree of mental trauma to be suffered by those closely associated with J.B." The responsibility was the greater because he knew that Mrs. Ralph, for one, would judge his abilities against those she had seen her husband display. Further, J.B. would be going to his grave in a blaze of publicity: while it was uncertain whether NBC's "living color" cameras would actually show the open casket, there was every likelihood reporters would view the body before the lid was finally closed. Hoover knew J.B. would be the center of attention at the funeral, and no amount of pomp and trappings would conceal careless or improper preparation on his part. The mortician had always worked by a golden rule of his profession: "Prepare each subject as though he or she were about to be the guest of honor at a very important social function."

The key to his success now, as always, was the final facial effect he gave to J.B.

Gowned and gloved—looking uncommonly like a surgeon—Hoover had embalmed J.B.'s body with chemicals, buffed and polished his nails, and used a cream-base cosmetic on his hands. Next he had dressed J.B. in the suit Mrs. Ralph wanted him buried in. He had spent some time giving a neat appearance to the cloth, nipping and tucking and, where necessary, snipping the fabric to get just the right fit.

Then J.B. had been carefully transferred to the very expensive casket his mother had bought.

Immediately Hoover saw a problem if he was to achieve his ultimate illusion, the appearance of peaceful relaxed sleep—J.B.'s bald head looked too prominent on the pillow. Hoover cut a hole in the cushion and eased the back of the head into it, so hiding from view the rear portion of J.B.'s clean-shaven dome. Then he fiddled with the body, depressing the right shoulder a bit, making sure the head remained on the same level as the hands. He again attended to the clothing, tightening the collar and tie, adjusting J.B.'s suit to give the best shape.

Now it was time for the final Hoover touches.

Using a makeup pencil, he drew in the faintest of lines under each closed eye. With a well-used painter's brush he dusted makeup on either cheek to give a delicate pinkish bloom to the skin. Using a light plum-colored lipstick he touched up J.B.'s lips.

Then something else caught his attention: J.B.'s paunch was too noticeable. He raised J.B.'s feet and placed a support under them. The paunch receded. Another illusion had been effected.

He turned back to the face, studying it from all angles. The nostrils were neatly blocked off, the eyes were just closed, and the scalp was free of that troublesome "gnomish syndrome." Hoover had achieved this by stretching the skin tightly and fixing it firmly at the back. It was entirely without wrinkles and had been slightly powdered so it would not shine under lights. But J.B.'s bristle moustache still troubled Hoover. He had already carefully trimmed it. He decided the problem was not the moustache but the lips. They looked too dry and so gave the moustache an artificial look, as if it had been stuck on.

Working very gently, he imparted to the upper lip a slight sheen of wetness, achieved by dipping the lipstick in turpentine. This wet look brought the desired result. The moustache blended in perfectly.

J.B.'s brain and heart were now down near his bowels; his lungs had been sliced and placed beside his kidneys and liver. Inwardly J.B. was an anatomical shambles. Outwardly he appeared in the full bloom of health—so much so that Dale Hoover genuinely believed J.B.'s family and friends would say he never looked better.

Only when he peeled off his gloves did the mortician remember the way the needle had punctured his skin. Once more he became anxious. But his hours of intense concentration had tired him. He would have a good night's sleep and then go to the doctor.

Fraser doubted any of the doctors in the large basement area would get much sleep this night. While Bachman had managed to remove the media from the room, the spate of telephone calls continued unabated.

As others dealt with them, Fraser concentrated on the task of finalizing the questionnaire his EIS officers would use in the morning when beginning their statewide interviews of legionnaires. Many of the questions concerned what had been eaten and drunk—including whether any homemade liquor was consumed.

Increasingly, Fraser saw that the disease was not going to be easy to classify. There was a common denominator in that it struck swiftly with headaches, muscle and chest pains, fever that shot as high as 107—as in the case of Jimmy and J.B.—and terminated in pneumonia. But from what so far could be deduced from the symptoms and X rays, it was impossible to know whether the cause was bacteria or viruses or something else. The sudden high fever was characteristic of bacterial pneumonia; the patchy inflammation of both lungs—rather than a concentration in one lung—was more typical of viral pneumonia.

Following the press conferences they had held during the day, the published statements of Bachman and Polk seemed to contradict each other, reflecting not only the uncertainty in the situation but also the lack of communication between the two spokesmen. Bachman thought it "likely the disease is viral in origin rather than bacterial" and went

on to say that the new cases suggested to him "the disease has not leveled off, although there is no reported secondary spread." Polk believed
the disease "to be airborne and transmitted person-to-person," indicating that secondary spread was occurring.

Both men were to be proved wrong.

Throughout the evening a number of new theories had been quickly
advanced. Could the epidemic be caused by the *Brucella* or *Shigella*
bacteria? Or the herpes or enteric viruses? And what about toxins?—
the highly specialized CDC laboratories were already gearing up for an
intensive search for traces of poisons in the tissues of victims. Fresh
samples of brain, lymph nodes, kidneys, liver, heart, and spleen had
been requested by Atlanta for toxicological testing.

Fraser knew that since the number of potentially poisonous substances was almost beyond count, the first tests would focus on those
known to cause fever, malaise, pneumonia, or other respiratory symptoms. Among the possible chemical culprits to be considered were
paraquat, ricin, and ethylene glycol; chromium, mercury, and other
heavy metals—many of which are found in pesticides and disinfectants
—were also under suspicion. Even arsenic would be looked for by the
CDC labs.

The results might be a long time in coming. Such highly complex
studies could take at least a couple of weeks to complete, and even
then there was no guarantee the cause of the epidemic would be found.

Yet Fraser's mind kept coming back to the suggestion made to him
just before he left Atlanta: the legionnaire outbreak was remarkably
similar to an unsolved one that happened in 1965 at a hospital in
Washington, D.C. The clinical symptoms then were also an abrupt
fever, lethargy, and nonproductive cough. The acute-illness phase lasted
about four days, often progressing into a pneumonia, which proved
fatal in fourteen of eighty-one cases. No agent could be found to have
caused the disease. Although there were many similarities between the
two outbreaks, there were also differences: the hospital had no air conditioning, and a nearby excavation site had been epidemiologically
implicated, suggesting that whatever caused the sickness came from the
soil. Did the outbreaks have something, yet to be discovered, in common which would solve them both?

It was another question to nag at Fraser during his developing investigation.

By eleven o'clock that night—having been traveling and working nonstop for eighteen hours—he had finalized the all-important questionnaire. Fraser asked the EIS team to assemble for a briefing. Each
epidemiologist would be responsible for following up eight of the reported cases. At the end of every interview they must telephone him
with their findings.

Only when he was satisfied each person knew exactly how and why the questions were to be put did Fraser send them to bed.

Thacker stayed behind to be specially briefed on his role with the media.

Fraser was blunt. "If you find it a hassle, let me know. I'll call them off. Don't let anybody get between you and your work."

Thacker was leaving the room when a thought struck him: Could he share a cab with Fraser to his hotel?

Fraser looked blank. Then he smiled ruefully. He had been too busy to book a room—and seemingly nobody had done it for him. He said he would sleep in the office.

Thacker shook his head. "No sweat. I've a couple of beds in my room. We can share."

Fraser hesitated. "I still have work to do. I don't want to keep you awake."

Thacker grinned. "I sleep like a log. Ask my girl friend."

"Perhaps I'll do that." Fraser laughed.

An hour later, as Thacker slept, Fraser sat at the small bureau in the bedroom writing up a record. Then, at 2 A.M., he telephoned the director of epidemiology at the CDC in Atlanta and began the first of the discussions he would have with him at about this hour every night he was in the field. These incredibly long days would tax Fraser both physically and mentally—severely testing his ability to make the sort of judgments that were his alone to make.

10

Interruption

He was dying. His lips covered with the same ugly blisters which had mushroomed on Jimmy's lips, and which Dale Hoover had carefully concealed, slowly and horribly he was dying. Joyce and the children were also dying, their lungs filled with blood, their skins burning with fever. His friends were dying. So was everyone else in Williamstown. The whole countryside was being devastated by a pestilence so contagious that whoever touched the sick and dead was immediately infected. The CIA had sent in a team to try and find out who was killing the legionnaires. And in the cities the Army had orders to shoot to kill any infected person who tried to move out of the cordoned-off ghettos where countless thousands were dying. Death, the aweful specter, stood waiting at the entrance to the Post Everlasting where all legionnaires hoped finally to go, and Death was beckoning him.

Dicko awoke, sweating. Something had disturbed his nightmare. He lay quite still, listening to the steady breathing of his wife, Joyce. The house was silent, the children asleep.

It was not only the strain of the past few days that had jerked him awake.

He looked at Joyce. Close and happy though their marriage was, he doubted she fully realized the impact the deaths of Jimmy and J.B. were having on him; he was reacting automatically, unaware of his emotions. Last night, in the slumber room of the Ralph Funeral Home, he had not felt the tears running down his cheeks, nor could he now remember what he said. Dicko was in deep shock.

Only much later would he realize how well he had organized matters, ensuring Jimmy would be buried with full Legion honors. Ten flags would be suspended from twin pillars by the main church altar; legionnaires from all over Pennsylvania would serve as a color guard; there would be a twelve-gun salute at the graveside in the presence of Adjutant Edward Hoak and other senior officers. And he had reserved for himself the final mark of respect he could pay to Jimmy: a hand salute before the silent mourners.

Nobody, everyone kept saying, could have done more. Dicko displayed not only love but high professionalism in the way he had gone about the funeral arrangements. People marveled at his rocklike strength, his calm, the assurance of his orders. What was doubly impressive was that the post commander was simultaneously making identical preparations for tomorrow's funeral of J.B. Even those who knew Dicko well were astonished by his iron control and imperturbability.

Yet something more than his nightmare had disturbed him early this morning of Wednesday, August 4.

Dicko looked toward the open window. The sun was up, promising another hot day. Not at all a good day for a funeral. Sacred Heart would be stifling, although Dicko suspected it would not stop Father Simpson from delivering a lengthy homily; the pastor had made it clear Jimmy's funeral was "special" and that, for his part, he was going to make it a memorable occasion.

Jesus, thought Dicko, listening again for the sound, *everybody wants to get in on the act*. He personally thought it ironic that the Church, which had dragged its heels over producing the dispensation necessary for Doris to marry Jimmy in Sacred Heart, should now be so anxious to display its pomp at his death.

It was also strange, he thought, the way people were reacting: he had a vague feeling he was being avoided. Joyce said the same thing; for some reason people just did not want to come too close to him or his family since Jimmy and J.B. had died. Even Doris was acting "sort of peculiar": she spent her time either alone or with her own family; there had been no sharing of grief with the Dolans. Perhaps, he mused bitterly, this was the way Doris wanted it. Jimmy was dead: her relationship with the family was dead. Feeling his anger rising, he forced himself to think of other, more pleasant, things.

Lying in bed—his ears still cocked for the sound that awakened him—his mind conjured up memories of Jimmy. There were those times they walked together in the woods, listening to the coons and woodchucks, returning home filled with a feeling of well-being; there had been those momentous episodes when they got gloriously drunk together, danced jigs during St. Patrick's Day celebrations, and those evenings they sat together in quiet fellowship and talked about all sorts of things, political and personal, global and local. They'd been closer than

twin brothers, sharing everything except Jimmy's love for Doris. Sometimes they had argued violently and fought over that, but those had
been short-lived interruptions in their relationship.

Dicko wrenched his mind back to the present and the sounds outside
his bedroom.

Far down the road an engine was revved: probably a car carrying an
early commuter to Harrisburg. Every year more people moved out of
the cities, smitten with the romance of country life, tearing up pastures
to erect their modular homes. It would only be a matter of time, he
suspected, before they took over Williamstown. Then things would
change, irrevocably, and for the worse.

But Dicko knew it wasn't that commuter's car which had awoken
him.

It was something else.

He slipped out of bed and walked to the window. The Dolan home-
stead had a commanding view of Market Street. The long road—
potholed, rutted with mud in the winter and spring, dusty in the summer and fall—ran on up into the town, past a succession of two-storied
colonials, painted white, with tacked-on porches, balconies, and out-
buildings. Between the houses were the business premises, nestling
back off Market in the streets running in one direction down to the
disused railroad, and in the other petering out on the slopes of the valley.

In the last few days any number of people had walked from their
place of work or home to come and sit in the Dolan kitchen, drinking
one of the endless cups of coffee Joyce served, smoking and talking in
low voices and offering their condolences. Among the first were
Franklin Levy, who ran Partners Factory, which made ladies sports-
wear, Carl Shomper from the service station, and Dan Derr, the plant
manager for AMP, the electronics factory Dicko had helped bring to
the town. Arthur Grubb, Williamstown's mayor, had stayed awhile,
reminiscing with Russell Wecker, the grocer, and Billy Adams, who
owned the shoe repair shop. Everybody had a story to tell about
Jimmy: George Kriz, who ran the George M. Kriz School of Dance in
the basement of his home, remembered what a good dancer Jimmy had
been; Edna Savage from the stationery store recalled his interest in
books, and Elizabeth Whitehead from the Pixie Greenhouse remembered how Jimmy liked to buy flowers for Doris. Walter Radichok,
who owned the Bear's Den, said he would have had Jimmy tend bar
any day, while John Washbourne, the town plumber, bet Slup Miller,
the blacksmith, that Jimmy would have worked in their occupations
with distinction. Even Flix Williard, who owned the Poodle Parlor,
had a memory of Jimmy: he had always been kind to animals.

The endless procession of callers continued late into the evening;

many people were too stunned to speak. And yet some of those Dicko most expected to see had not come to the house. They preferred to telephone instead. And Mrs. Ralph reported the same thing. Dicko did find it strange.

He continued to stare up the street. Nothing was moving, though outside some of the homes flags were flying at half-mast.

Then, from the far end of Market, coming up out of a dip in the road, he saw Robert Seip's patrol car slowly approaching. That, too, was unusual: Williamstown's police chief was not normally about at this hour of the day.

Dicko remembered the disturbing story he'd heard about Seip's teen-age son. Only a few hours after Jimmy's body was brought back to Williamstown, the youth had fallen suddenly ill with symptoms very similar to those presented by Jimmy and J.B. The boy was now under observation in Harrisburg Hospital. Dicko had heard Seip's wife was also unwell, as were a number of others in the town. He swore softly: his nightmare was beginning to come true.

He shook his head doggedly. There *had* to be an explanation. Yet no one could answer the one basic question everybody in Williamstown was asking: Although others might be sick, why were only legionnaires dying?

Maybe that was why Seip was out so early, looking for clues, a lead to what was killing the veterans. The TV and radio people, as well as the scores of reporters who had already been on the telephone to Dicko, spoke of a "mystery bug." But how had the bug got there? And how could something so lethal be so selective? Dicko recalled what Jimmy and J.B. had told him about "subversives." There had been that stark warning in the Legion *Journal*. And what about the strange story of the man in the blue suit whom George Chiavetta saw in the lobby of the Bellevue Stratford? It was all beginning to add up. Some reporters had asked whether he noticed any problem with the air-conditioning unit in his Holiday Inn suite. Dicko told them about the leak and the soggy carpet. Under the reporters' probing, other questions formed in his mind. Could the leak have been deliberate? Had "something" been secreted into the suite through the air-conditioning system? If so, why had not he, too, been struck down, along with the visitors who came into the room? Maybe a different method had been used. "Something" in certain of the foods? Perhaps a poison that affected some and not others?

He would not yet go as far as Virginia Anne had. J.B.'s sister had publicly proclaimed to *Time* and *Newsweek* that this was "sabotage" by some rabid anti-American organization: the legionnaires had been murdered en masse.

There was no evidence to support such a theory. But it was all very ominous and frightening.

Dicko's eyes followed Seip's car as it drove past the house. And there at last, at the other end of town, near the Sacred Heart Cemetery, he saw what had awakened him from his nightmare. Television cars and trucks of NBC, CBS, and ABC were arriving and parking by the grave-yard. Technicians were choosing camera positions; reporters were sur-veying the location. Even as he watched, more transport drove up, bringing to Williamstown the representatives of the world's press. It was the distant muted roar of their coming that had interrupted Dicko's dream.

The sight of the media moving into position galvanized Dicko. He had work to do. Showering and dressing quickly in his uniform of post commander, he rushed downstairs to the kitchen and began making and receiving calls on his wall telephone.

"This is going to be Jimmy's finest day," said Dicko to a caller. "He didn't get married, but he's going to have one helluva funeral."

Al Gaudiosi, to all those who contacted him, personally or by tele-phone, seemed single-handedly to have taken full and sure control of the immediate destiny of Philadelphia. His office was now the es-tablished clearinghouse through which all civic decisions relating to the epidemic were routed. To him came a mass of information, much of it in advance of what most people heard about the ever-widening ramifications of the outbreak.

Gaudiosi had been one of the first in Philadelphia to learn that Fraser had taken effective control of the medical investigation; he frankly did not care who ran the hunt so long as it got results. In spite of all expectations to the contrary, he was not interested in making po-litical capital out of the situation. He knew of and resented reports that certain of "the Shapp crowd" in Harrisburg were suggesting he was attempting to turn the outbreak to his and Rizzo's advantage, using it as a means to gain personal publicity and as a ploy to bolster Philadelphians' sagging confidence in their mayor. Politically ambitious though Gaudiosi was—he also knew of and equally resented his media image of being simply the mayor's Svengali—Gaudiosi felt he had a greater duty: to Philadelphia itself. He was willing to sacrifice anything —even his own political future—for the city.

That, above all other reasons, was why he had taken almost total control of the way City Hall responded to the crisis. His instinct told him the outbreak would have more far-reaching repercussions than the majority of people realized. The signs he was receiving confirmed this.

In Washington, spurred on by events in Pennsylvania, the Secretary of HEW was urgently completing a new plan for Congress that would

break the legal logjam surrounding the swine flu immunization program. The plan had the full backing of President Ford, who requested
that Congress approve it immediately, thus virtually ensuring it would
become law within days. Under the proposal the federal government
would accept responsibility for the safety of the vaccine and stand as
defendant in any damage suits resulting from its use, thereby completely protecting the drug and insurance companies that were holding
up distribution of the vaccine. While enough flu vaccine was on hand
to produce between 115 and 120 million doses, it would take weeks to
package and distribute it. Not before the end of December could the
last of some 200 million Americans receive their shots—much too late
to protect them if the legionnaires' outbreak proved to be the beginning of the swine flu epidemic predicted by CDC Director David
Sencer. The answer to that terrifying possibility could not be given by
the labs before the early hours of tomorrow morning, though Gaudiosi
had been somewhat reassured to hear of Sharrar's promise that in Philadelphia "we've got our guns, our syringes, our schedules. We've even
got a stockpile of cotton swabs."

But if the labs showed the outbreak not to be swine flu, then
Gaudiosi intended that not only Philadelphia's health and police departments be involved, but also personnel from the engineering and
water departments—and all their subdepartments—as well as university
and commercial research facilities; the tough city representative made
it clear he wanted results—and wanted them fast. Gaudiosi had found
unenlightening the statement uttered by Sencer on breakfast TV this
morning: "the most likely cause is a virus, a fungus, or a toxic substance—what we know is really what we don't know."

What Gaudiosi *did* know was that, by a blend of persuasion, logic,
and charm, he had already won some important concessions. After consulting with Fraser and Sharrar, he had played a key role in deciding
that the Eucharistic Congress should continue to its conclusion in four
days' time, on Sunday evening, virtually settling the issue with a decisive "There's no way to move a million people out of the city without
causing a national panic." He had also successfully argued with the Secret Service at the White House that President Ford should not cancel
plans to speak at the closing session on Sunday, clinching the matter
with the thought that the possibility of panicking the entire nation
held even greater danger than a possible threat to the President's
health. The presence of the President, he believed, would help restore
confidence and add something of the glamour the city had lost when
Philadelphia's "First Lady," Princess Grace, and her husband returned,
perfectly fit, to Monaco, having made their Congress speeches on Monday.

So far as Gaudiosi knew, no one from the congress was feeling unwell. But he also had his disappointments: a couple of conventions had canceled their coming to the city; a few baseball and football stars and musicians announced their intention of avoiding Philadelphia in the immediate future.

Gaudiosi feared this might be the tip of the iceberg. Unless there was a dramatic breakthrough soon, other cancellations could be forthcoming. Consequently the bulk of his time was taken up with keeping a watching brief over the local medical manhunt. He was probably better informed on all aspects of the investigation going on in Philadelphia than any other layperson in the city. This, he felt, confirmed him in his position as an expert on the epidemic. He realized he was treading on toes, and didn't care. He was determined to be, when necessary, totally ruthless, to fight with every weapon at his disposal to save his city.

He knew that the spiraling caseload and the splashy headlines it generated were causing widespread apprehension. Summer colds and sniffles drove strong men sheepishly to their doctors. In one city suburb a woman who had stopped for a few minutes to buy gas at a station owned by a legionnaire had called the health department to complain of chest pains. And victims turned up all over America among people who had been in Philadelphia during the Legion convention. A truck driver from New Jersey who delivered meat to the Bellevue Stratford was now in the hospital. A woman bank teller, taken ill with the mysterious symptoms the very day the convention convened, had just died. She had worked directly across the street from the Bellevue.

Most baffling of all was the case of Andrew Hornack, the forty-seven-year-old, 300-pound bus driver whose autopsy Bob Craven had supervised in Pittsburgh, and whose lung specimens—numbered E-76-19—were already being studied at the CDC in Atlanta. Hornack, Craven had now established, was only in Philadelphia for a very few hours and spent most of his time in his bus, leaving it briefly to stand by the Bellevue and watch his passengers, the forty-five teenage members of the Keystone Cadets band, marching in the Legion parade.

More worrying for Gaudiosi was that no fewer than ten of the youthful band members were now ill; all of them had marched around the Bellevue's Grand Ballroom on the last night of the Legion convention, after taking part in the parade. But publicly Gaudiosi was sticking to his stated position in this morning's newspapers: there was nothing to prove *any* of the city's hotels were implicated in the epidemic. Inwardly he was not so sure. There was an accumulation of facts which taken singly did not amount to much but when laid together presented cause for concern: complaints of a dank miasma seeping from the air-conditioning vents in rooms occupied by legionnaires, reports of "unusual" moisture on carpets, of "acidity" in bloody marys mixed in cadmium-covered water pitchers. Such criticisms were made of all four hotels where the legionnaires stayed.

Yet so far, in spite of inquiries by the squad of homicide detectives, city health department specialists, and the Philadelphia-based EIS officers, nothing—or nobody—stood out as guilty.

Worse, the ugliest possibility of all refused to go away. Still more people were beginning to wonder whether some madman had selected the Legion convention as a target of opportunity for sabotage. Others favored a radical organization, foreign terrorists, even a KGB-inspired act.

In Harrisburg, Bachman was trying to dispel similar rumors by telling reporters, "It stretches my imagination anyone could be that diabolical—or subtle."

Gaudiosi wondered whether the health secretary was really so disbelieving. For his part, he would continue to hammer away for an expert on chemical-biological warfare to be sent to the city. Only he might have the answer to one of the strangest characteristics of legionnaires' disease: its seeming selectivity.

The appalling prospect that the epidemic had been triggered by a human hand was only one of the possibilities facing Fraser. While accepting a CBW connection as conceivable—he had already requested superiors in Atlanta to contact the Department of Defense—Fraser resolved he would not deviate from the strict rote and example of his calling, that he would not allow himself or his young EIS officers to become sidetracked chasing individual esoteric ideas, however enticing. By definition, epidemiology was the study of populations, not individuals; it was searching for trends, looking for what was common to a group of similarly sick people that was not found in those who remained well.

Apart from issuing instructions on which specimens should be taken, and how, from the dead, the dying, and the seriously ill—later, inanimate environmental samples would also be needed—Fraser's main preoccupation was, by a process of deduction mixed with instinct, to discover the source and mode of spread of the actual agent causing the disease. Isolating and identifying that agent was a job for the laboratory scientists who, even now, were analyzing specimens in Atlanta to see whether a virus, a bacterium, or some poisonous substance was causing the outbreak.

As yet, Fraser was not sure of the agent's source—although it certainly seemed to be in Philadelphia somewhere, perhaps at a hotel or restaurant or other place where legionnaires congregated—nor did he know whether the agent spread through air, water, or food, or by some quite different means. And there was the tantalizing chance that it might have more than one source or place of abode and more than one means of spreading.

To narrow down the range of possibilities, Fraser was devising questionnaires to discover which drinks were consumed at the convention, and where; what food was eaten, and where; which functions were attended, where, and for how long. One of the surveys was today being conducted by EIS officers who were fanning out through Pennsylvania, seeing patients in hospitals and the relatives and friends of the dead in their homes. Fraser wished he were with them. For a doctor, nothing was quite so satisfying as the "laying on of hands."

Some questions his colleagues were putting resulted from suggestions forwarded by legionnaires and a public now fully aware of the basic signs of the illness. The answers would flow back to Fraser's desk for analysis, pieces of a puzzle he and his team must fit together to produce a sound, scientific theory about the source and subsequent mode of spread of the disease-carrying agent.

Fraser was seasoned enough to know that, in the end, he might produce the most plausible of theories but unless the labs successfully isolated the agent it would appear he had failed: the cause of the outbreak would seem to be unsolved. There were a number of such examples on the CDC files.

But the knowledge of what was expected of him and his colleagues helped make the investigation so challenging; being fully stretched, pitting the sum total of his epidemiological skills against the unknown, was more exciting than he cared admit to anybody.

His lack of sleep; snatched meals washed down by tasteless cups of coffee out of Styrofoam cups; the hot, fetid atmosphere he worked in; the relentless demands for decisions which only he could make and which could affect an untold number of lives: Fraser almost reveled in it all because, finally, there could be a victory—an objective heady enough for him to put aside the pressures and any feeling of personal vanity.

Nor had he time for prima donnas, though he had heard rumors there were some among his people in Philadelphia. He would look into that later. For the moment he concentrated on cementing his Harrisburg team into an effective, cohesive unit, exploiting to the utmost the individual strengths of its members while making little allowance for their personal weaknesses or foibles. And he was pushing himself even harder than those he was leading. In many ways he was like a cross between Sherlock Holmes—remote, alone, a law unto himself—and a police chief commanding a highly charged squad of plainclothesmen working on a baffling murder. Everything he did or said required the most careful consideration: encouragement, guidance, the occasional reprimand—each was delivered with clarity and, above all, brevity.

For himself, he needed time to think, to avoid a rush to judgment. There was no way he could, or would have wished to, withdraw from the frenetic activity he generated around him; the entire operation resembled a newsroom coming up to edition time. But now at least his actions would no longer be instantly jumped on by the press.

Since midmorning this Wednesday—at about the time Jimmy's funeral cortege was moving through Williamstown under the watchful stares of the media—Fraser and his expanding team became totally free of demanding reporters.

Earlier in the day, Bachman had peremptorily ordered him to move his headquarters to a spacious area adjoining the health secretary's offices near the state capitol. Fraser's instant reaction had been one of anger. He had bitingly told Parkin that he did not want "to be located so close to the political action where Bachman could look over my shoulder and those of the EIS officers during our moment-to-moment activity." In the end he had been persuaded the move was the only way to insulate himself and his team from the press.

Now that he was settled into his new offices, Fraser was pleasantly surprised by how well the setup worked. No reporter could penetrate the sealed-off area; media calls were effectively intercepted by the capitol switchboard and diverted to Bachman's press officer.

The base of operations Fraser now commanded was furnished exactly as he required: ample desks, chairs, telephones, and even easels on which the line list could be joined together sheet by sheet. The list told a grim story. By early afternoon it was over twelve feet long, a series of columns detailing the medical histories and movements of almost one hundred and fifty cases.

Fraser had laid out his headquarters with care. There was a large conference room containing two tables cluttered with telephones and manned around the clock by health department personnel. This was the receiving point for all incoming information; through these phones also flowed many of the orders Fraser gave.

Close to this was the EIS officers' War Room, dominated by a large circular table. The room's ample wall space was beginning to be covered with the paper work of the investigation; in some ways it looked like a busy brokerage office crossed with a betting parlor.

Leading off from these two focal rooms were a number of smaller ones that Fraser and individual epidemiologists could use to pursue their work in comparative peace.

The conference room, in addition to being the center where medical information was received and collated, also served as an administrative clearinghouse for the entire investigation; it was here that secretarial services were available, bills paid, expenses authorized, and all the time-consuming demands of a bureaucracy attended to.

Fraser had paid special attention to the telephone system. He insisted the phones be interlinked so anyone anywhere in the complex could cut in on or be connected to a caller. He also arranged that the phones in the EIS War Room, where he based himself, remained silent. To Fraser this was "critically important—we couldn't have phones ringing in the room when we were trying to think." But the system allowed for any "hot call" to be immediately transferred to the room.

Bachman's own office adjoined the complex. Yet the health secretary had, so far, stayed away from the area. His conspicuous absence was seen by those working there as a deliberate decision to show his total confidence in the way Fraser was running things. Bachman also placed at Fraser's disposal a senior administrator whose task it was to cut through the red tape that normally bound Pennsylvania's tightly run health department. The man had already worked wonders, freeing Fraser of any number of potentially irksome issues arising from an investigation costing $25,000 a day.

Having established his headquarters, Fraser spent time explaining to the nurses and other non-EIS personnel answering telephones in the conference room how they should make use of the case definition he and Thacker had devised. At the back of his mind was the realization that the public might find the concept of a case definition hard to understand. They wanted a simplistic definition that would tell a person whether he or she was at risk. Yet Fraser knew no definition could satisfy that requirement; for instance, it would only create confusion, and perhaps unnecessary apprehension, to suggest that anyone who had developed a bad cold during or just after the Legion convention actually had the disease he was investigating.

Equally, there was the danger the definition could cause trouble with the media, eager as it was for clear-cut answers to questions about precisely how many persons had died from the illness. Fraser knew the number of "official victims" would frequently change as people were added to or removed from the list, depending on whether their symptoms fitted the case criteria. Still, until he had more information, he was satisfied his preliminary definition was workable: fever of at least 102 degrees and a cough, or a fever allied to chest X-ray evidence of pneumonia, plus some association with the Legion convention.

This definition allowed those manning the phones to decide whether the information a caller provided was worth following up. If symptoms did not conform with the case criteria, the person was deemed not to be part of the present epidemic and therefore no concern of Fraser's; if the symptoms matched the criteria, the information was passed to the War Room for action.

Touring his headquarters—mostly listening and only occasionally giving an order—Fraser could see the system was working as well as could be expected. In the conference room every phone was constantly busy, receiving a flow of thousands of facts, requests, suggestions, offers, and the inevitable rumors. Each was noted and flagged for action or filed. Fraser had never faced such an input before; he doubted any officer at the CDC had ever been so besieged with information, coming in to his complex alone at the rate of almost six hundred calls an hour from all over the United States.

Apart from ordering all suspected cases be followed up, Fraser quickly came to the conclusion that he, too, would have to be selective when deciding what further leads to pursue. Inevitably, he tended to favor suggestions made by those he knew, however slightly: Parkin, Tsai, and Thacker, Sharrar in Philadelphia, the indefatigable Craven in Pittsburgh, his superiors in Atlanta. It was not a sort of nepotism or self-interest that made him adopt this attitude. He was guiding a growing team of doctors, scientists, technicians, and nurses, most of whom he had never met before. Until they proved themselves, he had no real way of knowing what weight to give what they said.

Fraser also had no firsthand knowledge of what those in Philadelphia were doing. He hoped that uneasy situation would improve once Walter Orenstein, a third-year EIS officer who would be senior to those already there, arrived in the city. But how would Orenstein relate to Sharrar, and would he be able to control the irrepressible Goldberger and Graitcer? Intuitively, Fraser felt his Philadelphia team were "doing their own thing." Yet it was impossible for him to oversee their actions from a distance.

Fraser was also sniffing the whiffs of grapeshot beginning to fly between the government authorities in Philadelphia and Harrisburg. He had no interest in the internecine warfare being waged over the epidemic between the Rizzo and Shapp administrations, unless it muddied the waters of his inquiries. Nor indeed did he want to tangle with Wecht; the prickly coroner, according to Craven, was continuing to "grumble" about the way the investigation was conducted. Well, let him grumble. Nor would Fraser become embroiled in the jockeying for media position; there seemed to be a great deal of that going on among many of those involved in the daily management of the state's health. He had expected no more or less. It was just another hassle.

Yet he had to admit the medical hunt he was masterminding, which so resembled a police dragnet, was well under way. Around him shirt-sleeved workers transferred information onto large sheets of paper; on a wall of the War Room was a map pierced with colored pins for deaths and reported illness. In the conference room a team was systematically telephoning the state's 265 acute- and general-care hospitals, trying to determine the total number of deaths and the circumstances surrounding each case. It was all part of the attempt to find a common denominator or set of experiences that would link all of the victims.

Everywhere he could hear the careful questioning and cross-referencing.

A nurse was identifying herself: "Hello. I'm with the medical team investigating this weird disease."

A state health doctor was talking to a patient: "Who did you room with? Which hotel? How long were you there? What did you drink?"

A physician at another phone was being even more specific: "What time did you first feel sick? What did you eat and drink that day? The day before? When did you arrive in Philadelphia? When did you leave? Did you go to the testimonial dinner? The Friday morning 'Go-Getter's' Breakfast? What did you eat there? What did you drink there? Did you visit any of the hospitality rooms? Which ones? When?"

Another doctor was broaching a more delicate issue: "Did you meet anybody in the city . . . party a little . . . with a girl . . . ?"

The possibility that a prostitute had introduced the infection was being actively considered. A discreet but determined search had begun to locate Maria Reeves and her fellow hookers.

A nurse asked a question her caller thought peculiar: "Did you have any contact with pigs before you became ill?" She was looking for evidence that could implicate hogs, the animal carrier of the swine flu virus.

Over and over again the endless questions were put and the answers carefully recorded.

And somewhat to Fraser's chagrin, throughout the country distinguished doctors were starting to state publicly what they thought had caused the epidemic.

A much respected former chief epidemiologist at the CDC studied newspaper reports on Martha's Vineyard while recuperating from a heart operation, and then said he felt positive the disease was psittacosis—"parrot's disease." The chief epidemiologist of the New York City Health Department announced, "The symptoms, the fact this is obviously a common-source outbreak, the fact there has been no secondary spread of the disease: all these point to ornithosis, a disease transmitted by bird droppings—and ornithosis is very hard to isolate."

Across America, other armchair experts were also rushing into print and onto the air to offer solutions that often only confused and almost invariably compounded the fear escalating from coast to coast.

And now a doctor had talked his way past the polite but firm women on the capitol switchboard and gotten through to Parkin, who wanted to pass him to Fraser.

"It's about treatment. Says it's important—"

"They all do."

"Says he's looking after six cases already."

Fraser decided to take the call.

The voice on the other end was crisp and businesslike. "I am speaking to you from the Sacred Heart Hospital in Allentown, where I specialize in infectious diseases. Many of the legionnaires who attended their convention live in this area. On Monday we admitted four patients who have remarkably similar symptoms. All of them attended the convention."

"Go on."

Fraser sensed the physician knew exactly what he wanted to say and nothing would stop him from saying it.

"They may well have psittacosis."

"Could be."

"Many of their symptoms suggest psittacosis—fever, chills, pneumonia."

"Those symptoms can also suggest other diseases."

"But they have high fevers and low pulse rates, classic symptoms of psittacosis. And it's not the usual kind of bacterial pneumonia. It's certainly not swine flu."

"How come you're so sure?"

"No secondary cases," said the doctor emphatically.

Fraser knew it was impossible to be certain it was not swine flu before the laboratory analyses were completed late tonight or more likely tomorrow. The man was reacting intuitively. Nothing wrong in that— the best doctors dealing directly with patients often had to be guided by guesswork—but in Fraser's situation, accepting anything without cast-iron proof would be dangerous.

"We have an infectious agent," said the doctor.

Fraser could tell his caller was coming to the nub of his message.

"It's obviously lethal. I think you should give an immediate recommendation for therapy."

"Uh-huh. What do you suggest?"

"You should publicly and urgently recommend all physicians use tetracycline."

The drug was a broad-spectrum antibiotic, effectively combating a wide range of infectious agents, including those causing psittacosis and rickettsial diseases.

"I'm afraid I can't do that," said Fraser. "I have no basis yet for recommending tetracycline in preference to the other antibiotics being used."

"No basis? What do you mean? People are dying—"

"I'm well aware of that. What I mean is I have no scientific proof tetracycline is more effective than, for instance, erythromycin or rifampin."

"I've tried tetracycline. My people are getting better."

"Good. But that could be the luck of the draw."

"Dr. Fraser, you're being irresponsible—"

"No, it is *you* who is being irresponsible. Please listen a moment. I have insufficient evidence to support your claim that tetracycline is the magic bullet—"

"I have six patients—"

"Will you please listen! Until I get clear-cut proof one antibiotic is better than another, it would be irresponsible of me to recommend anything. I am doing everything possible to get the information as fast as possible. That means systematically comparing case-to-fatality ratios of patients given tetracycline and those who got other drugs."

"You've got to recommend something. People are dying. Doctors want—"

"I know what doctors want. *I'm* a doctor! It's what we *all* want. The *right* antidote. But I'm certainly not going to recommend a drug simply on the basis of what you've told me."

"You've got to recommend something."

"For the last time, will you please listen. I do not have to recommend anything until I am certain of my ground. Your information is purely anecdotal."

"Is this how you do things in public health—?"

"What's that supposed to mean?" Fraser fought down his anger. He could imagine how frustrating it must be for physicians like this one to cope with the health bureaucracy of Pennsylvania. And he sympathized with doctors, faced with seriously ill patients, who were desperate to be told what to do.

"I honestly appreciate your calling. Please try to appreciate my position. For me to recommend any drug at this stage could be dangerously misleading. I need more data before doing that."

"Okay, Dr. Fraser. If that's the way you want it—"

"It's the way it is."

For the moment the issue was ended. In the weeks to come the Allentown specialist would take a close and active interest in all aspects of the epidemic, frequently talk to the media, and cling tenaciously to his belief in tetracycline and in the disease's being allied to psittacosis —no matter what the CDC said. But Fraser would refuse to be drawn, entirely rejecting advice or opinions not firmly based on epidemiological proof or scientific fact. It was his greatest strength.

The pandemonium was comforting. The shouts, orders, commands, and occasional tart reprimands were a balm, a reminder that here in the kitchen of the Bellevue Stratford nothing had changed. The tumult blotted out everything that had happened. It offered its own security. It was a defense against those unpleasant thoughts that surfaced whenever Frank Castelli had time on his hands. From the moment he was summoned to the executive floor, he felt abject misery. Nothing like this had happened to him in a long and distinguished career. What was more upsetting was that he knew the suspicion would linger in some minds; nobody would ever say anything, but it would be there, a tiny doubt that would not go away.

When the pressure of work eased, those thoughts returned more strongly than ever, increasingly troubling the executive chef.

For the next few hours, however, there would be no room for that to happen.

He didn't have to look at his watch to know everything was on schedule. His sense of smell confirmed what he could see: racks of lamb, noisettes of beef, the rice pilaf, *glace de viande*, and a score of other items were at just the right stage of preparation, part of the highly intricate business of readying meals for hundreds of guests who would tonight be dining in the hotel. The culinary demands of cardinals, bishops, and priests—along with those of the distinguished laity —were a constant challenge: the papal delegation, Mother Teresa, spiritual leaders from Asia and Africa, singers and musicians from around the world—all had special requests for Castelli.

The real pleasure of these past few days of cooking went some way toward lessening the hurt he felt at having his kitchen, his staff, and ultimately himself come under suspicion.

Chadwick, Varr, the serious-faced inspectors from various city departments, even the homicide detectives who had snooped around the basement area—each in the end told him to stop worrying, that they had found nothing serious to concern them.

But the thought wouldn't go away. He'd glance at a newspaper, switch on the television, listen to the radio—and it was there, the thinly veiled suggestion that the legionnaires had been deliberately poisoned by something they ate.

Looking around his kitchen, he knew it was unthinkable that anyone employed here could have committed such an unspeakable act. *He would have known.* Just as there was no talk in this kitchen of weights and timings—that was for cookbooks, he'd say derisively—so there was a great deal of tasting, fingering, looking, and sniffing: his eyes, nose, and ears were what told him whether a thing was right. They would also have alerted him if something was wrong. *No, he would have known.*

And yet, what had one of the detectives said? Something about how easy it would be to tamper with produce *before* it was delivered. The police had asked for a list of his suppliers and gone off to check them. Suppose a lunatic working for one of those firms had slipped something into the merchandise? How would they ever unearth him? The police would be looking for somebody with a motive. What possible motive could there be to poison a bunch of legionnaires? Unless a madman was on the loose. And psychopaths, he'd heard, were shrewd. How did you spot a psychopath? Or, for that matter, a thief—like the person who was snitching meat from his kitchen? He couldn't deny one thing: somewhere in this vast area of steel and concrete *was* a thief, perhaps several. Well, a person who could steal so stealthily could also have killed with equal stealth. The sudden realization shocked him. He shook his head; those damned thoughts were surfacing again.

Castelli fought them off by moving rapidly among his chefs, cooks, and assistants. Oblivious to the sudden gusts of steam from caldron lids being lifted or the waves of heat escaping from sizzling ovens, dodging sweating men hefting huge trays, pots, and pans or pulling laden carts from one station to another, Castelli conducted a continuous process of tasting, checking, ordering, changing, approving, and rejecting.

A trainee skimming a caldron of bouillon caught his attention. Earlier a chef had prepared the large vat of ground meat and whipped egg whites that had been brought to the boil and allowed to simmer for an hour, during which time the liquid absorbed flavor. The trainee's job was to ladle off impurities, but he was dipping his huge spoon too deep into the liquid. Castelli took the ladle from him and demonstrated the correct procedure.

He moved to where a cook was preparing espagnole sauce, a basic brown sauce made from wine, meat, and onions stuck with cloves. The cook was repeatedly straining and boiling the sauce until it reached the required thickness.

"Yesterday I boiled it five times. Today I need six," said the cook.

"And tomorrow maybe three. Maybe ten." Castelli grinned.

Even some of his more experienced men sometimes forgot that in many ways cooking was an imprecise art. No two sides of meat, no two ducks or chickens, no two fish were ever the same. Their age, their size, the weather, the latitude they were reared in, even the time they were killed—whether it was just before or after they had eaten—almost anything could affect the way they were when they reached Castelli's kitchen.

He paused to watch the *rôtisseur* preparing a chicken dish. A week before, when it was last on the menu, the chef had included the wings and legs. Now he used only the breasts. The dish would have the same name, taste the same, but it would be prepared differently, because by excluding wings and legs the chef had to adapt everything else to preserve the balance of the dish. It was like a sailor adjusting his sails to the wind—

Hell, thought Castelli with a start: could that be it? Could a sailor from one of those communist tall ships that had come to Philadelphia at the time of the convention—a seaman who drank with the legionnaires in their hospitality suites—could he have spiked the drinks of his hosts with one of those newfangled poisons the KGB were supposed to have? Perhaps the man had gone from suite to suite conducting some sort of deadly market research for his masters in Moscow? Castelli thought it over and then discounted the idea. It was just too fanciful.

He moved on, pausing to watch a chef changing attachments on the kitchen's massive electric mixer. The apparatus was capable of whipping, whisking, or grinding at the press of a switch.

Around him the clatter increased as dishes were positioned on steam trays ready for later delivery to dining rooms; "specials," ordered off the à la carte and room service menus, were being prepared by a small team of chefs who worked with astonishing speed, using their knives and cleavers with great dexterity while they boned, sliced, filleted, carved, and trimmed.

As the midafternoon room service orders were completed, waiters carried the food past women checkers seated behind billing registers. Nothing escaped their scrutiny. Their eyes constantly swept the kitchen. That was what made the theft of the meat so puzzling: whoever was taking it had to do so out of sight of the checkers. But even then, how did the thief remove the meat from the kitchen or past the security men? It really was a mystery.

Once more Castelli paused. A cook was reducing a sauce too quickly. Castelli took the pan off the flame, lifted it to his nose, sniffed it, dipped a finger in the liquid, and tasted. He shook his head and put the pan aside. The sauce was slightly burned.

"Never hurry, never hurry," he chided. "The sauce is the most important thing."

He reached for a clean pan and began to work.

Castelli was concentrating so hard on his task that the sous-chef had to tap him on the shoulder a second time.

"Chadwick wants you on the telephone."

Castelli continued to evaporate the liquid in the pan until it reached the correct consistency.

"He says it's urgent," said the sous-chef.

Castelli sighed. It was probably an early dinner order from a party of VIP's; it sometimes happened that some dignitary would ask Chadwick personally to tell the kitchen of a special requirement.

Instructing the cook to pour the sauce slowly into a boat, the executive chef hurried to his office.

"Castelli, we'll be coming down in a few minutes. Mr. Varr, myself, and Mr. Mallison."

"Who's he?"

There was a moment's pause. Then Chadwick's voice sounded suddenly very old and tired.

"Mr. Mallison's from the CDC."

11

Proliferation

Chadwick looked again at George Mallison. For once the hotelier did not hide the anger in a voice trained by years of framing soothing, unrevealing replies.

"You know what this could do, don't you?"

"It could, in the end, help to clear your hotel of any involvement."

Mallison's tone was polite but firm. George Mallison was the assistant director, Bacterial Diseases Division, of the Bureau of Epidemiology at the CDC. He rarely used his full title. It was not his style. Tall, lanky, his full-bearded face dominated by horn-rimmed glasses, Mallison preferred modestly to call himself simply a sanitary engineer. He had joined the CDC in 1951, coming directly from Cornell. His first job was to find a way to kill flies in the Savannah, Georgia, city dump. He had thought it a strange assignment for a highly qualified expert in his chosen field. But he had done it effectively enough for somebody in the CDC to spot his potential. He quickly became assistant to the director and moved rapidly through the agency's hierarchy—alternating between field and administrative work—before reaching his present position as one of the most respected investigators in the CDC. Essentially, Mallison's job was to "poke around in all those places others didn't look and try to find an epidemiological solution." He saw himself as "the nuts and bolts man," with qualifications mechanical rather than medical. Over the years his skillful probing had been an invaluable adjunct to the fieldwork of EIS officers. Ever since he first heard about the present outbreak, Mallison had daily badgered his superior officer—like everybody else in the CDC, he answered to somebody—to let him go to Philadelphia. Finally, on this Wednesday morning, he got his way. Now, five hours after leaving Atlanta, he was standing in what he thought must be a prime suspect in the investigation: the Bellevue. During twenty-five years with the CDC—Fraser had been a seven-year-old child when Mallison joined—the engineer knew he had never faced a more ticklish situation. From the moment he stepped into Chadwick's office he felt the man's hostility. Chadwick and Varr had been icily polite as he carefully explained what he wanted to do. Finally, after a great deal of discussion, Chadwick telephoned Castelli. Then, still in his office, he continued to question Mallison.

Now it was Varr's turn.

"How could it help to have you going around this hotel in the way you've suggested? That's bound to attract suspicion. The press will get their teeth into it. I can almost see the headlines."

Mallison looked at Varr. His eyes helped him make another judgment. Varr would be the more reasonable of the two, the one more amenable to persuasion. Despite Chadwick's carefully modulated voice, suggesting an iron control, Mallison suspected he might be "a screamer": something or somebody could make him snap at any moment. Mallison resolved to be extra careful nothing he said or did would provoke such a result.

"Mr. Varr, I'm here to help. I'm basically as interested in clearing the hotel as you are. I'll be delighted to tell everybody there's no problem once I've—"

"There *is* no problem!" Chadwick was becoming openly exasperated. He stopped, staring at Mallison, switching tack. His voice became soft and pleading. "Don't you see? It's one thing to go through the kitchen, but if you're spotted in the public areas, it's certain to cause speculation."

Mallison nodded, mustering all the tact and understanding he could in his reply.

"Let's try this. We'll go to the kitchen. And then, if that works, we can talk again."

"Talking's one thing. Doing what you propose is another."

Chadwick's anger was obvious.

Varr studied Mallison. When he had walked into the office, he had seemed a rather inoffensive middle-aged man. But now there was a change. There was a look of quiet determination about him; Varr suspected he would not be thwarted. He turned to Chadwick.

"Let's play it the way Mr. Mallison wants. At least for the moment."

Mallison relaxed. Varr had provided the opening that would allow him to get started. He was confident that once he was in, and had shown the hoteliers how he operated, their fears would go. He looked at his watch and smiled for the first time since arriving in the hotel.

"I guess it will soon be the chef's busiest period. Better not keep him waiting."

In silence they walked out of the office.

Mark Goldberger bounded into the Hahnemann Hospital, one of the finest in Philadelphia, with all the confidence of somebody who might literally be holding in his hands the answer to the epidemic. He was carrying an etiological package containing tissue samples taken from a legionnaire whose autopsy he had just left.

It had been the young doctor's first postmortem in Philadelphia; he would remember it for the speed of the pathologist and his remarks when the autopsy was over. The specimens, he told Goldberger, were to be rushed to the Hahnemann at the request of no less a person than state health secretary Bachman. The dead legionnaire, said the pathologist, looked like a perfect case for Katz.

Dr. Sheila Moriber Katz was thirty-three years old, but appeared ten years younger, and even those who envied her admitted she was deservedly ten years ahead of her position on the medical tree. The words most frequently used to describe her were "brilliant" and "ambitious." Following a succession of dazzling moves from one medical appointment to another, she was currently associate professor of pathology and laboratory medicine at Hahnemann; she was confidently expected to follow in the steps of the many other medical luminaries who had taught at the hospital. Perhaps because of the quiet intensity with which she expressed her views, perhaps because of her youthfulness (with her peaches-and-cream complexion, the tall, blond, and stunningly pretty scientist looked little older than her students), or perhaps because to anybody outside her closed circle she was cool, distant, and often dismissive—perhaps for any or all of those reasons there were some colleagues who said Sheila Katz was opportunistic, that in her quest for scientific answers she was willing to risk her reputation and even her life.

Goldberger's impression was more prosaic: she was a dish—pretty enough to play the heroine of any medical soap opera. With her welcoming smile and the way she swung those incredibly long legs, she gave the lie to the popular idea that women in science were short, dumpy, and unattractive. There were others who felt her strong feminist convictions were what really drove her to tackle new challenges.

But by eagerly involving herself in the legionnaires' disease drama, she unwittingly started a chain reaction that would eventually place her close to death as well as at the center of a scientific fire storm.

Stephen Thacker sensed the barely concealed anguish in Dicko Dolan's voice.

"You're too late. We've just buried Jimmy."

"I'm terribly sorry, Mr. Dolan, to have got you at this time. But could I ask a few further questions?"

The young epidemiologist lowered his voice, holding the phone closer to his ear, anxious none of the reporters and cameramen standing outside the phone booth would hear. He suspected one or two of them might try to make something out of the unfortunate timing of his contact with Dicko. During the past few hours, in his appointed role as epidemiologist-on-call-to-the-media, Thacker had learned a great deal about the ways and wiles of the press. On the whole, though, after the initial difficulty of trying to act naturally with a dozen film and still cameras trained on him and an equal number of reporters noting everything he said and did, Thacker was beginning to enjoy the experience. And in spite of the repetitious nature of his work—making appointments by phone and then putting to patients identical questions over and over in the same precise order—the press posse's initial enthusiasm for photographing and recording him had not diminished—even if it was just like "shoe-leather journalism," as one reporter had said in disgust to another, this going from person to person attempting to establish what had occurred.

Thacker consulted a checklist. "Can I ask you about J. B. Ralph?"

"You'd best talk to his mother. But not now. She's burying him tomorrow."

Thacker put a sign against J.B.'s name.

The voice in his ear became flat and hard. "Why are you bothering us today?"

Thacker explained, once more, how every available EIS officer in the state was crisscrossing Pennsylvania interviewing stricken legionnaires and their families and friends in an endeavor to unearth a common denominator, a clue connecting the victims. The only way to do this was by careful questioning and cross-referencing.

The voice softened. "Okay. But now's not the time—"

"Mr. Dolan. I am truly sorry—"

"That's okay. You're just doing your job." Dicko hung up.

Thacker glanced at the waiting pressmen. They too, he knew, were only doing their job.

He stepped from the booth, grinning.

"First the good news. Williamstown's out."

A ragged cheer came from the newsmen.

"Now the bad news. We're going to Chambersburg."

A collective groan greeted his decision.

"That's the back end of the world," protested an agency photographer. "People don't die there. They're born dead in Chambersburg!"

"You should be glad we're not going to McAdoo. I hear it hasn't even got a soda fountain!"

The photographer's capacity for chocolate malts was a running joke.

"Let's get this show on the road. I work for a daily, not a monthly," called the *Inquirer* reporter.

Led by Thacker in his hired car, the convoy of press vehicles drove into Chambersburg and parked beside the town's hospital.

Inside, Thacker first studied the patient's charts, then donned a yellow mask, gown, and rubber gloves and, followed by the media men, marched to the room of the ill legionnaire. At the doorway, the reporters stopped, frightened to enter for fear they would catch the disease from the man.

The veteran struggled to sit up and greet Thacker.

A film cameraman muttered, "I thought he was sick."

"He is sick."

"Then why doesn't he lie down and *look* sick!"

He thrust a light meter into the room as an electrician switched lights on from the corridor.

A nurse stepped forward to smooth the sheets. The patient held her hand and winked at the reporters.

"You're sick, remember? So *look* sick!" repeated the cameraman as he leaned a little farther forward from the doorway.

"And remember, Doctor. Keep your voice up. I want plenty of level," shouted a sound recordist in the background.

Thacker stood beside the bed, waiting for the cameraman to edge hesitantly into the room and settle into position.

"Sit on the bed, Doctor."

"Doctors don't sit on patients' beds."

"They do in the movies! Go ahead. There's nothing in the AMA rules that says you can't."

Another cameraman suddenly shouted, "You're blocking my shot! I can only see Steve's hands!"

There was a jockeying just inside the doorway as the watchers rearranged themselves.

"Jesus, will you guys hurry up?" shouted the *Inquirer* reporter. "I've got a deadline to catch."

Finally, after a couple of false starts—a camera jammed, there was a brief power cut—Thacker began to question the patient.

When did he first feel sick?

The Sunday after the convention, ten days ago.

Thacker wrote down the answer on his form.

Had he attended the Go-Getter's Breakfast in the Bellevue?

Yes.

Thacker checked a box.

Had he gone to the Testimonial Dinner the night before at the Benjamin Franklin Hotel?

Yes.

Had he drunk iced water from the galvanized containers in the Bellevue ballroom?

No.

A photographer moved closer to the bed, knelt near its foot, and, at arm's length, pointed his lens at the patient.

Concentrating totally on what he was doing, Thacker continued to take the legionnaire through the long list of carefully formulated questions on his pad.

"Hold it please, Doctor," ordered a film cameraman. "I've gotta reload."

His colleagues moaned good-naturedly, switched off their lights, and began an animated discussion among themselves about the length of this particular working day.

Thacker continued to talk quietly to the patient about the convention. Caught up in the spirit of the occasion, the man kept looking toward the press men.

"All set, Doctor," called the cameraman, who had placed a new magazine of film in his camera. "Let's try and get this in one take."

The interview continued for another five minutes. Then Thacker put his last question to the veteran.

Had he recently been in contact with pigs?

The patient shook his head. He didn't like pork.

Thacker said he had no more questions; the media men must now leave while he examined the patient.

"Don't move yet, Doctor," shouted a cameraman. "We need some cutaways. Look concerned. Like you've heard something important."

Finally the film cameramen were satisfied. They left Thacker alone with the legionnaire. He checked whether the man had any enlargement of the liver or spleen, looked for signs of pneumonia remaining in his lungs.

When he had finished the examination, Thacker thanked the patient, wished him a continuing recovery, and left the room to phone Fraser to report that although he was now getting a good feel for the illness, the interview had produced nothing that seemed especially significant.

Thacker then rounded up his press posse and headed toward Hershey, where he would see the last legionnaire on his list.

The heat in the kitchen made George Mallison perspire. The noise, thankfully, made it easier for him to avoid conversation with Castelli, Chadwick, and Varr.

Around him the tumult of hundreds of meals being prepared for serving continued. The tempo was so frenetic that few of the staff gave Mallison more than a quick, curious glance.

From time to time Castelli pulled himself away from Mallison to plunge amid the teams of cooks and helpers serving and apportioning, working with a machinelike rhythm that in a single moment filled a plate, slapped on a metal cover, and loaded it on a waiter's tray.

A chef, like a policeman on traffic duty, was stationed in the center of the kitchen, directing the flow of laden waiters past the vigilant checkers and out to the dining rooms.

And the air was filled with shouts: waiters questioning the progress of their orders, cooks barking at their assistants; demands for flour, sauces, pastry, gravies—an endless flow of words that at times threatened to drown the clatter of saucepans, caldrons, and trays being lifted and dropped.

A cart with three large fresh-baked hams was pushed at high speed across the kitchen, forcing Mallison and the others to back away.

Castelli stepped forward to help a chef who had begun rapidly to dissect the meat. Selecting and sharpening a knife, Castelli began to carve, ensuring each plate received the same portion, evenly cut and not too thick. An assistant whisked the plates to the nearby vegetable service counter. In no time only the ham bones remained on the cart.

Wiping his hands, Castelli rejoined Mallison, who was continuing to move slowly through the kitchen.

Eventually he reached the executive chef's office. After a careful look around the glass-walled interior, he turned to survey the kitchen once more.

The pace was slackening as the service to the restaurants began to wind down. Now busboys were streaming into the kitchen, carrying trays piled with dirty dishes. Only the cooks at the room service station were still fully occupied cooking.

Mallison looked to Castelli, smiling, and told him he kept a fine kitchen. The executive chef grinned, his relief visible. He excused himself and returned to his work.

Chadwick spoke. His voice was pleasant, but Mallison could detect the tension beneath. Nor was there any mistaking Chadwick's attitude: he wanted to assure Mallison the rest of the hotel met the same high standards as the kitchen, so what was the point in pursuing his proposal to inspect the entire building?

Mallison said nothing. He thought: *Why is he so anxious not to have his hotel looked at? Is it professional pride—or something else?*

Besides, added Varr, they were already cooperating with the CDC on another level: they had agreed to give Goldberger a list of Bellevue Stratford staff addresses and phone numbers so he could contact and interview whichever of them he pleased.

Mallison considered. *Why had they agreed to let Goldberger check out the employees while remaining so reluctant to have him examine the hotel?*

He spoke, addressing Varr, his words for Chadwick. Goldberger was concerned with a different segment of the investigation, more interested in the human factor—

Chadwick interrupted. He understood that. But *people* were dying, not a *building*. And there was no evidence they were dying as a result of staying in the hotel. How could the hotel conceivably be involved?

Mallison eyed him carefully. He sensed Chadwick's fuse was shortening. He didn't want to trigger his anger. It was time to soft-pedal, to patiently explain that the disease-causing agent had to have a home somewhere and all he was trying to do was ascertain it was not in the Bellevue; additionally, under his supervision, other sanitary engineers would be doing exactly the same thing at other hotels where the legionnaires stayed.

Once more Varr came to Mallison's rescue, gently suggesting to Chadwick that if that was the case it would look bad if the Bellevue was the only hotel that refused an inspection. And a clean bill of health from Mallison would be the best possible answer to give to the press.

Mallison nodded eagerly, admiring the way Varr had handled the situation. He did not know, of course, that Varr's concern to placate Chadwick was partially because he feared any untoward strain could precipitate a heart attack in his boss. On more than one occasion since the crisis began, Varr had noticed a stab of pain in Chadwick's eyes accompanied by a sudden shortness of breath.

Relieved now the matter seemed settled, Mallison said he would tomorrow be bringing a questionnaire for completion by the hotel's chief engineer. As for tonight, he would like permission to collect samples of the cooling-tower water on top of the building.

The two executives looked at each other. Then Chadwick agreed, with the proviso that Mallison be accompanied by Varr and remain totally inconspicuous when passing through the public areas.

Mallison left Castelli's kitchen, having been careful to give no hint of concern. While the kitchen would probably satisfy any public health inspection, he thought it imperative not only to return to the basement area but also to conduct a most thorough investigation of the entire hotel.

Though he had as yet no epidemiological proof, Bob Craven was also beginning to believe the Bellevue was somehow implicated in the outbreak; all his inquiries pointed at least a finger in that direction. It made it even more frustrating to be here in Pittsburgh, hundreds of miles away from where the "real action" was. Valuable as he knew the work was in Pittsburgh, he realized it would soon become peripheral to the main investigation; it must only be a matter of time before his contribution tailed off. Then either it would be back to Atlanta to reunite with his colleagues in the CDC surveillance team still anxiously watching out for swine flu—Craven had no doubt the present epidemic was not due to that—or, more likely, Fraser would request he join him in Harrisburg. Neither prospect was altogether appealing. He would much rather be with Graitcer and the others who had drawn Philadelphia as their fief. That possibility made him if anything the keener to wrap up his efforts in Pittsburgh. He continued to skip food and sleep and to devote every waking moment to thinking and determinedly pursuing everything that looked promising.

Like all the doctors engaged in the hunt who came into contact with the media, Craven had taken time to adjust to the relentless questions of reporters. But in the end he, too, realized they had a job to do and the best way he could help himself was to try and assist them. He was making something of a local reputation among Pittsburgh's press as one of the most cooperative EIS officers on the case. He spent time explaining to them why there could be no acceptable substitute for the slow process of scientific analysis, and speculation, however plausible or interesting, must not be seen as an alternative to proven fact. And he was always careful to give full credit to local health officials, taking particular pains to avoid saying or doing anything that might rouse the ire of coroner Cyril Wecht. As a result, Pittsburgh's media had presented some of the best-informed reporting on the epidemic.

That went some way toward making the city a little more bearable to work in for Craven.

But, he had to admit, even the hamburgers and coffee he was basically surviving on seemed to have the distinctive Pittsburgh flavors of coal and iron ore being melted and smelted in a process that lit the sky luridly and produced a giant's share of the steel to build America's automobiles and the ribs of its skyscrapers, along with mountainous quantities of electrical equipment, aluminum, and the by-products of coke— not to mention being home for the profuse products of H. J. Heinz. Craven had never known a city whose industrial eggs were so highly concentrated in one basket. And yet, despite this cornucopian industrial fecundity, Pittsburgh was not wealthy; it suffered from hardening of the traffic arteries and its government didn't take in enough money to provide the city with all the services it needed. In some ways Pittsburgh was a municipal plunderland, not a very tolerable place in which to live.

Could that be the reason, three full days after news of the epidemic had broken, the calls to the city's health department showed no signs of slackening? Did living in the kernel of the nation's industrial might make these people more nervous? Was it the incessant clatter of heavy industry, the endless process of puddling pig iron, which made them phone with fear in their voices to ask the same questions: Were they safe? What should they do? Was it spreading? Should they leave the city? The state? One person had even asked whether he should leave the country.

Craven, like those working with him, tried hard to ease their anxieties. But it was tough going, made more so because of his own lack of sleep. Since arriving in Pittsburgh he had managed only about ninety minutes of catnapping a night before he plunged back into the frenetic, freewheeling hunt.

And as everywhere else, the investigation was complicated by what Craven described as "the high number of nuts who crawled out of the woodwork."

The terrible disease—or whatever it was—that struck down the legionnaires had already spawned a degree of speculation that was almost certainly a record. Craven suspected this might be partly the result of what most Americans had painfully learned in the post-Watergate era: they were rarely told the total truth about anything. Before the epidemic was more than a few hours old, virtually everyone had a theory —and many were anxious to foist them on harassed health officials. While dismissing the great majority of the explanations as outlandish, Craven was forced to recognize something about current American society: it was preoccupied with the idea of conspiracies and believed that the truth, whatever it might be, was often concealed by powerful vested interests. In such an environment, even the most incredible suggestions were given a hearing and went public, becoming a straw to cling to or a reason for panic.

Since Monday a number of theories were going the rounds. Among them, the Republican Convention Dry-run Theory was based on the premise that the legionnaires had been a trial run for a left-wing group planning to release a poison at the Republican National Convention that would wipe out the GOP. The Ransom Theory argued that a group of European terrorists had used the legionnaires as a test and would soon publicly announce their capability to destroy New York/Los Angeles, et al., unless they received a multimillion-dollar ransom. The World War I Theory claimed that legionnaires who had served in that conflict were carrying a strain of deadly virus with a fifty-nine-year incubation period and that the only solution was to segregate all elderly veterans. The Outer Space Theory stated the epidemic was a warning from Mars and its inhabitants that the Viking lander was not welcome. The Great Salt Lake City Conspiracy Theory asserted the epidemic was part of a Mormon plot to take over the world. The Enemy Within Theory postulated that a U. S. Army germ warfare expert was really a Russian mole who had struck first in Philadelphia and was still in possession of enough biological agents to wipe out a dozen cities.

And now, early this Wednesday evening, Craven had a quiet-voiced man on the phone calmly explaining he, too, knew the cause of the epidemic.

"Dr. Craven, I've got an army training manual and it has a section on chemical warfare—"

"Does the manual have a serial number?"

The man gave a series of digits.

Craven tried a simple check. "Can you please repeat that? I didn't quite get it."

The man rapidly repeated the numbers in the same sequence he had first quoted them.

Craven stiffened. A lunatic might well have slipped up. Further, the man sounded so rational and matter-of-fact.

"Let me read you just a little of what it says here in the CW section."

"Read it slowly. I want to take notes."

The man read steadily, sending a shiver down Craven's spine: the epidemiologist had never heard of the agent mentioned in the manual —he wasn't even sure how to spell it—but some of the side effects it caused sounded very similar to those experienced by the sick legionnaires.

"Would you please spell the name of that agent?"

"I've told you enough already."

"Are you in the Army?"

"No."

"Where did you get the manual?"

"I just . . . just got it. That shouldn't interest you."

"Right." Craven was anxious not to lose him. He wondered: *Is there any way I can have this call traced? I just wish I had one of those homicide detectives they're using in Philadelphia.*

"Can I meet you somewhere? I promise, nobody will know who you are—"

"No, Doctor, you can't," said the man flatly.

"Look, this manual could be important—"

"That's why I called you."

"Can't you read me the entire section?"

"No. It would take too long. It's all about kill ratios and incubation time. I'll make a Xerox copy and mail it to you."

"I'd like to see it sooner than that," said Craven. Alarm mixed with his excitement. "Look, you were good enough to call and I can see you want to help—"

"Doctor, stop snowing me. I said I'll mail you a copy."

"Right, right." The thought kept crossing Craven's mind: *This is no nut, this could be crucial.*

"A day won't make any difference to you, Doctor. The damage has been done—"

"But the manual may give an antidote—"

"I doubt it. There's probably no antidote. There isn't for most CBW agents."

"My God," whispered Craven. "Do you know what you're saying?"

"Yep."

"Mister, I don't care who you are, or how you got hold of this stuff. But I need to see that manual immediately."

"For Chrissake, Doctor, I've told you. I'll put it in the mail."

The caller hung up.

Craven looked around the busy War Room that was the center of the epidemiological hunt in western Pennsylvania. Several of the staff were ashen-faced with fatigue, their voices hoarse from many hours of talking. What would they say if he told them: *I've just had a guy on the phone who seems to know far more about CBW than's good for him and who claims a CW agent killed all these people?*

He turned to a secretary typing up a report.

"You know anybody in the Army?"

"My husband's in the Reserve." The girl continued typing.

"Could you call him about a training manual?" Craven glanced at his notepad and repeated the serial number. "It could be important."

"Yeah? How important?"

"Maybe very, very important."

The girl looked at Craven. "Okay. I've got several friends here with husbands in the Reserve. I'll get them to call as well."

Twenty minutes later the return calls came in. The reservists had checked: the manuals with serial numbers either side of the one Craven had been quoted were readily available, but the manual with the serial number the man had given him was unobtainable—entirely missing from all the military libraries the reservists had tried.

Craven's sense of unease and excitement grew.

He racked his tired brain over what he should do next. He remembered he had an uncle who was an officer in the Army. He called him: could he urgently find out what the mystery manual contained?

An hour later, around 11 P.M., his uncle called back. The manual was strictly classified. There was no way even he could get a copy. Clearly its contents could not be revealed without breaching national security.

Craven let out a long, low whistle. His anticipation drove away his exhaustion.

He spoke quickly into the telephone to his relative. "You've got to find me someone at the Pentagon who's there at this time of night."

"Why? What's going on?"

"I don't know for sure. But it could be something big."

His uncle gave him the number of the duty officer at the Pentagon.

Craven put down the phone and sat lost in thought: *Oh boy, this is all we need, germ warfare!*

He called the Pentagon. The duty officer listened without interruption until Craven had finished.

"Is that everything?"

"Yes."

"I'm sorry, Dr. Craven. I can't help you."

"What do you mean?" Craven exploded; all the intense pressures of the past days finally caught up with him. He lambasted the hapless duty officer.

"Listen, Dr. Craven. I'll tell you this much. The manual is classified because it has a lot of secret things in it about basic warfare strategy. But I can assure you we're out of the CBW business. There's nothing in that manual relevant to what you're dealing with."

Craven sensed the duty officer was speaking the truth. The epidemiologist felt deflated and exhausted. Another promising lead had fallen through. The disappointment would be engraved forever in his memory.

Everybody carries pictures in their mind, thought Graitcer; images that remained, sequences joined together without rhythm or reason. This image, he knew, was one that would last: the city where he had grown up and spent most of his working life looked rotten and alien from where he now sat, in the passenger seat of an unmarked Philadelphia Police Department car.

The dark shape beside him interrupted his reverie, growling for him to roll up his window.

The faces of the men and women hurrying along the street blurred as the car picked up speed to pass quickly around a particularly large patch of rotting refuse that had spilled from the sidewalk onto the road.

A moment later the car's speed dropped.

The voice told Graitcer he could again lower the window.

His companion briefly turned luminous eyes on him: did he still want to keep the air-conditioner off?

Graitcer nodded, settling back in his seat, thinking. There were a lot of ideas circulating about how the disease was transmitted, air conditioning among them. The dentist had an uneasy feeling that when it was all over and the EPI-2 was written—the CDC form that would spell an official end to the investigation—air conditioning would be one of the named culprits. There was no way of proving it—not yet. But almost all the patients he had spoken to mentioned something unusual about the air-conditioning vents in their hotels. They had either been too noisy or expelled some sort of liquid or, as one man put it, "they just didn't seem right."

The epidemiologist kept his thoughts to himself. He had heard automobile air-conditioners frequently leaked and could produce a potential health hazard. Yet there was, he suspected, little chance his companion would feel any qualms about a possible malfunctioning cooling system in his car. The man seated beside him was a veteran homicide detective who never in his life had been bothered by illness. He had forcefully told Graitcer that as he hadn't the time to get sick, he wouldn't. Now he drove slowly for several blocks, easing the car down one street after another, moving effortlessly in and out of the late night traffic, all the time chewing on a cigar he did not bother to relight, his eyes constantly scanning the sidewalks.

Even toward midtown, the garbage filled the warm air with a sickly stench; piles of lacerated plastic bags were everywhere.

But now, after thirty-five days of deadlock, there was hopeful talk of a settlement to the dispute. A deal was being worked out between the Rizzo administration and the trash collectors' union that would give its workers what they had always demanded: more money.

The detective pointed at a heap of refuse and grunted that once the garbage was cleared, the epidemic would be over.

Rats, he insisted, they were the cause. Rats carried fleas. A flea had bitten a legionnaire. He passed the disease to his colleagues. Kill the rats and the whole goddamn thing would be over. They didn't need policemen and doctors driving through the night. They needed more rat collectors.

Graitcer said nothing. He knew there was no scientific evidence to support the theory that the source of the epidemic was in infected refuse. Like Sharrar, he doubted the garbage was much more than an eyesore. Eventually, of course, it must be shifted, but that would in reality be more of an act of civic cosmetology than anything else. And the rats, which he had occasionally glimpsed scaling the trash, could be dealt with quickly. Again, Sharrar had assured him their numbers were being kept to a minimum by the city's rodent exterminators, just as the Bellevue was regularly serviced by a pest control firm.

The hotel was a few blocks away, its massively solid shape blotting out the night sky.

Maybe Mark Goldberger was right: maybe the search for the source of the outbreak should be concentrated inside the hotel. Graitcer had been impressed by Goldberger. He was clever and funny—but he was also not altogether happy about the way the investigation was being run. And Graitcer, too, had his doubts. It seemed to him the lines of communication between Philadelphia, Harrisburg, and Atlanta were not at all clear and sometimes got crossed. The newly arrived Walt

Orenstein, who was rooming with Goldberger, now appeared to be in charge of the CDC contingent in Philadelphia. Graitcer was unsure where that left Sharrar, let alone Fraser. For himself, his loyalties still lay with his swine flu surveillance superior in Atlanta. He would continue from time to time to consult directly with him.

Graitcer glanced at his watch. It was almost midnight. He had now gone for almost three days without proper sleep. Yet he did not feel tired. In part the sheer momentum of the continuous pressure he had worked under since arriving in the city sustained him. It had also sharpened his already formidable powers of observation and recall. Forever committed to memory, or his diary, were whole incidents and conversations. His diary also reminded him of things to do. This very day he had called his mother to wish her happy birthday; she had asked him what he thought of Ronald Reagan's choosing Pennsylvania senator Richard Schweiker as his running mate against Ford for the Republican presidential nomination.

Although Graitcer was politically minded, more vivid in his memory now was everything his companion had said and done since they began driving together back and forth across the city. He guessed this was probably due to the sheer novelty of being chauffeured around Philadelphia by a black policeman who normally tracked down murderers and rapists. Shortly after Graitcer had received the negative report from the state labs on the swine flu serum test, the detective was assigned to escort him from one city hospital to another in order that Graitcer could question suspected cases and study their medical files. To date he had interviewed fourteen patients. Often the policeman barely waited for Graitcer to complete his questionnaire before he launched into his own interrogation. To the sensitive ears of the epidemiologist, the detective's approach sometimes seemed unnecessarily harsh—and so far it had produced nothing significant.

Nevertheless, the policeman now advanced another theory of how the outbreak was triggered: some subversive could have started it. Anybody in the police department who had ever attended a seminar on the criminal spreading of disease could confirm that the technology was frighteningly simple. It needed little more than to arrange for a person with a specific fatal and transmittable disease to spit into a vial and then, after only a little help from a lab technician, to aerosolize the sputum in a crowded place. And there would be the epidemic, swiftly and surely engineered.

Yet, countered Graitcer, no terrorist group had come forward to claim credit for the outbreak. Didn't that rule out the counterculture?

The detective shrugged. The talk at HQ was that additional surveillance had been ordered by the FBI on all possible terrorist suspects: Puerto Ricans, members of the Jewish Defense League, Cubans, known PLO sympathizers, communists.

Graitcer shook his head wonderingly. He had read about the paranoia of the Philadelphia Police Department: it was a subject of constant comment in the media. But he had never realized how deepseated it was. As the car headed across the city, he wondered what the policeman would do if they came across a holdup, an assault, or one of the other major crimes he had spoken about so laconically. Graitcer knew that if trouble came he would do exactly what his companion had ordered: lie flat on the floor of the car and stay there.

So far, apart from gangs of youths roaming aimlessly through the streets of the slum areas, nothing untoward had caught the attention of the detective.

Perhaps because of this, as the night progressed, he developed a theme that was threatening to try even Graitcer's patience.

This case had to be cracked quickly. It was like a murder hunt. The trick was to get to the scene of the crime fast, pick up all the available evidence, round up all the likely suspects, and squeeze them in a precinct interrogation room until the guilty one was obvious.

One problem with this particular investigation, reasoned Graitcer, was they did not know where the crime had occurred, who all the victims were, what was the *modus operandi*, or where the killer had gone —except seemingly to ground.

So what were they driving around for? Hoping to flush the goddamn killer into the open? What sort of way was this to run things?

They were driving around gathering information.

So if they were gathering information, Graitcer must have some idea what he was gathering information against. Right?

It wasn't quite like that, objected Graitcer.

Okay. How was it?

Graitcer began to explain how widespread could be the menace to public health, that the epidemic could have been triggered by any one of dozens of agents, that only recently the CDC had further broadened its programs of detection and control to include diseases that had just come to be recognized as potentially epidemic in nature. Often they were noncontagious diseases resulting from environmental factors, such as pollution, malnutrition—

Jesus, he wasn't suggesting starvation killed the legionnaires? Goddammit, he'd seen them in town. Hams of men, fighting fit—

No, said Graitcer patiently, he was not suggesting malnutrition was responsible, even though many of the legionnaires were not as fit as they looked. He was saying it was one of the many causes of illness in this day and age, as was pollution, and in trying to form a picture of what happened, everything had to be considered.

The detective grunted. So who was paying for all this theorizing?

The city, the state—but in the end the federal government would foot the bill; while the American health care system was one of the most advanced in the world, many regional public health authorities were understaffed and limited in the services they could offer by lack of finance.

The policeman growled. So what's new?

Graitcer's mouth tightened. He inhaled sharply, was about to speak, then stopped. Why should he expect this overworked and probably underpaid policeman to understand the problems of the nation's health service? Almost nobody outside the PHS did.

He grinned. What was that saying, about a nation getting the services it deserved?

The detective smiled back. He said Graitcer sounded like a cop, acted like a cop, so why not use a cop's rules and go and catch his killer?

Graitcer sighed. He would try one last time. He turned to his companion and began to speak. He asked him to imagine a murder hunt where he didn't know whether the killer was a man, a woman, or a minor; where he had no idea whether the weapon used was a gun or a knife or something else. How would he rate his chances of solving such a case—and quickly?

The policeman slowly shook his head, too bemused to reply.

That, Graitcer went on, was the sort of problem he and his colleagues now faced—only it was a thousand times more complex. The killer could be one of a multitude of viruses, bacteria, toxins, or fungi. To check them all out required more specialized laboratory backup and scientific skills than were ever used in any police dragnet.

So how did they hope to catch the culprit?

With patience, perseverance—and a lot of luck. And the sort of special sixth sense that all good detectives possessed.

The policeman nodded, pleased. That he understood. He gunned the car across Walnut and headed on up Ninth Street, past the U. S. Court House and General Post Office, thinking about what Graitcer had said. Then he broke his silence. Wouldn't it still be sensible to search for somebody who could have introduced the killing agent, whatever it was, and make him tell what he'd used?

Graitcer slumped in his seat. There seemed, after all, no way to convince this policeman that the mysterious disease need not have been introduced by anyone, that its agent might have been in the environment for ages. And that its disastrous effect had only become evident because of a unique situation—if it had not hit at the Legion convention, whose members were in close touch afterward, it might have gone on killing totally unnoticed.

Instead, Graitcer pointed toward the splash of light glowing half a dozen blocks ahead in the city's Chinatown. Maybe, he kidded, some death-dealing drug had escaped from there?

The detective grinned. Now Graitcer must be joking. Everybody knew nothing had any chance of surviving in a Chinese stewpot.

Laughing, the detective was about to relight his cigar when Graitcer spoke again.

Eggs, he said solemnly, the answer could be in the egg harvest.

The policeman bit his cigar butt. What sort of crazy statement was that?

Graitcer did not bother to explain. He looked at his watch, wishing he could order his companion to drive to the state laboratories instead of the next hospital. *The eggs could hold the answer.*

Robert Sharrar had deliberately ignored the passage of time until the opening minutes of this Thursday, August 5. He knew the isolation of a virus required slow and invariably highly complex procedures that could involve hundreds of man-hours spread over an exasperatingly lengthy period, often caused by the laborious need to rerun the laboratory tests. The process had a ritual of its own that could not be hurried.

That was why he had fought off the temptation to call the state laboratories to find out whether the promise Graitcer had received held true: that the specially prepared eggs would be ready for harvesting in the early hours of this morning—and would then reveal whether the hoped-for colonies of flu viruses were growing inside their shells.

Even after that, Sharrar knew, the work would continue, involving among other things the preparation of further tissue cultures, statistical correlation of data, the use of ultracentrifuges and electron microscopy. Yet the questions might never be totally resolved; scientists did not always agree even on how to define a virus. It was a microorganism, but of what kind? It was coated in protein but, depending on its type, the covering enclosed a strand of either RNA or DNA. Its shape could vary from a spherical glob to a geometric triangle. And the scale of the problem facing the state lab scientists could be gauged by the fact that a billion times a billion viruses would easily fit into a small salt shaker.

Yet, despite everything, Sharrar was quietly hopeful the harvested eggs would solve a mystery that for the past days had meant he hardly moved from the second floor of 500 South Broad Street. In the stark overhead light the area now looked dingier than ever, the baseboards more scuffed, the floor covering shabbier, the windows grimier. Everywhere there was a litter of Styrofoam cups and overflowing ashtrays. Permeating it all was the distinctive smell—a blend of sweat and stale perfume—of hard-pressed men and women in wrinkled, soiled clothes, working through the night, adding new data to the wall charts and maps or trying to make sense of the scraps of information cluttering every available surface inch of their scratched desks: scrawls they had taken down over telephones that continued to ring. Each piece of paper held some fact, name, or number that just might offer a clue. As the night advanced, these desperately tired workers also kept an eye on the time.

At 1:15 A.M. Sharrar finally yielded. He phoned the state lab and spoke to Graitcer's contact.

The microbiologist said it was still too early. She would call the moment the results became available.

Sharrar sighed. In an otherwise anxious situation there was at least one bright spot: his assistant, Mitch Yanak, whom he had sent home with symptoms that now looked like those of legionnaires' disease, was showing signs of recovering as quickly as he had become ill. Yanak would not have to wait for the slow process of developing a vaccine which would follow the discovery of a new disease-causing virus. That could take months, even years—assuming, of course, it was such a virus that was causing an epidemic in which so far no less than twenty-two lives had been lost and some one hundred and fifty persons hospitalized.

At about the same time, Parkin also telephoned the state lab from the War Room in Harrisburg.

The microbiologist repeated what she had told Sharrar. It was still too early.

A voice cut in on the call: he wanted this telephone link kept open until the results of the egg harvest were known.

The woman hesitated. She did not know whether she had the authority to spend departmental money keeping an open line. The voice became raspingly familiar. It was Bachman ordering her to stay on the line to relay the results the instant they were known.

In the War Room, Fraser looked toward Parkin and said nothing. He, too, had listened in on the call. Like everybody else, Fraser knew the health secretary was driving himself hard. But Bachman was much older than almost all the others involved in the investigation. Fraser had seen him catnapping on his office couch and wondered whether the physical strain was beginning to tell. He hoped not. In many ways the health secretary was a godsend, able to circumvent and cut the bureaucratic red tape so often associated with an emergency. And Fraser had continued to be pleasantly surprised how well they were working together; in fact the whole Harrisburg-based team was now a smoothly functioning unit. That, he recognized, was due in large part to Parkin's willingness to work with, even for him. His early fears that he would have a running fight with the state epidemiologist for control of the investigation were no longer there.

Bachman shouted for Fraser and Parkin to come into his office. As they did so, people in the War Room found excuses to drift closer. The office door was open and they could see the health secretary's telephone receiver lying on his desk.

The woman's voice carried clearly as she said the process of candling the eggs was well under way.

Her colleague examined another egg under a bright light to locate the tiny hole she had originally made in its shell. She found the opening and daubed it with iodine to sterilize it. Next she carefully pierced the egg's air sac. Then she used an eyedropper to suck up some of the semiclear liquid. Concentrating to keep her hand rock-steady, she moved the dropper toward a test tube. This was a critical point. One mistake, the slightest inadvertent squeezing of the dropper, *anything* at all that would allow the tiniest droplet to escape could release a deadly virus into the air. She made no mistake. The liquid was safely deposited into a vial.

She turned to a tray containing tubes filled with the red blood cells of chickens and guinea pigs. She added a measured quantity of red cells to the liquid she had put in the test tube. If an influenza virus was present in the liquid, its protein coating would attract the red blood cells, causing them to clump and settle in a distinctive patch at the bottom of the tube. If no viruses had grown in the egg, the cells would clot neatly together in a single red pellet.

When all the tubes were prepared, they were placed in a refrigerator. The settling process—which would produce either a patch or a pellet— needed about forty minutes.

The time would be up at 2:00 A.M.

Waiting for the results, drumming his fingers nervously on the desk top, clamping the telephone to his ear as the deadline approached, Bachman asked Fraser how accurate the test was.

Fraser chose his words carefully. The test was reliable under ideal conditions. But like everything else, if rushed it could be less than conclusive.

Bachman grunted and barked into the phone: How much longer?

There was a moment's silence. Then sudden excitement drove the fatigue from the woman's voice as she reported that the vials were being taken from the refrigerator.

Another pause.

In the War Room, those who were themselves talking on other telephones ended their conversations and looked expectantly toward Bachman's open office door.

The silence stretched.

Then the microbiologist broke it, her voice quivering slightly under the strain. All the vials contained pellets. There was no clumping, no sign of any virus.

Bachman shook his head and slowly replaced the telephone on its cradle. "It's negative. Not just swine flu negative, but negative influenza, period. We're up against something much tougher. It's not going to end like I'd hoped—happily ever after."

People at the doorway began to move back into the War Room, not bothering to hide their feeling of defeat and dejection.

Fraser rose to his feet, towering over the health secretary. The report, he said, clearly indicated one thing: the most obvious diagnosis had been ruled out. They would virtually have to begin again from the start.

"The press isn't going to like this," said Parkin. "And what about the *Daily News?* They've got a deadline to meet before the ten o'clock press conference."

"They can wait to hear until then like everybody else," barked Bachman. "Maybe the governor will come over and make the announcement."

Fraser looked steadily at the two state health men: there *had* to be an answer.

He went to a private office and dialed Atlanta. Early though the hour was, CDC director David Sencer must be told swine flu was no longer likely. Yet despite—or perhaps because of—the new challenge, professionally speaking Fraser was "relieved, delighted, and excited." Had it been swine flu, continuing with the investigation would have had little interest for him. He would probably have asked to be replaced. Now it was different.

Any concealed doubts he might previously have harbored about his own ability to lead the investigation now vanished. Fraser felt ready for whatever lay ahead.

Personal relationships, Ted Tsai thought wearily to himself, were what the success of the investigation would largely depend on. But they were so delicate, so diffuse, and often, like the characters in a Chinese parable, so vague. He accelerated past a truck, concentrating for the moment totally on his driving, squinting his eyes against the dazzle of oncoming traffic and looking for the exit to the next all-night coffee shop on the highway between Pittsburgh and Harrisburg. He drove fast for a mile or so, forcing his senses alert. The warm middle-of-the-night air rushed through the car, making his eyes smart. He reduced speed, eased into the slow lane, and started to think again about the many-faceted relationships the investigation had produced.

It was an intellectual exercise, which Tsai found was the best way to stay awake. He had been on the road for sixteen solid hours—or was it eighteen?—driving from one tiny hospital to another, sitting at the bedsides of a succession of elderly and very ill legionnaires, taking samples of their blood and sputum, asking them identical questions in the same order, writing their responses in the neat hand a Chinese astrologer would undoubtedly have said was part of Tsai's astrological makeup. It went with his compassion, his deep sense of integrity and dedication to the service of others. If Tsai hadn't become a doctor he would have made a good priest in a temple, or perhaps even a philosopher, explaining the troubled history of his people to succeeding generations. Instead he had chosen a path that presently placed him, around four in the morning, on a Pennsylvania turnpike, heading for Harrisburg with the specimens and data from eight widely dispersed patients.

His mind drifted back over the relationship he had tried to establish with them. There had often been a look of surprise in their eyes when he'd come to their bedsides; he supposed it wasn't every day a Chinese doctor turned up in the boondocks. Yet hadn't he read somewhere the Chinese played a part in building the railways that carried Pennsylvania's products across the nation? And didn't they run the best laundries in the state, as they did everywhere else? Perhaps that was it —the looks of quickly suppressed surprise were really because the legionnaires had not expected to see a Chinese *doctor*: perhaps they associated his people with takeouts, starch and steam, and laboring?

Maybe it was a throwback to World War II, which several of those patients had fought in; perhaps subconsciously they compared one oriental race with another, mixing Japanese with Chinese. Or maybe it was the Korean War that had left the legionnaires with a collective image of Red Chinese hordes rushing toward the 38th Parallel. Tsai didn't know—just as he did know he could never bring himself to tell any of them his own father was now a general working in Washington, D.C.

In turn, he had also been totally surprised by the legionnaires. Almost to a man they told him, often in some detail, that they were the victims of what one called "diabolical sabotage." They had been deliberately poisoned. They couldn't tell him how, they just kept insisting that was what happened. They differed only in their choice of poisoner, offering either a communist or another subversive group. He'd written it all down. But when he probed further, looking for evidence of poisoning, they became wary. To some at least, Tsai supposed he was just another foreigner. He didn't think there would have been any point telling them he was as patriotically American as they were. And there simply wasn't time for that sort of contact. Under the conditions he had worked—where minutes often counted—there was no opportunity to build a relationship slowly. It had to be established swiftly—rather in the way he had behaved when the newsmen had homed in on him in Harrisburg. He remembered how Fraser had also quickly established his presence among those around him. It was tremendously impressive. But what about the relationships between individual members of the entire team? How well had they been established? He wasn't sure. Perhaps, at a lower level, it didn't matter so much.

Tsai spotted the exit sign. Five miles. Ten minutes. Then more coffee but no food: eating would make him sleepy. There were still another hundred miles or so to go, adding to the four hundred he had already driven.

In the War Room, he remembered, some of his colleagues had been rather abrupt when dealing with patients over the phone, jumping in with questions and not always listening, as if they wanted to keep moving forward. With often no more than a word or a glance, Fraser showed that was a mistake. He was the key, no doubt at all: every other relationship stemmed from him. Tsai had never known anybody, not even his own father, who could be so decisive, so aggressive, and so stimulating to work for, as Fraser. He'd spoken to him several times during his lonely drive around the state. At the end of the last call, Fraser had said: *Ted, take it easy, don't push yourself too hard.*

Another leader might have urged him to hurry. But partly because Fraser had not done that, Tsai now felt compelled to drive through the night. It was a measure of the man, the way he could draw out new strengths in others when exhaustion seemed close.

Tsai saw the neon signs ahead and drove off the highway. The coffee shop parking lot was virtually empty at this hour. Through its brightly lit windows he could see a counter hand talking to a waitress. He envied them and, for just a moment, wished he was back home in bed with Sherry. He'd phoned his young bride several times since coming to Pennsylvania. Sherry had been understanding and supportive and gently teasing about his brief appearance on network TV: she'd glimpsed him amid the hurly-burly in Harrisburg.

Tsai parked the car. He'd sit for a moment, willing the stiffness in his neck to go away. It was pleasant and relaxing now that he didn't have to drive. And it was easier to think further about relationships. There was the difficult one between Parkin and Bachman. It was really much more complex than most people realized. When this was over and the CDC gone, what would happen then? What would Parkin do? And Bachman? Where would his future lay? The question was . . .

Ted Tsai never found the answer to that question. He fell asleep behind the wheel of his car.

12

Obliteration

Dicko glanced back. A quarter of a mile behind him, Williamstown looked pretty enough to qualify for one of those *Saturday Evening Post* covers he remembered from his youth. The town shimmered in the full splendor of a summer's day: a blend of white-painted buildings framed in dark green foliage. Almost every house displayed a flag at half-mast. He turned to peer again in the other direction, continuing to stare down the road that led from the town and into the valley. He stood alone, away from the others, waiting.

Less than two weeks ago, J.B. had driven along that road into Williamstown, newly bald and filled with melancholia, but alive. Now, in a short while, Dicko would watch J.B.'s ornate coffin being lowered into the ground.

Dicko quickly blinked his eyes and concentrated even harder on the road, trying to blot out the memory of J.B. in the casket. Jesus, thought Dicko, if J.B. could have seen himself with all that paint and powder on his face, he would have died laughing. Yet somebody—Dicko couldn't remember who—had whispered in the Repose Room that Mrs. Ralph was delighted with the way her son looked. And Dale Hoover murmured that he had striven to reproduce the thoughtful, formal look J.B. had assumed when editor of the *Echo*. For Dicko's part, he had been glad when the coffin lid was lowered for the last time. The sight of that cleverly composed face, so smooth, so serene, and so unlike the J.B. he knew, was not the one Dicko wanted to remember of his friend.

He glanced toward the Milk Barn. Some of the reporters talking among themselves were eyeing him curiously. He swore softly and turned quickly away. At least, Dicko thought, they had the grace to leave him alone for the moment.

His first close encounter with the world's media had left him bewildered and often angry. As post commander he willingly took the brunt of the media assault. He had lost count of the number of reporters since Monday who had knocked on his door; all he knew was that for every caller a dozen others telephoned, often late at night. He tried to answer their questions with his customary thoroughness, but soon realized many of them didn't want his details: they merely wished him to confirm information already in their possession. He found it a puzzling way of doing things. Some of the newspapermen—notably those from the New York *Times* and Washington *Post*—were courteous and apologetic for intruding at such a time. But many were brusque and insensitive. A nadir had been reached the day before when Jimmy's funeral was turned into a tawdry circus, with cameramen clambering over graves and reporters badgering mourners. Dicko accepted that the media had their job—he had even been persuaded all this publicity might help solve the salient mystery of why the legionnaires were still dying—but he also felt the media should show some respect.

Earlier this morning Dicko had spotted reporters going from door to door in the town—like brush salesmen, he thought contemptuously—trying to pick up photographs of Jimmy and J.B. and bits of information about the dead men. He doubted they would glean much. Williamstown folk had a way of clamming up in the face of nosy outsiders.

A photographer had snapped him getting out of his car as he arrived at the Milk Barn; now a TV crew was slowly moving around him, filming him standing ramrod straight in his uniform, his legionnaire cap fixed securely on his head. He blinked his eyes again, glad of the sunglasses that hid the wetness on his lashes. Jesus, these TV people were tacky. And what about that reporter, the one who claimed he was from *Newsweek*? What had he said—something about the town becoming divided and filled with fear? Dicko had told him flatly he was talking crap. Yet now he wasn't so sure. There *was* something going on. People, men and women he had known for years and on whose reaction to any given situation he would have been willing to bet, had begun to behave oddly. Where he expected them to rally around, they now kept a distance. After Jimmy had been lowered into the ground, Doris whispered to him she felt like a leper, the way some people avoided her. She asked him point-blank whether the disease was catching. He gruffly told her not to be foolish. She had hurried away; later she sent word she would not be at J.B.'s funeral. He could understand that. When Doris left Jimmy's grave she was on the point of collapse. And he himself had to draw on almost the last of his reserves to come through that dreadful experience and prepare for today's funeral for J.B. But a number of people who attended Jimmy's committal would not be present for the interment of J.B. Some had telephoned to say they felt unwell; he had heard reports that there were now half a dozen people in the town with symptoms of the disease that killed J.B. and Jimmy. Perhaps that was why so many reporters had arrived in Williamstown—to wait for more deaths?

Dicko felt a flush creep up his neck. It was caused not only by anger but by fear. Even in his shocked state he was well aware of rumors that the disease could be as deadly as any known to modern man—and there seemed to be no agreement on an antidote. Forcing himself to think of other things, he looked again toward the Milk Barn, this time ignoring the reporters, remembering the little details J.B. had imparted to convey the full impact of the day he walked into the bar with a black go-go dancer on his arm. Jesus, that must have been a sight. But who could blame J.B. after the way he had been treated by Carol?

Nobody yet knew whether Carol would show up for the funeral. If she did, Dicko was sure he would recognize her even after all this time: no matter what Carol did to her hair or face, there was no way she could disguise that swinging walk, the way she moved on those slim, shapely legs, drawing every man's eyes. He remembered how J.B. had stared after her, pride and fierce possession in his face. And after she left him, J.B. never again looked at any woman quite like that.

If Carol came, would she bring the boys, J.B.'s sons? Dicko had overheard Mrs. Ralph and Virginia Anne whispering when they were viewing J.B. in the Repose Room. Mrs. Ralph had somehow persuaded Carol not to change the boys' last name. How ironic, thought Dicko, that J.B. had not lived to see his one wish realized. But Mrs. Ralph had told her daughter that Carol might still keep the boys from the funeral.

Suddenly a line of cars appeared down the road. Dicko looked at his watch. They were early. Standing in the at-ease position, he waited for the convoy to approach.

The cars conveyed senior officers of the Legion from its state headquarters near Harrisburg.

As the first car stopped, Dicko stepped briskly forward to open the door for Edward Hoak. The adjutant looked sternly at the newsmen; some of their colleagues in Harrisburg had begun to suggest the legionnaires might unwittingly have poisoned themselves with the home-brewed liquor or the food they took to the convention. Hoak believed he recognized the beginning of a campaign to shift responsibility onto the Legion. Equally troubling were reports from all over the state that legionnaires and their families were being ostracized. But what really upset Hoak was the knowledge that many sick legionnaires were having serious problems paying their hospital bills; some were already under pressure from certain hospitals to do so immediately—or their treatment would be stopped. Hoak knew few veterans carried sufficient cover to meet the costs of a battery of unexpected tests and intensive-care nursing. He had been horrified to learn of one hospital administrator who was "closing in on a patient, even threatening to take his house." The adjutant was attempting to stop such harassment by organizing a fund-raising campaign that would ensure no legionnaire had to forgo treatment through lack of finances.

The issue would remain a festering sore, causing considerable bitterness and anguish in the coming weeks. In the end, under Hoak's driving persistence and with support from the teamsters' union, the money would be found to help pay individual bills, which were as high as $22,000. Typically for Hoak, he would also underplay his own role—just as now he insisted to newsmen he had come to Williamstown simply as one legionnaire saying farewell to another.

Dicko was visibly moved and relieved. One of his doubts had been that the presence of "this top brass from State could give the occasion the wrong flavor." More than anything, he wanted the funeral to be Post 239's good-bye to J.B.

Hoak took Dicko aside and began quietly to question him. Was there enough money to pay for Jimmy's and J.B.'s hospital bills and their funerals? Were their dependents taken care of? Dicko satisfied Hoak on both counts. What about the attitude of the townspeople: were they beginning to avoid the legionnaires and their friends? Dicko told Hoak what Doris and the *Newsweek* reporter had said. The adjutant frowned. If this continued, it could seriously damage the whole Legion.

Dicko gritted: To hell with that.

Hoak grinned. Dicko had always been a loner.

One of the officers with Hoak said he was thirsty.

Dicko nodded toward the Milk Barn.

The man went into the bar and asked for a glass of water. As he turned to leave, the barman pointedly smashed the glass.

Jesus, breathed Dicko, when the shaken officer told him what happened, it was as if the plague was here. In somber mood, Dicko got into his car and led the convoy into Williamstown.

Long before they reached the Ralph Funeral Home—from which the burial service would proceed—they drove past scores of cars, trucks, and vans: mobile studios and telecommunications vehicles were parked the length of Market Street.

Almost every TV and radio station in Pennsylvania had either sent a crew or made other arrangements to have the funeral covered. All three national networks had dispatched large teams. Every major newspaper in the state had sent journalists. So had the nation's major metropolitan newspapers. All the national and foreign wire services were there, as were the weekly news magazines. A number of specialist photo teams had arrived, along with the foreign press and overseas broadcasting services. In all, close to two hundred journalists were jostling the mourners trying to get into the funeral home.

Dicko parked his car. Using his elbows, he began systematically to carve a pathway for Hoak and his followers toward the door of the funeral home.

Then he glimpsed her: a flash of ash-blond hair, carefully coiffeured. For a moment she was gone, lost in the melee. He shouted. She didn't hear him. He plunged on, taking Hoak and the others in the direction he had seen her. He wanted to thank her for coming, to tell her he was sure J.B. had thought of her right up to his death. But Dicko was too late.

Clutching tightly to the hands of her two small sons—oblivious to the stares of people who had once been neighbors, shrugging off any attempts by reporters to question her—Carol reached the door of the funeral home.

Shortly afterward Dicko led the others into the building's chapel.

Seats beside the flag-draped coffin had been reserved for Dicko and Hoak; the other officers stood at the back of the chapel.

Dicko glanced across the aisle at Carol. She was seated with her sons separating her from Mrs. Ralph and Virginia Anne. All three women stared ahead, frozen-faced. Dicko sensed the hostility between J.B.'s mother and Carol. He felt immeasurably sad. He realized he had been hoping that if Carol came there could be some sort of reconciliation; somehow that would have been an appropriate tribute to J.B. Dicko remembered how once his friend said he was almost willing to die to get Carol back and have the whole family together again. Looking at the three unflinching women seated on the same pew yet alienated by so much bitterness, Dicko realized it could never have been.

On that discordant note the burial service began, the prayers and hymns competing with the noise from outside.

A number of TV reporters had chosen the funeral home as a backdrop for their camera statements—the introductory and bridging remarks that would link the film footage being shot around the town.

NBC's correspondent rehearsed a passage about the struggle of a small community to accept mysterious death. The CBS reporter was declaiming that while Williamstown buried its dead, scientists had ruled out swine flu and were beginning to concentrate on toxic substances. ABC's correspondent was using one of the telephones that linked his van to the network's headquarters in New York; the reporter was trying to get clarification on the endless flow of information coming into his mobile control van. Bachman had announced a dramatic drop in the number of new cases—none were reported yesterday— while claiming it was too early to say whether the trend would continue. The health secretary had also got into what appeared to be a public dogfight with CDC director David Sencer over the total number of cases. Sencer put the figure at 153; Bachman insisted there were only 108. And Bachman also said the emphasis of the investigation was definitely shifting toward toxins, although he had not ruled out the slower-moving viruses. The ABC reporter groaned. What the hell was a slow-moving virus?

In another truck a radio producer was monitoring an optimistic report from the CDC stating the cause of the disease was expected to be known within twenty-four hours; no reason was advanced for this belief. From Washington came a flash: the federal plan to protect children against polio, measles, and mumps was threatened by the same insurance problem that had dogged the swine flu vaccination program. In adjoining control trucks, still other news was being received. Much of it was conflicting, often confusing, and sometimes without basis. It added to the problems of newsmen in Williamstown trying to scale down the amount of information and eventually incorporate it into the framework of J.B.'s funeral. The epidemic would again lead the evening news on all three networks with huge blocks of time, the fourth day in a row the outbreak was the nation's top story. As a media event it was already ranking alongside the death of President Kennedy and Watergate.

While the closing prayer was being said over the coffin, Dale Hoover slipped out of the chapel, blinking his eyes against the brightness of the day. His reaction would be interpreted by one reporter as evidence that "even those only professionally involved wept at this funeral." If anything, Hoover was, "professionally speaking, happy—all the arrangements went clockwork smooth."

And, surveying the street scene, the undertaker was certain the media turnout was greater even than for Jimmy's funeral. A number of reporters who had developed that easy familiarity common to their trade began to shout questions at him.

How long to go, Dale?

A couple of minutes.

The cameramen began to focus on the door behind Hoover.

How much did the casket cost? A lot?

That was a private matter.

Was he scared—knowing how J.B. had died?

No, he had taken precautions.

What about his finger—what was the story there? What had his doctor advised?

Hoover flushed: how did they know about *that*? Nothing could be hidden from these reporters. Well, he would tell them the truth. He was still scared despite his doctor's reassurance; he was keeping a close watch on his finger and continuing to have daily checkups.

The reporters wrote it all down. The story of Hoover's mishap while embalming Jimmy would ultimately appear in a number of publications, a macabre footnote to his role in the drama.

Cameramen shouted for him to move as the door opened and the bearer party emerged with the coffin.

Hoover felt "both proud and deeply moved." Half-blinded by the camera lights, he thought wonderingly: *The whole world is going to see J.B.'s casket.*

Perhaps it was understandable for him to regret that the world would never see the artistry he had on display inside that coffin. Given a chance, he was sure his workmanship on J.B. would have considerably advanced the cause of the American way of death. He had also at first regretted that the pomp and ceremony for J.B.'s funeral had been cut to a minimum. Mrs. Ralph had vetoed plans for a color guard and graveside rifle salute. Now, as he helped place the casket in his hearse, Hoover was glad there was nothing to distract attention from the immense coffin.

Hundreds of people had gathered at the Fairview Evangelical Cemetery at the west end of town by the time the cortege arrived.

Mrs. Ralph walked proudly behind the casket. People marveled at her composure. A pace behind came Virginia Anne. She was followed by Carol and the boys. At the graveside the two groups divided, the Ralphs to one side of the bier, Carol and the children to the other.

Dicko glared at the phalanx of still and movie cameramen, who were not only in danger of trampling on the floral tributes but also of actually falling into the open grave.

Hoak and the other senior Legion officers stood at the foot of the grave. A contingent from Post 239, made up of J.B.'s closest friends, was at the head.

Dicko stepped forward to deliver a final short prayer.

He paused. Mrs. Ralph was looking intently at her two grandsons. Almost imperceptibly, her hand reached out, as if to beckon the children to her.

The boys looked at their mother. Carol pulled them close to her side.

Mrs. Ralph mouthed something. It might have been a plea.

There was no mistaking Carol's reply. Low, but clear to all those around the grave, she uttered one word: *No.*

Mrs. Ralph lowered her hand and looked steadily at the coffin.

Choking with emotion, Dicko uttered his prayer.

Nothing broke the silence except the whine of film cameras recording the final salute Dicko gave the casket, and the poignant moment when he folded the flag and presented it to Mrs. Ralph.

Adjusting her glasses, she peered at the emblem for a long moment. Then she raised her head, touched Virginia Anne's arm, and walked steely-erect from the graveside.

She turned just once to give her grandsons an understanding look while at the same time totally ignoring Carol.

Within an hour J.B.'s mortal remains—apart from what had been sent to Atlanta—were interred and covered with dark earth. Then, as a final gesture, the elderly cemetery caretaker placed a small flag in a bronze standard where J.B.'s headstone would be.

Slumped in an armchair in a Manhattan high-rise, Maria Reeves stared at the TV screen, the throbbing in her head driving out what the doctor on the noonday news show was saying. She poured another glass of ice water, her shivering rattling the cubes in the pitcher, the third she had drunk since staggering out of bed at breakfast time. It was turning out to be a mother of a bad idea to have come to New York. There she had been, up in the Catskills breathing clean country air, when one of those impulses that always governed her life told her to call Cheryl, a friend from the days both girls had been hookers on and off Broadway. In no time Maria was persuaded to abandon the resort hotel—where she was resting after her strenuous stay at the Bellevue Stratford—and come to New York to stay with Cheryl. On the very night she arrived, her friend had been badly injured by a hit-and-run car and was now in the hospital. And, groaned Maria, the way she felt, she would soon be there herself. The vague impression of malaise she experienced at the Bellevue had developed to the point where she now felt as unwell as she had earlier in the year.

She groped for the ice cubes in the pitcher and, sucking on one, used a handful to rub her face to try to ease the burning sensation in her skin.

The blurred voice from the screen seemed to be personally addressing her: a feeling of tiredness, weakness, and a general run-down condition was followed by slight headaches, chest pains, and muscle aches; then chills would set in and intensify, accompanied by sweating, a dry cough, and ferocious headaches.

The picture cut to the show's hostess, who asked the doctor what advice he had for anyone suffering from such symptoms.

His face filling the large screen in a corner of Cheryl's living room, the doctor smiled a first-the-good-news smile. Most people with those symptoms probably had a bad case of flu. They should not be alarmed; a few days in bed and a mild sedative would usually suffice. Except— and the smile vanished—if a person had been in Philadelphia for the Legion convention or in contact with somebody who was there. Then, enunciated the doctor, those symptoms could signify something serious, even fatal.

Maria used the remote-control button to switch to a quiz show. The doctor was just trying to frighten her.

As she moved toward the kitchen to refill the pitcher, she felt a sudden stabbing pain in her abdomen that forced her to drop the jug and, on all fours, crawl to the bathroom, where she was violently sick. For a while, too exhausted to move, she lay on the carpet, clutching her stomach. At last the pain eased and she was able to pull herself to her feet.

She looked in the mirror. Her face was waxy and white, her eyes burning with fever.

A shower, she decided: that would cool the fire scorching her body. Too dazed to care, Maria stood under the spray in her kimono and drenched herself in cold water. Then, dripping, she staggered back to bed.

Sometime later—time, for her, had ceased to have meaning—she awoke with a start.

From outside, the sounds of the city drifted up and through the open bedroom window.

Maria turned her head toward the curtains and groaned. The ache was worse than ever. Her throat seemed to be closing. Pools of hot moisture lay under her arms and in the small of her back. Her thirst raged on. Yet her teeth were chattering uncontrollably.

She knew, then, that she must seek help. The thought filled her with dread. But the doctor on the TV show had been quite specific: anybody with symptoms like hers who had been in contact with legionnaires could be in deadly peril. Even so, she believed that to get medical aid would mean having to face awkward questions. The truth might emerge and precipitate a sequence of events that could shatter the subterfuge of the life she had so carefully constructed. Her doctor might break his professional oath and pass on the word that she was a whore. A few years ago a physician had done just that. She had consulted him about a sudden hemorrhaging after an illegal abortion—the legacy of a misbegotten romance. The doctor informed the police. It took a lot of lying to extricate herself.

Maria moved her head, sending fresh stabs of pain through her skull. She sank back on the pillow, counting slowly—as she had done when a child—up to fifty, mouthing after each number: *Pain, go away*. She tried again, sat up, and gradually eased herself out of bed. Her feet were cold and wet on the carpet.

She shambled to the kitchen and poured cold water down her parched throat. She began to feel better, strong enough to go back to the bathroom, towel off the perspiration, and spray herself with deodorant. Then she went back to the bedroom and dressed.

An explosion of vigor seemed to have gripped her. Forgotten now was the idea of consulting a doctor. Instead she would go out, have her hair done, buy some new clothes, return, pack, and catch the early evening Metroliner to Philadelphia. She could be home in time for dinner. A good night's sleep and she'd be better.

A sudden bout of coughing convulsed Maria, almost doubling her up with its force. Tears streamed from her eyes.

Shivering uncontrollably, she again began counting: *Pain, go away.*

Now she knew. It was something in this apartment that was making her sick. She had to get out of here. The pain was shooting through her entire body, stabbing, burning shafts of hurt that traveled from her head to her toes and back again. She went to Cheryl's closet, removed a winter coat, wrapped it around herself, and staggered from the apartment, clutching her purse.

For a time Maria walked in a trance around midtown Manhattan. She had a vague memory of slumping in the seat of a taxi and being unable to tell the driver where to take her. He threatened to call a cop and hauled her out of the cab, cursing her as a drunk or a dopehead. She started to wander in and out of department stores, her progress marked by bouts of unrelieved coughing. People looked askance at her. She was past caring. She just wanted to be left alone. In that wretched condition she reached Macy's. Wet-faced and shaking, she moved through the store. Passing by the radio department, her ears heard a familiar voice. It was the doctor who had been on TV. Here he was again, uttering another of his dire warnings about something he was now calling legionnaires' disease.

Legionnaires' disease: the words stunned Maria. Now she knew what she had and how she had got it. Terrified, she lurched from the building.

Shortly afterward she was spotted by the crew of a police patrol car who were watching out for her, having been alerted by a detective in one of the stores she had shambled through; she had been categorized as another of those New York winos who sometimes attempt to seek shelter in big stores. From time to time the police rounded them up.

The patrolmen, experienced in such matters, recognized that Maria was not a drunk or a junkie. They took her to the nearest hospital. She was barely conscious when admitted.

Later, she would remember a jumble of impressions: hands undressing her under bright lights, masked faces peering down, muffled voices, her mouth prized open, footsteps, new faces and voices, urgent commands, movement. She was being lifted, wheeled down a corridor and into an elevator. Another corridor and more voices. Eventually she was alone in a small empty room. There were bottles above her bed that led to needles in her arms. There were wires running from her body to machines. Then sleep.

Maria was totally unaware of the battle going on inside her between the deadly invader and the defenders of the intricate structure of cells, tissues, organs, and systems that had kept her alive from the moment she was conceived. Powerful though these were, by themselves they could not stop the marauder, which penetrated farther and was now fighting with the white blood cells, specially trained to monitor, challenge, recognize, and engage alien organisms. The invaders reached the fertile area of tissue and the streams of blood that could feed and help transport them through Maria's body. At each stage her natural defenses came into action. The lymph nodes mobilized their own vast armies of white cells. The bone marrow, spleen, and liver worked relentlessly to produce still more white cells. And temporarily the enemy's progress was halted. Then it gained sufficient strength to seep into the tiny blood vessels in her lungs, relishing the womblike warmth of those sacs, rich in sugar and oxygen, the ideal environment for colonization.

At that point outside forces had joined in the struggle: medical equipment and medication were mobilized for the battle. Burning with fever, Maria was barely aware of what was being done in the hospital: expert fingers slipping another needle into her arm, regular listening to her lungs, gauze cleaning her mouth, collection and analysis of bodily samples—the constant checks and monitoring of intensive-care nursing for what had been diagnosed as a severe case of pneumonia. And leading her fight for survival was one of the most powerful of modern antibiotics: erythromycin.

Slowly at first, hardly perceptibly even to the sophisticated medical equipment surrounding her, the organism was driven from the ground it had held.

The fight would last days; then, though still weak, Maria insisted on discharging herself, right up to the end evading the questions of her doctors and nurses. They, being busy people, did not persist. Perhaps because they were so occupied with other crises, it was also understandable that—in spite of the intense publicity—nobody connected Maria's illness with what was happening in Pennsylvania. After leaving the hospital, she returned to Cheryl's apartment, collected her belongings, and traveled to Philadelphia. At the back of her mind the conviction was growing that her life had been spared as "a sign from God."

Eventually Maria would experience a religious conversion and give up her profession.

None of this could she have foreseen the Thursday afternoon she slipped into exhausted, chemically induced sleep in that intensive care cell. Least of all could she have guessed that if her connection with the legionnaires had become known she would have been of great interest to those searching for the cause of the outbreak.

It was caused, the voice explained, by a condition known as oxygen sleep starvation—OSS—stemming from what he would call, for simplicity's sake, biological nuclear solvent—BNS—in which biological elements in the blood were atomized by an induced chemical trigger. Ordinarily benign, those elements were then lethal. A small vial of BNS would have been enough to create OSS; a single drop placed on the pillow of each afflicted person would have been sufficient.

Sharrar sat quite still, trying to switch his mind to what the caller was saying. A moment ago he had been talking to his wife, managing to snatch a few words with her at her office. Karen had just been to see her obstetrician, and the baby was in the right position, its fetal heartbeats strong and regular. It looked like an early September delivery. Before then, Sharrar promised Karen, the pressure would be off. He would have time to be more supportive, to do those domestic chores which he was now forced to neglect because of the demands of the investigation. Perhaps there might even be a chance for a few days' break before their baby was born. Talking quietly to Karen, he had almost forgotten about work. But he had barely replaced the receiver when this authoritative voice was put through, jarring him back to the present, and was confidently explaining to him how the epidemic was caused.

Though he said he was a researcher, neither the man nor his New York institute was familiar to Sharrar. That, in itself, did not matter. What was puzzling was that while his caller used professional terminology—moving easily from hidrosis to the effect of oxygenic cells and the need to run basophilic tests—a lot of what he said was foreign to the city epidemiologist. Until now Sharrar had never heard of OSS and BNS.

The man laughed indulgently. Research in the United States, apart from the work at his institute, was nonexistent—but the Soviets were well advanced.

Sharrar stiffened. Was his caller a *medical* researcher? Was his institute recognized or funded by any state or federal agency?

The man did not hesitate. Hadn't Sharrar heard what he said? Didn't he know that, when the Russian Sputnik orbited the far side of the moon, its crew had made contact with Venusians who passed on the secrets of OSS and BNS to them? And wasn't it lucky for America he and his institute, using a process even the CIA did not know about, had been able to electronically filch those secrets from deep within Mother Russia?

Sharrar groaned. Another nut had penetrated the defenses around 500 South Broad Street. Firmly but gently—even after five days of such nonsense, he had not lost his innate good manners—Sharrar freed himself from the call.

Coping with cranks, he reminded himself, was now part of the job. Harder to tolerate were those in authority who, for one reason or another, were starting to muddy the waters of what was already an opaque situation. Many of them seemed unable to appreciate, let alone understand, that the aim of epidemiologic investigation was *precise* re-creation. The process took time and clear thinking. Barring a breakthrough—always a real possibility—Sharrar knew the footslogging fieldwork of Fraser's "shoe-leather epidemiologists" would continue unabated.

Backing them up, scientists at the CDC laboratories were turning to more sophisticated procedures. Experiments with mice, guinea pigs, and even monkeys were being conducted in an attempt to detect any of a multitude of microbic agents.

Additionally, the possibility of poisoning was being actively pursued. But again, none of the voices beginning to criticize the conduct of the investigation appeared to have any understanding of the problems scientists faced in attempting to find a toxic agent.

For a start, there was the all-important incubation factor. The symptoms of legionnaires' disease, Sharrar believed, did not become evident until about three days after the original infection. And usually another three days passed before the patient sought medical aid. That meant almost a week had elapsed from the onset of illness before any samples were obtained for toxicological analysis. Specimens taken at autopsies were even older. Consequently there was every likelihood that, if a toxic substance was responsible, it would previously have been excreted or metabolized into a different form.

During Sharrar's phone conversation with Fraser—the two men were in frequent contact, exchanging ideas and information—he had discussed another problem. It was probable some of the samples obtained so far were, in a toxicologic sense, contaminated and unsuitable for scientific study. Though later some uninformed people would argue the contamination was due to incompetence, the truth was toxicological analysis required somewhat different postmortem procedures from the usual. A pathologist normally regarded a specimen as "clean" if it had been taken in an aseptic environment using sterile utensils. But "clean" to a toxicologist could mean the specimen had to be free of such contaminants as metals, chemicals, organic compounds, and, in

some cases, even plastic. It all depended on the test the toxicologist intended later to conduct. For instance, any pathologist cutting into tissue with a steel knife had very probably transferred microscopic slivers
of metal onto the samples; unless the samples taken were so large their
contaminated surfaces could be cut off in the labs, they were virtually
useless for certain metal poison tests. The same thing could have happened to tissue placed in stainless-steel bowls or on autopsy trays. Even
metal morgue tables could cause toxicological contamination. Sharrar
had himself been surprised to discover that the only sure way for
pathologists to work from now on was to use glass scalpels and bottles
previously washed with acid to remove any trace of metals. And the
bottle stoppers should be made of Teflon as a further precaution.

But even though now instructed to do so, how many of the state's
pathologists—renowned for their strong-willed independence—would
bother to follow such troublesome procedures?

And there was still another problem. It was emerging that, for some
toxicologic purposes, insufficient tissue had been removed from the
corpses.

The majority of the scientists at the CDC required only a minute
amount of tissue to prepare microscopic slides and run their tests; the
equivalent of a sliver of fingernail would usually satisfy the needs of a
virologist or bacteriologist. But a toxicologist often had to run many
more tests, and sometimes with large specimens, thus requiring samples
of greater size. Put at its simplest, the toxicologist could want specimens weighing several ounces, and also from different parts of the
body, including areas that did not normally concern his colleagues,
such as muscle and fatty tissue.

These specialist requirements, it now transpired, often had not been
fully catered for, because when the first autopsies were performed—
including those on Jimmy and J.B.—the possibility of toxicological testing had not yet arisen. Fraser, Sharrar knew, had recently issued instructions ordering all EIS officers attending postmortems to ensure the
new criteria were met.

Even so, with some 100,000 potentially toxic agents to choose from,
it might take years to weed out only the most likely suspects—and
years more to nail the one agent responsible.

Again, how to convey all this to newsmen driven by deadlines, and
to Legion officers whose fears Sharrar could understand and sympathize
with—but whose anger, when directed at the health department, he
found hard to accept?

Joseph Adams, commander of the American Legion in Pennsylvania,
was complaining that the means for notifying Philadelphia's health authorities of a problem were inadequate. Adams told friends that on the
previous Sunday night—the evening before the outbreak officially be-

came known—after hearing from Hoak about the first wave of sick and dead, he had "grabbed a phone book, looked up under 'Emergency,' found a number listed in the book, and I got the morgue. I talked to the man in the morgue. He said, 'You better call the switchboard and ask for the medical officer in charge for the weekend.' I called. I told the operator who I was and what had happened. She told me to hold on. The next one I got was a lady. She told me I would have to wait until nine o'clock in the morning. I could not tell anybody anything—the place was closed. I said to her, 'Do you realize what is happening?' She replied, 'You do not seem to realize we are not open'!"

Sharrar did not doubt the story was true. He simply wondered whether Adams had any idea how tight was the health department budget; it did not allow for a round-the-clock service at weekends. Yet Sharrar also knew Adams' complaint would have to be fully investigated, a time-consuming exercise that might provide some suitable sacrificial lamb from the local bureaucratic fold while achieving very little else—except to confirm again that without sufficient funds the department could not function properly.

As it was, much of Sharrar's time was spent dealing with requests from those occupying the rarefied heights of the Rizzo administration. And there were others, too, who tried to influence him one way or another to declare the end was in sight. Hoteliers such as Chadwick offered gentle persuasion, pointing to the drop in bookings already noticeable; airline executives claimed passengers were refusing to fly into the city; the Chamber of Commerce tried to preempt the issue, its president suggesting the legionnaires might have poisoned themselves through their own food or drink.

Gaudiosi, surprisingly, had hardly ever called. The city representative was much too busy talking to the media and offering Philadelphia's health commissioner the benefit of his advice. And Polk himself, some people thought, was beginning to show signs of becoming increasingly "twitchy." Sharrar did his best to placate his boss, regularly passing information up the health department ladder.

But nothing seemed able to satisfy some of the Legion hierarchy; it floated the idea that "a conflict of interest" had arisen between the Bachman and Polk administrations. In some ways, as Sharrar knew, there was nothing new in *that*; but at the epidemiological level, the relationship between Harrisburg and Philadelphia was good.

Yet the more he studied the inflow of data, the more was Sharrar convinced what he was seeing might be only the tip of an epidemiologic iceberg. He feared there could be many more cases in the city than the present methods of detection had identified.

It was a very possible hypothesis. And it was one that would soon disrupt the smooth working relationship between himself and Fraser.

Graitcer did not have to look. The tinny bump and grind music flooding through the sleazy back-street bar not far from the Bellevue was once more reaching its climax, signaling that another stripper was about to divest herself of the tassels attached to her nipples and pluck off her G-string just as the lights on the tiny stage momentarily blacked out.

The EIS officer had lost track of how long he had been sitting in the smoke-laden room while his companion, the hotel's air-conditioning repairman, repeatedly broke off what little conversation passed between them to watch one girl follow another across the stage, each vying with the next to be more suggestive.

Yet the repairman appeared a promising lead. His symptoms fitted the case criteria and he had been in the Bellevue for part of the crucial period.

With the help of Goldberger—who had assumed the responsibility for surveying the hotel employees—Graitcer had tracked down the repairman. He had adamantly refused to meet Graitcer at the hotel. Then he insisted he would be interviewed only if Graitcer bought him lunch. The repairman had chosen the strip bar as the venue.

The food was as tasteless as the parade of flesh that passed before their stageside table. After a few minutes, with a deafening screech the recorded music reached a crescendo and the lights flicked off.

"Can't we try and wrap this up?" pleaded Graitcer. "I've an autopsy to go to."

"Yeah?" The man squinted at him. "You get to some exciting places."

"Yes."

Graitcer peered at his note pad, aware the music had started again, the prelude to another girl in skimpy undergarments coming on stage.

"You were on and off work for nine days. You took your own temperature. It reached one-oh-two on several occasions. You had non-specific body aches and a cough. Right?"

"Yeah."

The music was building.

"Look. Your kids were ill. Same thing as you. Now your wife is sick."

"She's getting better."

"Good. But I'd like you to see a doctor and have some blood taken—"

"No."

The man turned toward the stage.

"It's only a pinprick—"

"No blood. I'm not having any blood taken. Period."

The music crashed into an overture. Onto the stage stepped a lithe black stripper.

The repairman was concentrating so hard he did not even notice Graitcer get up and leave, paying the tab on the way out, briefly wondering how he would itemize it on his expenses. By the time he reached the door he felt confident of one thing: from what he had gleaned, it was almost certain the repairman and his family had experienced only bad attacks of flu. Another lead had come to nothing.

The homicide detective was waiting in the unmarked police car, parked by the curb outside the club.

"Had a good time, Phil?" he growled pleasantly as Graitcer slid in beside him. "Those girls wind you up?" He winked slyly. "I could ask my friend in Vice to lay on something special—"

Graitcer sighed; he still wasn't quite used to the detective's heavy-handed humor. "The only thing I would like you to ask your friend is how to get in touch with any hookers who worked the Bellevue during the convention."

"Hey, Phil. You're really into this girlie thing, man. You wanna be careful."

"Okay, okay. Let's cut the comedy and head for the morgue."

"Anything you say, boss, suh." The policeman grinned, puffing on a new cigar and easing the car into the traffic.

Fifteen minutes later, Graitcer joined the pathologist and his assistants in the basement necropsy room of the mortuary to oversee the removal of specimens from a dead legionnaire. Everybody was masked and gowned and handled the body with unaccustomed caution. Within an hour the samples and fluids had been bottled and labeled. First they would go to the state laboratories to be apportioned, and then half would be flown to the CDC in Atlanta.

Graitcer was barely back in the car before the dispatcher at police headquarters was ordering them to drive immediately to the Pennsylvania Hospital and collect another batch of samples, which had been cleared to go directly to the CDC. A courier was already waiting at the Philadelphia airport to carry them on a Delta flight departing at five-thirty.

"How far's the hospital?" Graitcer looked at his watch. It was five o'clock.

"Quite a way."

"We'll never make it."

"Not in this car." The detective grabbed the handset and spoke to the dispatcher.

A minute later a wailing police siren drew closer. Weaving in and out of the traffic, a patrol car raced toward them, lights flashing.

"He'll get you there," shouted the detective, pushing Graitcer out of the car.

Graitcer leaped into the patrol car, which was moving even before he closed the door, its siren carving a path through the rush-hour traffic.

He looked at his watch: 5:04—twenty-six minutes until the plane took off.

The car careered through the streets, swerved to avoid a delivery truck, and roared on, traffic miraculously opening and closing around it.

Three minutes later it reached Pennsylvania Hospital, at the corner of Eighth and Spruce streets. Graitcer charged across the sidewalk and in through the main door. A doctor thrust a cardboard box into his hands, apologizing that there had been no time to pack the tray of test tubes in a proper container.

Running at full tilt, sidestepping startled onlookers, Graitcer returned to the car and tumbled into the front. The car accelerated so violently he was hurled back in his seat, his hands tightly clutching the box, his knees braced against the dashboard.

By the time the car had driven four blocks down Spruce and was crossing Twelfth Street, it was traveling at over sixty miles an hour.

At the intersection with Broad, Graitcer spotted policemen holding up the traffic. With a squeal of tires, the car turned right, heading up the wide thoroughfare.

"They're clearing our route," shouted the driver above the sound of the siren. "It's just like you're the President—or the Pope!"

Ahead, by the Bellevue, yet more policemen held back the traffic so they could turn west into Walnut.

Graitcer hardly gave the hotel a glance. He looked at the speedometer. It was climbing again, nearing the 80 mph mark as they continued their nerve-tingling dash through the center of the city. At every intersection police waved them through. He looked at his watch: 5:12 P.M. They were still in the downtown area.

"Call Delta," suggested Graitcer. "Tell them we're coming."

"They already know," yelled the driver. "Stop worrying! They won't have to hold the flight!"

"If you keep driving like this, we'll be in Atlanta before the plane!"

Graitcer sat tight. There was nothing he could do but pray he would survive this pell-mell race down the length of Walnut Street.

"Hold on!" The driver spun the wheel and barely shaved between two vans. He gunned the car across the junction with Twenty-third Street and roared across the Schuylkill River. With a screech of tires, the car turned south onto Interstate 76, heading toward the airport.

"Are we going to make it?" asked Graitcer, glancing again at his watch. It was 5:17 P.M.

The driver didn't reply. Traffic was bumper to bumper on the expressway. He forced his way into the middle of the lanes, driving down the dotted line, pushing cars off to either side.

"Oh hell," he shouted at Graitcer. "Now we have a real problem!"

Road construction work was going on ahead. Detours were in operation. There were tangles of traffic everywhere.

The driver grabbed the handset and began to talk swiftly. He turned and winked at Graitcer.

"Okay, we got help coming."

Thrusting his way through the traffic, using his siren almost like a physical tool, the driver reached the Penrose Avenue Bridge.

Waiting by the bridge were two blue Cherokee Jeeps of the airport police force.

They pulled out from the side, one positioning itself in front of the patrol car, the other behind. At the end of the bridge, the leading Jeep turned off onto an adjoining emergency road.

Traveling now in a three-car cavalcade of flashing lights and blaring sirens, Graitcer suddenly became aware of a personal problem. The dash to and from the hospital had affected his leg, still healing after his running mishap. It was beginning to throb painfully.

The airport came into sight. Graitcer thought: *I'll never make it through the terminal. Not with this leg. Not in time.*

The leading Jeep took them past the terminal entrance.

"Hey!" protested Graitcer.

"Relax," said his companion, grinning. "You're gonna make it."

Graitcer looked at his watch. It was 5:29 P.M. He stared despairingly out of the window. Away in the distance he could see the Delta plane.

Suddenly the lead Jeep seemed to be driving straight at the high wire fence surrounding the airport. Even as the procession approached, a policeman swung open a gate in the wire and they passed through at full speed.

Graitcer looked boggle-eyed at his companion. The three vehicles were now driving flat out down a taxiway.

A minute later they reached the plane. Graitcer eased himself from the car and walked stiffly toward it.

A side door to the jet was opened. The plane's captain stood waiting at the top of the steps. Graitcer handed him the box, telling him it was for the CDC courier sitting at the front of the first-class compartment. He turned and went back to the patrol car, its siren now stopped but its lights still flashing.

Only when he was again seated in the car, the policeman lighting a cigarette, did Graitcer realize he was trembling—and not only from excitement.

13

Coarctation

His normally benign face flushed with fury, William Chadwick glared at the spread on his desk of all the newspapers available in Philadelphia this Friday morning, August 6.

Watching Chadwick with compassion, his own anger expressed in the way he continued to pick up, scan derisively, and then discard one newspaper after another, Harold Varr thought: *The media has finally struck with a vengeance—it's even worse than I expected.*

All week he had prepared himself for the onslaught he feared must follow that outlandish incident when those two reporters burst into his office with their wild statements about the legionnaires being poisoned.

Day after day the media had skirmished with the Bellevue, "making hit-and-run forays, testing our defenses with their nasty little questions," as Chadwick saw it. At first nothing appeared in print to link the hotel with the outbreak; it seemed to Chadwick his appeal for local editors to act responsibly had paid dividends. Then references to the Bellevue's having been the convention headquarters began to appear. Gradually, sometimes edition by edition, the hotel had become increasingly featured in the developing story. Often it appeared to Varr that the Bellevue's name was dragged in needlessly, perhaps to provide glamour for a scenario that already contained all the other ingredients necessary for a major media event: mystery, tension, death—possibly murder—the sort of unfolding drama that sold newspapers.

Varr was also critical of the television coverage, regarding some of the network reporting as "highly irresponsible" in its suggestion that, for many, Philadelphia was now "a place to avoid." Although not imbued with the paranoia the outbreak was beginning to produce in others, he nevertheless wondered whether the networks, based in New York, were not subconsciously displaying "that city's desire to put down Philadelphia."

Late the previous afternoon—spurred by a statement that the hunt was "narrowing" to focus on the four hotels where the conventioneers had been housed—the reporters chose to converge on the Bellevue, virtually ignoring the three other establishments. They swamped the hotel's switchboard, swept through its public rooms, cornered its staff, and buttonholed its guests. There was no way Varr could stop them.

The brunt of their insistent questioning fell on him. Chadwick was refusing to talk to the media and was in any case spending much of his time at boardroom meetings with the Bellevue's owners, trying to decide what could be done.

It had been, remembered Varr, pandemonium. When he had tried to qualify a reply to a reporter, he was rudely told to be brief; when he attempted to provide background, he was asked whether he was making excuses. And when eventually he had finally protested, the journalists read him the City Hall statement by the deputy health commissioner, issued with the approval of Gaudiosi. Varr had now heard the statement so many times—even this morning it was still being read on the breakfast news shows—he felt he could repeat it word perfectly. Since no bacteria or virus had been isolated, the search for other agents had begun. Hotelkeepers would be questioned about air conditioning, ice-making machines, water purification systems, exterminators and pesticides, equipment breakdowns and repairs, new cleansers, and recently purchased eating and drinking utensils.

In vain had Varr pointed out that the Bellevue was only one of the hotels where the legionnaires had stayed, only one of a score of public places they visited. Shouldn't the reporters ask the same questions of employees at the Phillies' stadium? At the museums and art galleries? Or the restaurants, bars, and cafés the conventioneers frequented? Why pick on the Bellevue?

His questions were brushed aside.

Deeply shaken by the experience, Varr had finally retired to his suite and braced himself for what he sensed was coming. Now the display of newspapers on Chadwick's desk confirmed his worst fears: it seemed to him the hotel was being inextricably associated with the outbreak.

An eye-catching headline in the New York *Daily News* stated: FEAR SIGNS THE REGISTER. Perhaps, mused Varr, it was prompted by an earlier banner in Philadelphia's *Daily News*: A GUEST NAMED FEAR CHECKS INTO THE BELLEVUE.

Varr turned to the local paper and began to read tonelessly: *The four bellhops talking in hushed tones in the lobby of the Bellevue Stratford Hotel yesterday afternoon didn't think "it" was over.*

Who, demanded Chadwick, had given staff permission to talk to the press?

The reporter, said Varr, had likely either eavesdropped on the bellhops' conversation or obtained the information by posing as a guest. He continued to read: *The lobby of the Bellevue Stratford is usually a clearing house for the political gossip in this town. The chatter is usually about City Hall, the ward leaders, the judges and the deals. Yesterday's discussions were much more grim.*

Varr paused. Did Chadwick want to hear more?

The managing director slumped in his chair, nodding.

Varr read out the damning phrases describing mysterious illness and death and the frightened attitudes of staff. Woven into the text were observations about business being affected, the Hunt Room and Stratford Garden restaurants at lunchtime "only 60 percent filled."

Chadwick took the newspaper from Varr, scanning the story, his lips working soundlessly, his eyes unable to believe what he read. When he spotted his name his fury exploded. Because he had refused to speak to the *News* he was now being pilloried in print for his silence. He ran his hands through his hair. And what if some nosy reporter learned what Mallison was doing?

Varr smiled briefly. There was no need to worry. Mallison had said the last thing he wanted was publicity.

Another worrying thought surfaced in Chadwick: just suppose Mallison found something wrong, some minor defect. It might have no bearing on the cause of the outbreak. But if it got out, that could be enough. Then it would be no good saying all the finest hotels in the world sometimes developed small running faults.

Like the main air-conditioning cooling unit, ventured Varr. It was still leaking. The chief engineer had told him he would have to add about 200 pounds of replacement refrigerant this very day.

But, countered Chadwick, they both knew there was almost no real risk involved. The Carrier Corporation—which serviced the unit—had made it quite clear that the hotel's decision to run the faulty machine through the hot summer months in preference to stopping it for repairs, while not exactly desirable, was safe. The company, continued Chadwick, understood very well the need to provide full air-conditioned comfort for guests while taking what they all agreed was a risk so minimal it could be discounted. Anyway, most air-conditioning units leaked vapor a little—even those used in automobiles, and no one complained about them. Adding refrigerant today could not possibly mean there was an increased hazard to health. Yet, concluded Chadwick, to a re-

porter the leak might appear dangerous and even provide the basis for
a sensational story.

That was the trouble with reporters, concurred Varr, they jumped in
without knowing all the facts.

Together the two men continued to read the newspaper reports carefully. Chadwick grew increasingly gloomy: the damage had been done
and things could only deteriorate.

His newfound pessimism worried Varr. He feared it might influence
the staff and have a scarring effect on Chadwick himself. Consequently
he tried to extract from the reports what little comfort was available.
He pointed out that none of the stories stated any of the victims were
taken ill or died as a result of staying in the hotel.

The implication was there, insisted Chadwick, and in many ways
that made it worse. People would read what they liked into the stories.
It was bound to have an adverse effect on business. In the long term
the results could be disastrous. Left unsaid, but clearly understood by
them both, was that well before then the future of the hotel might be
put in the balance. Even without the outbreak, Chadwick could not be
altogether certain the Bellevue's owners entirely shared his belief that,
within six months, the hotel could be well along the path returning it
to its old glory. Until now they had been prepared to back him. But in
these circumstances, how long could he expect them to continue? The
epidemic and its attendant publicity could not have come at a worse
moment. It was not beyond the bounds of possibility, repeated Chadwick, that the media could make or break the hotel.

Varr looked at his superior sympathetically. Was the strain beginning to be too much? Chadwick, like Varr, had been working eighteen-
hour days since Monday. And each man knew the newspapers were
right in one respect: already trade *was* down, bookings *were* being canceled, guests at the Eucharistic Congress *were* trying to check out of
the Bellevue and into other hotels.

This oblique criticism of the Bellevue, Varr knew, Chadwick took as
a direct personal attack on himself. For him, the hotel and he were
one. The Bellevue was his life. He had hoped the media would leave it
alone. That hope was now dead. It was a devastating blow to an intensely proud man.

If anything, Varr was a pragmatist. By the time he had finished reading the reports, he saw it as inevitable—given the hotel's place in Philadelphia society and its reputation around the nation—that the press
would continue to zero in on the Bellevue. And the extent of the coverage showed the epidemic was already considered one of the major
American media events since Pearl Harbor; indeed, the press had
alluded to the irony that some of the legionnaires had survived World

War II only to be stricken down in the very cradle of the freedom they had fought to preserve.

Continuing in his attempt to extract what little cheer there was, Varr pointed out that the New York *Times* had given prominence to the belief the outbreak was "slowing down." Indeed, it must be over, said Varr, for President Ford had stated he would be coming to the city on Sunday to attend the closing ceremony of the Eucharistic Congress. He certainly wouldn't do that if his life were endangered.

Chadwick brightened. Maybe the President would say something to help the situation?

Varr privately doubted Ford would want to become involved in further medical controversy. He was still drawing intense fire over the swine flu vaccination program. Some commentators were beginning to wonder—given that Ford had successfully beaten Reagan for the Republican nomination—whether the issue would not seriously damage his chances of reelection in November. As it was, Jimmy Carter was shaping up as a serious threat. One of the key moments in their campaigns was planned to take place in Philadelphia, where both candidates would come together in a few weeks to debate their policies on network television.

It could, mused Varr, be the perfect antidote to all this wretched publicity if both the President and his challenger stayed at the Bellevue.

Chadwick beamed: that was a very fine idea. He would try and set it in motion. He reached for the telephone to call first the White House and then Governor Carter's campaign manager.

Quietly, Varr began to gather up the newspapers.

Riding upward in one of the hotel elevators, George Mallison appeared to be concentrating hard on the paper he had bought from the newsstand in the lobby. The *Inquirer* could tell him little about the outbreak he didn't already know, but he hoped reading it would effectively discourage questions from any of the staff who were becoming curious about his continual presence in the hotel.

Mallison could have reassured them on one thing. Following his visit with Chadwick and Varr to Castelli's kitchen, he had returned and after careful examination come to the conclusion that there was no evidence to suggest it was in any way related to the epidemic. Mallison only wished he could be as confident about the hotel's cooling and ventilation systems.

He had examined the two Carrier refrigeration machines that chilled the water for the air-conditioning system and noticed the leakage of the R-11 refrigerant. Like Chadwick, Mallison saw no need to inform the press of the problem. He knew R-11 was a very stable compound and, in normal operating conditions, nontoxic. But under other, very specific, conditions it could decompose, causing symptoms very similar to those the legionnaires displayed. But for that to happen, the R-11 would need to be subjected to very intense heat in a pyrolytic, oxygen-free environment, the sort found at the tip of a burning cigarette. Yet people smoked in cars whose air-conditioning units were leaking and there were few, if any, reported cases of their becoming sick or dying as a result. And how could the vapor have reached the hotel's public areas in the first place? Air from the engine room was vented directly into the street. If it then somehow found its way back into the hotel, and then somehow become pyrolyzed, how could it have been so selective, afflicting only legionnaires and their guests? Some of them had not even entered the hotel. The chiller unit was still leaking. Why was it not continuing to cause people to become ill?

Mallison shook his head. It didn't add up. He was willing to place his reputation against the leaking refrigerant's being the cause.

Yet it was possible the disease-carrying agent—whatever it was—had been distributed by the hotel's ventilation system. That was why he had been methodically collecting the first of hundreds of samples of dust, water, air, ice—*anything* he thought would interest the biologists and toxicologists in Atlanta. In some ways he was like a human vacuum cleaner, sucking up the droppings of life. It was never easy for him to explain what he did; that was another reason for avoiding the press. And from what he had glimpsed during his frequent elevator trips, the perky little operator now taking him to the eighteenth floor was also no great lover of the media. She had been on the point of boiling over the previous evening when the press armada swept into the lobby.

Anna Taggart continued to glance speculatively at her solitary passenger. At this time of the morning, the up elevators were almost always empty, the flow of passengers downward to the lobby. She *knew* he wasn't reading the newspaper, just hiding behind it. And despite his conventional dress and bulky briefcase, which made him look like a middle-aged executive heading for a sales meeting in one of the hotel's conference rooms, he had not fooled her. She had caught him out several times yesterday: once, on the tenth floor, when she'd opened her cage he was kneeling by the elevator door carefully sweeping dust into a plastic envelope, which he put with the others she glimpsed in his case. He had smiled sheepishly and walked off down the corridor. Next a maid, a friend of Anna's, told her she saw the tall, gangling stranger in a storeroom transferring rug shampoo into a small bottle. Later Anna spotted him again, this time on the fifteenth floor, holding a little glass vial under a leaking ice-making machine.

It was those envelopes and vials which gave him away. Anna had seen homicide detectives use them on the late-night movies when they were collecting evidence to nail a killer. She badly wanted to ask him what progress he was making. But the way he pretended to be reading the newspaper as well as his forbidding manner stopped her. And she was sure he was no local policeman. She could recognize them all. Besides, during a brief conversation she overheard him having with Varr, he had said the "agency" now had hundreds of its people involved in the hunt. Anna didn't have any difficulty in interpreting "agency" to mean either the FBI or the CIA.

Mallison got out on the eighteenth floor. In many ways it was one of the most elegant parts of the hotel with its Rose Garden, Oak Room, and smaller reception rooms. At this time of the morning the area was deserted. Mallison was glad. He didn't want to draw undue attention to himself or where he was going. He climbed a flight of service stairs to the floor above and entered the hotel's cavernous loft. He put on his coveralls. There was barely enough light for him to see, to continue his painstaking study of the air-conditioning system, identifying each of the pipes that carried water to and from the refrigeration units in the subbasement through a maze of pumps, feed tanks, converters, and safety valves. Using a flashlight, he located the pipe leading from the huge water tower on the roof. He traced the route of other pipes located in the loft and eventually reached the area around the two tanks that provided the hotel's drinking water. All seemed in order. He continued, climbing up to inspect the nearby chilled-water expansion tank. In the beam of his flashlight he immediately spotted a faulty float. It meant the tank was not being automatically refilled and consequently was not feeding chilled water into the system. He climbed down and picked his way forward. Then he saw it, a hosepipe connected at one end to the water supply from the tower on the roof and at the other to a pipe leading to the air-conditioner unit serving the Rose Garden. This makeshift arrangement overcame the problem of the faulty float in the expansion tank. But if the valves at both ends of the hose were left open or leaked and various check valves malfunctioned, it was conceivable that roof tower water could be fed into the drinking water tanks. And the water from the tower had been treated with powerful corrosion-controlling chemicals.

It was clearly a highly undesirable, possibly even dangerous, situation. Could it, in fact, be the cause of the outbreak? The potential cross-connection between the hotel's drinking water and that from the tower, which was suitable only for the air-conditioning system, was undoubtedly illegal. But Mallison presumed that since the potable water system was probably under higher pressure than the chemically treated water, it was unlikely there had been any appreciable contamination. Still, it made his collection of water samples all that more important. And he would be obliged to let officials of the city water department know of the potential cross-connection he had found. They would doubtless wish to make further investigations.

He climbed more steps and out on the roof. The first thing that caught his eye was the pigeons. They and their droppings were everywhere, including on the huge water tower.

"Oh boy," he said to himself. "Now, this is interesting."

Back in Atlanta, before he became involved in the outbreak, the forty-eight-year-old chief environmental engineer of the CDC already suspected pigeons. He thought the legionnaires' flu-like symptoms were very similar to those of histoplasmosis and psittacosis, two respiratory diseases spread by sick birds. Over the years Mallison had become something of an authority on psittacosis. He knew if it was acquired from some birds, including turkeys, it was generally more severe than when contracted from ducks, chickens, pheasants, or pigeons. Even so, psittacosis derived from pigeons could be fatal.

Everything about the outbreak suggested psittacosis: the way the mysterious disease had seemingly traveled via the respiratory route, rapidly entered the bloodstream, and produced a systemic disease involving the lungs. Even the incubation period—seven to fifteen days—appeared to fit. So, too, did the insidious onset of the illness, the chills that suddenly swept to a full-raging fever, the headaches.

Standing on the roof, wrinkling his nose against the faint but unmistakable smell from the large colony of cooing pigeons, Mallison could clearly remember how, five years ago, he was called in on an outbreak involving several hundred schoolchildren in Ohio who had become sick soon after Earth Day, the day dedicated to promoting the need for a clean environment. The children had developed severe flu-like symptoms. From the outset Mallison had suspected they might have histoplasmosis, but he could not understand how the disease could have spread so quickly in so many children. Then, after several days of patient investigation, he discovered the outbreak was linked to the children's Earth Day activities. As part of the observance, some of the pupils had helped clean their school yard, kicking up clouds of dust that contained the droppings and feathers of diseased birds. The dust was sucked into the school's air-conditioning unit and spread through the classrooms. Mallison had demonstrated how this was done by setting off a smoke bomb in the yard. Its fumes were drawn into the air-conditioning unit and carried to the classrooms.

Looking at the pigeons roosting on the roof, he could not help but wonder whether something very similar had happened here. He peered over the hotel's parapet, looking down nineteen floors. There were pigeons perched on the windowsills of guests' bedrooms and a huge number picking at refuse in a nearby street. He turned again to the roof tower. Apart from the probability of droppings being sucked into and spread by the hotel's air-conditioning system, there was also the distinct possibility that sick pigeons had fouled the water in the tower. If they had, and if that water had been transferred into the hotel's drinking water supply through the hosepipe he had just seen, the way would be open for the legionnaires to have been infected by two separate, and complementary, routes.

George Mallison decided that, in a surprisingly short time, he had found a most promising lead.

As in everything he did, David Fraser took trouble to prepare himself before he began to write. He knew this questionnaire was critical.

He had moved into one of the "think tanks," the name Jim Beecham gave to the small rooms just off the main conference room and War Room, and positioned the desk so he was clearly visible to anyone passing the door, which he left open as a further reminder that, although he did not wish to be disturbed, he was instantly available to deal with any sudden development. Fraser did not expect one today. Indeed, his "good outbreak" looked likely to continue for some time. When he had left Atlanta with only a few dollars in his pocket and clothes for a few days, he had confidently told Barbara he expected to be home by the end of the week. Early this morning he had telephoned to say it could be weeks before he returned. The case, he confided, was the toughest he had tackled. Barbara had murmured sympathetically. She could hear the tension in his voice. She told him how the children were missing him and had become used to his appearances on TV and in the papers. Fraser made his wife laugh when he described how he was washing his own underwear in the bathroom washbasin.

He didn't tell her he was managing on only about four hours' sleep a night while directing one of the biggest epidemiologic field forces ever assembled, that many of its members were sometimes fractious and often needed the firmest of handling, that when dealing with them he had not always been successful in containing his anger, that he had undoubtedly bruised egos and would continue to do so, that the relentless pressure he personally was under, arising from the sheer size and diversity of the investigation, made him at times feel ready to pull out his shaggy mop of hair by the roots. Above all, he did not tell her he was desperately tired but would continue to drive himself until he dropped.

Barbara intuitively understood her husband's unsaid thoughts. She knew her man. It was rest, not sympathy, he needed. She told him as much before they ended their call.

Now, deliberately pushing any thoughts of home from his mind, Fraser concentrated on the crucial questionnaire he had decided must be prepared and sent to the 1,002 Legion posts in Pennsylvania. The

Legion, with the help of state police patrol cars and even helicopters, would distribute and return the completed forms to him. Fraser had taken soundings from many of those working on the outbreak on what questions should be asked. He had yet to incorporate their suggestions with his own into a sensible framework, properly presented.

For a time he sat at the desk, silently reviewing all he knew about the Legion. In his mind he had formed a basic composite of a legionnaire: blue-collar, plain-speaking, God-fearing, with clear-cut values and views free of any intellectual frills or fancies—always allied to an abiding belief in military power. With his Quaker background and sincere belief in pacifism, Fraser had expected to have little in common with the veterans. But in his contacts with them he had come to admire the way they had coped with a tragedy that could well have caused lesser organizations to collapse. The Legion remained steadfast and entirely cooperative. Its members, he decided, would want questions put in plain, unvarnished words, rather like a military order. Fraser was used to framing inquiries that way.

He settled in his chair and began to write the questions in his sloping left-handed script. First he requested brief biographical details. Then he moved to the meat of the questionnaire, asking each recipient to place a check mark beside the hotel he had stayed in: *Bellevue Stratford; Holiday Inn—Midtown; Ben Franklin; Holiday Inn—Penn Center; Sheraton.*

Fraser reflected. He was not sure legionnaires had stayed in each of those hotels, nor whether some of them might have stayed elsewhere. He added to the list to be checked: *Home; Other—Specify.*

He paused briefly, then wrote a simple question designed to ascertain which days were spent in Philadelphia by each conventioneer. Next he decided to ask two questions to find out how many hours on each of those days each recipient had spent specifically at first the Bellevue Stratford, then the Ben Franklin. Whatever Fraser's private opinion, he had as yet no convincing data—let alone proof—that either hotel was implicated. Those two key questions would help clarify his thoughts. Fraser stood up, stretched, and strolled out to the War Room.

It was, as usual, a hive of activity. All his EIS officers were back from their stint in the field. Although he himself badly wanted to see patients, he wasn't at all sure how much useful information was gleaned in that way. Nevertheless, it was reassuring for him to have physicians close by who had recently dealt directly with the sick. And he was pleased by reports of how they had conducted themselves. Thacker and Tsai, in particular, had worked under trying conditions: Thacker coping well with the media—despite having allowed himself to be photographed sitting on a patient's bed, which led to much ribbing from his friends—and Tsai tactfully overcoming the one or two difficult moments when he had been insensitively asked about his ancestry. Fraser could see both doctors were continuing to work hard, chasing leads by telephone and adding to the line list.

Parkin, too, was proving a magnificent support, cutting his way through the local bureaucracy, getting results with a mixture of firmness and joshing. He seemed to know everybody. That might be an invaluable asset, mused Fraser, when his Legion census was being circulated.

Sipping a coffee, he returned to his office and began again to write steadily, framing each question with care, making sure that whenever possible the answer would be a clear yes or no. This would greatly facilitate the computer analysis of replies, which was to be done in Atlanta.

He reached the point in the census where he wished to deal with what each conventioneer had eaten and drunk. He devised a series of interlinked questions: *Did you drink coffee at the Friday morning "Go-Getter's" breakfast? Did you eat pastry at this breakfast? Did you use ice in soft drinks? Did you use ice in mixed drinks? Did you buy ice from outside the hotel? Did you buy block ice? Did you buy ice cubes? From which store did you buy ice? Did you get a free beer mug at the Friday morning meeting? Did you drink anything from the free beer mug?*

Fraser paused to review what he had written. There was another matter that had yet to be raised. He was beginning to believe the disease-causing agent was airborne-transmitted. Apart from through the air-conditioning—and he knew Mallison was checking on that—there were a number of ways it might have been spread. Although the thought was still far from complete, he was coming to wonder whether the agent had been carried through the hotel by that most mobile of all its services, Anna Taggart's elevators.

To test the validity of the hypothesis, Fraser framed a question: *On Friday the 23rd how often did you ride the main elevators (front door) in the Bellevue Stratford?*

He repeated the question to cover the elevators at the hotel's Walnut Street entrance, allowing in each case for four possible answers: *Did not ride; 1–5 times; more than five times; don't remember.*

Fraser's final question was open-ended: *Describe anything unusual which you think may be related to the illness.* He hoped the responses he received might clarify some of the rumors flying around the state about "subversives," poisons, and other hellish possibilities.

His CDC superiors, he knew, were now having urgent and highly confidential discussions with the Defense Department and FBI about chemical-biological warfare. Both the Bureau and the Army were remaining as tight-lipped as ever, but it was emerging that the CIA had the capability of making deliberate death look like the result of natural causes—using one of a long list of chemically created toxic agents that could mimic perfectly the deadly diseases of nature. Such toxic agents, as Fraser well realized, were not the poisonous products of bacteria but chemical substitutes. While they could make people sick or dead, they could not reproduce themselves. Was that why the laboratory tests to isolate the disease-causing agent had so far failed—because it was no longer there to be found? Fraser didn't know. But the news filtering through from Atlanta was chilling. A couple of decades ago scientists working on CBW had, for instance, perfected aerosols filled with anthrax, a potentially fatal disease that closely resembled pneumonia in its presenting symptoms. Officially, all these deadly discoveries were said to have been removed from harm's way. Yet who could say for certain that the enormous search for weapons from drugs had really come to an end?

Fraser preferred not to think further about the subject. As he began to check through the twenty-three headings on his two-page questionnaire, Parkin appeared at his door.

"Walt Orenstein's on the line. Says it's important."

Fraser knew Orenstein would never interrupt him unless it was urgent. In his view the third-year EIS officer was "a very bright, very capable guy." That was one reason he was acting as Fraser's deputy in Philadelphia. He reached for the phone.

"Dave. Can we talk?" asked Orenstein cautiously.

"Hold on." Fraser closed the door of his office. "Okay, shoot."

"There are serious problems down here."

"What sort of problems?"

"Attitude problems. Work problems. All kinds of problems."

"Like what? Like who?"

"Graitcer, for a start. He's been reporting directly to swine flu surveillance in Atlanta."

"Nothing wrong with that until we ruled out swine flu. But it's got to stop now."

"I'm rooming with Goldberger," continued Orenstein. "I can tell you he's not happy either. Nor is Sharrar."

"Sharrar?" Fraser could not hide his surprise. "Surely you're not having trouble with him. Sharrar's a savvy epidemiologist."

"Sharrar's not the problem. It's the question of who's in charge here. You're a hundred miles away. Everyone's getting into the act. Sharrar's got ideas, his bosses have ideas, Goldberger and Graitcer and the other guys have ideas, you've got ideas. I try to push yours, but it doesn't always work."

"It's mine that matter," said Fraser flatly. He paused. "Walt, I'm going to come to Philadelphia. I'll be there tomorrow. Have everybody ready."

Fraser put down the phone. He was angry. Not at individuals but at the bureaucratic muddle that had led to this mess. Until the time came he would think no more about it. He switched his mind back to Harrisburg and the activities surrounding him.

For the rest of the day, fueled by coffee and sandwiches, Fraser continued to study and supervise the collation of the extensive line history of clinical and epidemiological information on some one hundred and fifty cases. It was, in many ways, the most rewarding part of his work. All the data so far collected suggested that the majority of victims were legionnaires who had attended the convention and visited the Bellevue Stratford. The questionnaire would help to confirm whether or not that was true.

It also appeared likely a typical illness began six days after arrival at the convention. As well as chills and nonproductive coughs, there were often abdominal pains. By the time the typical patient saw a physician, his fever was usually between 102 and 105 degrees. Apart from pneumonia in the lungs, there was usually little else obviously wrong—although many victims seemed to have been previously physically debilitated for some reason.

That broad clinical picture was being analyzed and added to by Fraser's team in the War Room.

One member was establishing the median age of hospitalized patients; they seemed to be significantly older than those being treated at home. Again, the fatality rate was highest among the hospitalized, of whom almost one person in five died. That evidence suggested the elderly were at considerably greater risk from the disease than the young.

Others of Fraser's doctors were comparing the medical records of patients to try to establish which signs and symptoms were common to all. In most cases their blood showed a slight increase in the white cell count; there was moderate hypoxemia—a lack of oxygen in the arteries —and also hypocapnia, indicating a diminished carbon dioxide content. Just before death, the majority of victims displayed a rapid increase in the pulse and respiratory rate.

X rays of patients were now being studied at the CDC and the results forwarded to Fraser. He was not altogether surprised to learn that nine out of ten showed abnormalities, but he guessed it would be a long time before the radiographs could be fully evaluated. Even to the center's skilled radiologists they were already puzzling. In those so far received, while pneumonia could be seen in both lungs, it was not evenly distributed—it seemed at first to concentrate in small patches and only later disperse through the structure of the lungs.

Fraser thought the findings fitted a rapidly progressing interstitial pneumonia. But what caused it? And equally important, what was the best way to treat patients?

In pursuit of an answer to that question, another of his epidemiologists had began the laborious analytical task of evaluating the relative efficacy of the wide variety of drugs that doctors were using. Reportedly over twenty different antibiotics and four species of steroids were presently being prescribed—administered in varying dosages, through various routes, and even in differing combinations. As yet the officer's calculations did not clearly indicate which should be the preferred choice for treatment.

Seated at a separate desk, a statistician was charting the demographic characteristics of the outbreak, listing the afflicted by age and sex, noting whether they were official delegates to the convention, members of legionnaires' families, or members of the Women's Auxiliary. The information necessary to finalize the study was far from complete. Even the total number of legionnaires who had been to Philadelphia was unknown. Estimates ranged from 2,274—the number of delegates who had cast votes at the convention—to 10,000.

Fraser hoped his questionnaire would provide a more accurate figure. When it was distributed over the weekend, each Legion commander would be asked to ensure a copy was given to everyone connected with his post who had gone to the city.

All through Friday afternoon and late into the evening, the flow of incoming telephone calls continued. They brought information for adding to the line list, supplementary data for the many individual projects being pursued, and frequently news of further possible cases. Those whose description passed the screening case definition were added to the line list, instantly initiating yet more inquiries and analysis.

Toward midnight the pace in the War Room slackened, and the EIS officers and other staff gradually departed. Around one o'clock Fraser and Thacker drove to the hotel where they shared a room.

Thacker was too tired even to think of calling his girl friend. He was asleep the moment he fell into bed.

Fraser, as usual, telephoned his superior at about 2 A.M. to deliver an update. He found nothing unusual in the nocturnal timing of this regular call. He mentioned he was going to Philadelphia in the morning but did not say precisely what he intended to do.

Soon afterward, at the end of another nineteen-hour working day, he fell asleep thinking about how the disease-carrying agent might have traveled.

Sometime later a startled Thacker was roused by Fraser's shouting and sitting bolt upright in bed.

"That's it! That *must* be it!"

"David, you okay?" asked Thacker, switching on the bedside light and looking anxiously at Fraser.

"Never felt better." Fraser grinned. "Steve, it's the elevators. It has to be!"

He jumped out of bed and began to pace up and down, barely able to contain himself.

"I think, Steve, I've solved it. The way the agent spreads. It's by the column of air that's displaced every time an elevator goes up and down the shaft."

"What elevator?"

"The ones at the Bellevue Stratford. Look. We're pretty sure this outbreak has a common source. Let's assume that source is somewhere in the Bellevue. We haven't found one particular room or anywhere in the hotel where every single victim went. And that's the point. Everybody goes in elevators and nobody thinks about it! Now do you see?"

Thacker pushed back the bedclothes, rubbing his eyes, banishing the last vestige of sleep.

"David, you could be right! Everything suggests the agent's airborne. Elevators work like pistons, pushing air up and sucking it down." Thacker frowned. "But how did it get into the shafts in the first place?"

"There's a little air-conditioner unit on top of elevators. Maybe they're leaking refrigerant. Or say something toxic was put there. The gas could be getting into the elevators themselves—"

"And then let out through the elevator doors when they stop at each floor."

Fraser finished: "That's why only guests seem to have been hit. There haven't been any deaths reported in the staff. And you don't find staff using guest elevators."

Thacker raised an objection. "But what about the operators? And the elevators that room service waiters use?"

"Yeah." Fraser continued to pace, thinking hard. "Maybe, for some reason we don't know, they've built up a resistance. Or maybe staff elevators don't have air-conditioning units."

They continued to discuss the matter for over an hour. The more they talked the more convinced both became. When they again fell asleep, each was sure a solution had been found to one of the most important questions associated with the epidemic.

Around seven o'clock, Fraser got up, shaved, showered, and dressed in his green suit to travel to Philadelphia.

First, though, he had to make an important telephone call to one of his peers, the director of the Influenza Surveillance Center in Atlanta. When the epidemic was thought to be swine flu, it was the surveillance director who had chosen Graitcer and Craven to send into the field.

Through them he had maintained a continuing involvement in Fraser's investigation, even dispatching a computer terminal and statistician to Philadelphia. Fraser felt the time had come to end what he saw as meddling.

He decided to telephone from one of the think tank offices. Fraser didn't want to embarrass his colleague by being overheard; it would be easy for what he was about to say to be seized upon by one of the local health department workers.

The lines to the CDC were constantly engaged. Even this early in the morning the agency was receiving 3,300 calls hourly from all over the country. So heavy was the traffic that director David Sencer was among those manning the phones.

After several attempts Fraser eventually got through to the surveillance director.

"How's it going, Dave?" the man asked pleasantly. "I'm reading and seeing a lot about you all on TV—"

"Look, I want you to stay off my turf. We both know this has nothing to do with swine flu anymore. So it has nothing to do with you. And I didn't request that computer terminal you've sent to Philadelphia."

"But Graitcer and Craven are trained in remote information processing—"

"I don't want a computer terminal. More to the point, I don't want you and your unit in Atlanta analyzing my data. I'll arrange for that myself."

"We could be helpful. We're used to computers in my outfit—"

"So are we in Special Pathogens. I don't want you doing any more work on this thing. Don't interfere."

Fraser put down the telephone.

Bachman was waiting when he came out of the office.

"I hear you're going to Philadelphia?" he asked quizzically.

"Right."

"Gonna ride shotgun?"

"Maybe."

Bachman grinned. "You've got my support to shake the whole city apart to solve this thing."

Fraser nodded noncommittally. He wasn't going to be drawn into the war of words flying between Philadelphia and Harrisburg; nothing would make him go to the ramparts for either the health secretary or Gaudiosi, who had begun to stalk each other through the media.

Equally, in the relatively short time they had known each other, Fraser had come to like and respect Bachman. He was true to his word, hadn't meddled, but was always on hand to offer support. Fraser had yet to make contact with Gaudiosi. From what he had heard, the city representative was as tough as Bachman and could be even trickier.

"How long you gonna be away?"

"Most of the day. Parkin will oversee things while I'm gone."

"I'm not worried about Parkin. I'm worried about you," said Bachman, his voice softening. "You're tired. You're running yourself hard. I don't want you to drive—"

"I'm okay—"

"I'll give you my car and chauffeur. You can sleep on the way down. He knows the city. He can take you wherever you want to go."

Fraser smiled, grateful for the offer. Bachman could be full of surprises.

During the journey, Fraser was too wound up to sleep. His mind constantly moved back and forth between the serious staff situation Orenstein had outlined and the possibility that the elevators in the Bellevue Stratford were involved.

Seated in the air-conditioned comfort of Bachman's limousine, he reviewed some of the factors which led to that belief. Although it was now certain the illness was not confined to people who had been to the Legion convention, it did appear that all the victims, for one reason or another, had been in the Bellevue. And there was some evidence—so far based largely on the data the EIS officers gleaned during their forays through the state—that legionnaires who had stayed overnight at the Bellevue had more often become ill than those who stayed elsewhere. Further, among the latter, it seemed those who became ill had spent more time at the hotel than those who remained well. Fraser hoped his latest questionnaire would clarify whether these apparent trends were true. He also believed it likely the census would rule out the most obvious suspect—food and drink. That left the likelihood the disease was spread through the air, quite conceivably by the elevators.

He put the thought from his mind when he walked into 500 South Broad Street and entered Sharrar's second-floor office.

Orenstein was waiting with the city epidemiologist. Fraser thought both men looked tired, especially Sharrar, who also seemed tense and apprehensive. Fraser felt a twinge of sympathy, remembering that behind his shy and diffident manner Sharrar was an intensely proud man. He normally possessed a great deal of autonomy; in the past, even Polk seldom interfered. Now Sharrar was hearing from Philadelphia's health commissioner almost every hour. And Fraser guessed his own presence must inevitably threaten Sharrar's independence. He would go carefully. The last thing he wished was to upset a man he admired professionally and liked as a person.

"Where do you want to start?" asked Sharrar.

Fraser smiled. "It's your territory, Bob. Why don't you just lead me over it?"

It didn't take Fraser long to realize Sharrar was viewing the epidemic from nearly the opposite perspective to his. One of the main thrusts of Sharrar's investigation was to try to establish whether the outbreak was only the tip of an even larger epidemic. Sharrar feared that even now the disease might be surreptitiously sweeping through the city without anyone knowing; its victims might believe they had pneumonia and flu, their physicians might be trying to treat them for such ailments while not recognizing the symptoms for what they were—the manifestation of a disease that could be spreading inexorably. To determine whether this was so, a great deal of effort had gone into collecting the names of everyone who had a fever or a cough, not just those who had some loose connection with the Legion convention. Sharrar reasoned that if the city was in the grip of an unrecognized epidemic, then hospitals in the area would be treating more cases of pneumonia-like illness than usual. Consequently he had assigned six physicians to visit three major local hospitals and plow through the scribbled medical records of everyone treated in the emergency rooms from July 1 onward.

"It's a big job, David, reviewing that many medical records. Even the writing is often hard to read." Sharrar spread his hands. "You know how it is. Those doctors are always in a hurry. And the amount of medical information they place on file varies enormously."

"What have you found out so far?"

Sharrar showed him the epidemiologic graph that plotted the daily number of respiratory disease cases since July 1. If there was an epidemic it would show as a jump in the line, probably in the immediate aftermath of the Legion convention.

There was no jump. The curve remained essentially even.

But Sharrar had not abandoned this line of inquiry. He meant to order a check on the other hospitals in the metropolitan area.

"Sixty hospitals will tie up a lot of manpower," said Fraser mildly. "I'd rather my people didn't pursue that."

"We've already analyzed the death certificates of everyone who's died in the city since July," reported Sharrar, "comparing the number of flu and pneumonia deaths with figures for the last couple of years."

"And?"

"Nothing significant yet. But it has to be done," concluded Sharrar.

There was silence in the room.

"Bob, I don't think you're going to find your hidden epidemic," said Fraser at last. "I think we should only be looking for cases that fit our case criteria."

He turned to Orenstein. "What about the EIS officers? What are they working on?"

"Goldberger's started to survey some of the Bellevue Stratford employees."

"Only some? Is he checking the lobby personnel?"

"It's a random sample," explained Orenstein.

Sharrar continued. The intention of the Bellevue survey was to establish whether any of the employees were ill, and particularly whether they showed symptoms similar to those of the stricken legionnaires. It would also be interesting to know whether the disease had attacked other guests at the same time. They were now dispersed throughout the country. It was difficult to trace them.

Fraser nodded sympathetically. "I know. But what we have to do is try and make this a concerted effort. Otherwise there's a real danger of fragmentation." He looked carefully at Sharrar. "Maybe it's a problem of organization. I'm up in Harrisburg. You're down here. . . ."

"We can talk on the telephone."

There was another silence.

"What's Graitcer doing?" Fraser asked Orenstein.

"He's busy. Never stops. Has lots of ideas. Some good."

"*Every* idea we pursue has got to be good. I don't want epidemiologists running all over the place chasing their tails." He turned to Sharrar. "How have they worked for you?"

"Okay. They're very enthusiastic."

Fraser paused, then made up his mind. There was, after all, no way to soften the truth. "This is a statewide investigation. We have twenty-eight EIS officers in the state. There's only room for one person to be in charge of them. For better or worse, that happens to be me."

Sharrar stared at him silently. He knew Fraser was right. He himself was exhausted. Finally he nodded his agreement.

Fraser smiled back gratefully at the men who had originally helped select him for his CDC post. He spoke again. "There's no doubt about one thing, the focus is switching to here. How'd you feel if I moved the whole team down to Philly? Pulled in everybody for a blitzkrieg."

"You got a target?"

"None in particular. But the Bellevue does look interesting."

"Why the Bellevue?" asked Sharrar. "I've already had people go over it."

"They ride in the elevators?"

Sharrar looked blank. And then, as Fraser expounded his idea, a slow smile crossed Sharrar's lips.

George Mallison didn't smile when, thirty minutes later, Fraser quietly explained his theory of the leaking air-conditioning units on the elevators. As they stood in the Bellevue lobby, surrounded by the swirl of religious dignitaries attending the Eucharistic Congress, Mallison shook his head. There were no such units on the elevators.

"Okay," continued Fraser, "but if you wanted to poison everybody in the building, what would be a good way of doing it?"

Mallison didn't hesitate. "You're right. The elevators. A bottle of noxious substance attached to the top of an elevator would be a very efficient way of mass poisoning." The engineer's eyes widened. "You don't think that's what happened?"

Fraser looked serious. "I don't know." He motioned toward the elevators. "Let's go for a ride."

For the next forty-five minutes they climbed over and rode up and down in the elevators, to the total mystification of Anna Taggart, Harold Varr, and Bill Chadwick. Afterward Fraser and Mallison agreed that what would become known as the Elevator Theory was definitely a possibility.

At four o'clock in the afternoon, Fraser addressed the EIS officers in a conference room at 500 South Broad Street. He made it bluntly clear that, from now on, things would be done strictly his way. There would be no need to consult with anyone in Atlanta, there would be no more going off on esoteric tangents. While he was prepared to listen to everyone's ideas, he would be the final arbiter of what would be done. If anybody didn't like it, they could quit.

ISOLATION

14

Collaboration

Instinctively, as the hostess announced that the Delta flight from Harrisburg to Atlanta would be landing in a few minutes, the CDC courier reached protectively for the cyclindrical package with its label proclaiming in bright red letters that it contained etiologic agents, followed by a printed request in slightly smaller type to notify the director, CDC, in the event of the parcel's being damaged or leaking. In theory that couldn't happen; ever since certain airline staff were thought to have become exposed some years back to samples of polio virus that had been inadequately packaged, the law required that etiologic agents sent by air should be so securely packaged that, like a plane's flight recorder, the container would survive a crash intact.

Sometimes, during the repeated shuttling between Pennsylvania and Atlanta, the courier had pondered what David Sencer might actually say if somebody phoned him and announced: *Excuse me, Director, but one of your little packages is damaged and leaking and people are getting sick all over the place.* Assuming, that was, a caller could now actually get through to the agency, let alone contact Sencer. In his years with the CDC, the courier had never known the organization to be so embattled. The selection of newspapers he had read during the flight on this Monday morning, August 9, told part of the story.

Unsolved previous outbreaks were being dragged back into the headlines. Among them were the baffling 1968 epidemic of "Pontiac fever" in Michigan and the even more lethal outbreak at St. Elizabeth's mental hospital in the District of Columbia, which had killed fourteen out of some eighty patients and staff.

The press was also giving space to scientists who were not directly involved in the investigation but who were nevertheless prepared to postulate in print the most bizarre propositions. These included the possibility that a madman had squirted the legionnaires with a spray gun or dropped tiny time pills full of poison into Philadelphia's air-conditioning systems.

Such suggestions would be enhanced by legionnaire George Chiavetta, who, at about the time the Delta jet was descending into Atlanta, was calling a friend, a detective, to tell him all about the strange man in the royal-blue suit with that ominous-looking contraption who had haunted the vicinity of the Bellevue. Chiavetta's account would produce another angle to the story of a disease that this morning's Washington *Post* confidently claimed had ousted Jimmy Carter and the Olympics as a topic at any social gathering.

And perhaps sensing the CDC's medical detectives were no closer to solving the case, normally cautious scientists were discarding their inhibitions to raise the sort of questions the Washington *Post* said sounded like Sherlock Holmes reading Agatha Christie novels. Why had some victims been struck down with the disease the day after the convention and some not until a week later? Why was there an absence of what all epidemiologists looked for in any outbreak—pattern? Why should roommates and spouses of dead legionnaires remain perfectly healthy? Why did it seem hotel employees were immune to the affects of— *what?* And there the questions came thick and fast. Was it a toxin? A fungus? A bacterium? Was it native to the United States? Could it have been brought from Vietnam, the by-product of all the chemical agents which had been used to try and subdue that country? Was it from China? Russia? Was it, in fact, from anywhere on Earth? Or could it be from somewhere out there in space? Dr. Richard Traystman, one of the nation's leading specialists in lung physiology, had just cheerfully announced that "in my most ludicrous dream, it could be somebody landed on Earth, came into contact with these people and inadvertently exposed them to a new organism. Maybe he landed in that hotel and shook their hands. No explanation anybody else has is more valid."

Comments like this made the courier glad he had been given a row to himself and was seated well apart from the others. Even so, the cabin crew looked pointedly at the clearly labeled package beside him. Nobody said anything, but it was not difficult to imagine their fears.

As the plane banked for its final approach, the courier had a spectacular view of Atlanta, the sun glinting off the gold leaf on the dome of the state capitol and shimmering the windows in the forty-one-story First National Bank Building. As they flew over the city at this height, there was nothing to show that 112 years ago Sherman's torch had left

Atlanta in ashes and condemned it to decades of slum torpor. Even in
the relatively recent past, for many Atlanta had been no more than another stop on the southern baseball circuit. Twenty years ago there was
no building over fifteen stories; now the city housed the world's tallest
hotel and was headquarters for Jimmy Carter's presidential campaign.

The jetliner continued to descend toward the airport; the Hyatt
Regency—its glass-walled elevators like Christmas tree ornaments slid-
ing up and down the outer shell of the hotel—fell away, leaving time
only for a glimpse of the soaring architectural splendor of Peachtree
Plaza, and then the plane was landing.

Even before it stopped, the courier was on his feet and standing by
the door.

A hostess held back the other passengers until he had left the plane
and hurried to a waiting car. He got into the backseat, nursing the
elongated package across his knees.

From the ground there was ample evidence to confirm the truth of
Atlanta's civic boast to be "the world's next great city." With its
megastructures, which contained a dazzling network of offices, restaurants, shops, and theaters; its delicate lattice of glass bridges in the sky
linking one elegant tower to another; its imaginative design and layout,
integrating highways with plazas: in so many ways Atlanta was already
a supercity.

None of this presently concerned the courier. He was much too involved in what he was doing, and why, to let his concentration stray
from the container in his lap. The very fact he hand-carried samples
from Pennsylvania was, he knew, a measure of both the importance of
his duties and the seriousness and urgency the CDC attached to the
outbreak. The CDC, somebody had written, was now the laboratory of
last resort.

It had always been so. Every year more than 170,000 specimens from
all over the world came to the CDC for disease diagnosis. Some, such
as smallpox, were virtually extinct. Other viruses, such as those responsible for Lassa, Marburg, Ebola, and South American hemorrhagic
fevers, were new and threatening. With its massive serum bank containing more than 250,000 samples of almost every known disease, the
CDC was like a zookeeper riding herd on quarantined cultures of
deadly viruses, a library of recent human afflictions: malaria from
Trinidad, cholera from Italy, encephalitis from Texas, as well as polio,
typhus, and influenza strains from all over the world. Each sample was
cross-indexed and labeled "open stock," "restricted," or "posterity."

The courier was certain that part of the samples he was carrying
would end up with only the last label.

He liked working with the CDC. It *was* a federal bureaucracy, but one
that allowed casual dress and freedom to challenge and dissent. Even

among the high-level personnel he occasionally came into brief contact
with—the directors of laboratories and heads of divisions—there was
little self-importance and almost nothing at all to suggest the CDC was
a stepchild of probably the biggest bureaucracy in the nation—the Department of Health, Education, and Welfare. Many of its employees
felt the CDC's unique position within the federal hierarchy largely rose
from its role as family physician to the American body politic.

At this particular time, thought the courier grimly, the CDC was
also once more the nation's coroner—trying to solve one of the most
baffling spates of deaths in its entire history, and having to do so in the
full glare of the media just when the agency's credibility was already
being questioned. The swine flu vaccination program had been approved but was still being hotly debated. Critics within the CDC increasingly saw it as a costly and self-serving exercise in preventive medicine, hinting darkly that its implementation in a few weeks might
cause more immediate harm than good. The courier had heard during
visits to the serum bank, which dated from the fifties, that there was
no store of the flu virus that had caused the pandemic in 1918; consequently when the Fort Dix flu virus surfaced, the CDC had to make a
choice—to ignore it or to assume it was similar to the highly dangerous
organism that had caused the pandemic. The CDC, and particularly
David Sencer, had chosen the latter course. It was a gamble that some
staffers at the center were predicting would not pay off—either for the
CDC or for Sencer.

The courier felt sure Sencer's image was not being improved by the
way the most publicized epidemic in modern history was unfolding. So
far it seemed to be just one big question mark. Perhaps, he mused, the
answer could be in the container he carried into the complex of buildings that housed the CDC in Atlanta's northeast suburbs.

Since that meeting on Monday night, August 2, when Sencer announced Fraser was being put in charge of field operations, nearly a
hundred other Atlanta-based specialists had become involved in the investigation. The first of what would be 2,603 separate determinations
in toxicologic pathology had been made, the first of 5,120 tissue slides
prepared, the first of 990 serologic tests conducted in the search for possible infectious agents.

Yet the puzzle seemed as far as ever from being solved. Throughout
the maze of interconnected buildings at the CDC headquarters—in
the administrative offices in the East Wing of Building 1; in the audi-
toriums, classrooms, and cafeterias of Building 2; in Building 6, where
animals were housed in luxury and bred with care, frequently in order
to die in the cause of science; in the "hot lab" of Building 7, where
entry was restricted to only a very few research microbiologists and
where scientists sometimes worked in protective suits fed with filtered

air as a precaution against contamination from some of the most dangerous organisms on earth—in all of these places, everywhere in the CDC complex, the question in one form or another was endlessly repeated: *What* had caused legionnaires' disease?

Though the media had published little evidence of the fact, preferring for one reason or another to concentrate the "science" end of its reporting on what was happening in the Philadelphia laboratories, the CDC had tooled up to deal with the crisis in an astonishingly short time. Virologists, toxicologists, and bacteriologists had all been involved in the search from the moment the first specimens arrived; they would, understandably, resent later criticism that they had been slow off the mark.

Nowhere was this more true than among those working in the hodgepodge of clapboard buildings and Quonset huts housing the increasingly besieged toxicology division at Chamblee, eight miles from the CDC headquarters. Here the small staff of thirteen had been putting in such incredibly long hours, their chief had just ordered that the laboratory would be closed from the middle of that afternoon until the following morning: "We're totally spent, productivity's dropping, and people's patience snapping. We've got to get some rest before we can continue."

Though no one mentioned it, everyone realized that the risk of a serious accident increased when overtired scientists were handling potentially lethal specimens. As specialists dealing with exotic diseases, they accepted that they must always face certain calculated dangers. That was an occupational hazard: the art was to balance caution with the professional urge to go on. And even when fully rested and alert, many scientists still felt trepidation as they handled the deadly samples from Pennsylvania.

The first specimens received had gone to the virus laboratories. Although swine flu had been quickly ruled out, the search for other viruses continued. Tissue cultures were made from the CDC's huge stock of healthy, living cells. Under ultrahygienic conditions, attempts were made to kill those cells in various controlled ways with minuscule amounts of the infected legionnaire specimens. While the idea behind these experiments was simple—find the virus—their rendition was highly technical. Involved at certain stages were colonies of mice and other laboratory-reared animals; they were injected with specially prepared specimens and then carefully observed to see whether or how they were affected. Great care was taken to ensure that no extraneous or unnoticed factor had distorted the findings. To help overcome this possibility, there were control groups of animals living close to those being tested. As the experiments were concluded, the results were compared between groups. Then a new series of trials began, and those results compared. Nothing was ever taken for granted, and there was a built-in allowance for variables. It was painstaking and totally demanding work, the rote and example of all scientific research—and it was going on in dozens of laboratories throughout the CDC.

Sometimes the strain showed, as it had in the toxicology branch. There was an occasional angry word from a technician who was normally calm, a cry of frustration from a researcher not known for histrionics. And from the "front office"—the administrative wing—came polite but insistent requests for progress reports. Few of the lab workers realized the tremendous pressures being concentrated upon the management by the media and the public. Those who telephoned the agency seldom knew whom to ask for when they did manage to get through. As a consequence, the press office and Sencer's staff took the brunt of the calls. Even so, the phones throughout the sprawling complex continued to ring, with callers demanding an answer to the unknown.

In this intense, superheated, and highly competitive maelstrom of high science and low-keyed passions there now emerged, almost casually, two more researchers. One was Dr. Charles Carter Shepard, one of the most respected scientists in the entire CDC colony. Until this morning he had been far away from it all, alone on a hiking vacation in the Rockies. During his absence a relatively new collaborator, research microbiologist Dr. Joseph McDade, had been quietly running tests connected with legionnaires' disease. Separated by years, social background, and mores, the two men were nevertheless joined by a powerful intellectual bond. Both had the capacity to take a problem and think it through clearly, virtually isolating themselves in the process from whatever else might be occurring outside their individual laboratories. They had little knowledge of, or interest in, the wider ramifications of the Philadelphia outbreak; they were only interested in trying to solve a problem which, in some ways, now interrupted the orderly routine of their other endeavors.

Shepard was chief of the CDC's Leprosy and Rickettsia Branch. He had returned from vacation half-expecting the mystery in Philadelphia to be solved; instead, he found McDade and other staff still engaged in the hunt.

The tall, slim sixty-one-year-old had never lost his love for the backcountry. For the past few weeks he had been backpacking in the Grand Teton Mountains of Wyoming. He had first heard of the epidemic seven days ago when he briefly came out of the woods to replenish food supplies and buy a local newspaper. Shepard digested the few reported facts and concluded it was "obviously a pneumonia," possibly produced by one of the diseases his branch studied, Q fever, a febrile illness transmitted to humans from sheep and cattle. He had called the CDC and been told specimens would be delivered to McDade for routine analysis as soon as they arrived. Reassured, Shepard had loped back into the wilderness, putting the matter out of his mind, striding along one mountain trail after another, a gaunt, craggy-faced man, surprisingly youthful in looks and vigor, carrying a tent and everything else he needed to survive on his back. There was nothing to suggest to the occasional person he encountered that Shepard was a world-ranking figure in his highly specialized field. His long and distinguished career as a scientist-physician in public health research had been marked by achievements of such an outstanding nature as, for instance, to redirect the whole technique for treating leprosy: 15 million lepers presently benefited from his findings.

Now just returned and sitting in his CDC office, Shepard listened without interruption as McDade brought him up to date on what had happened while he was away. Tests had been started to check serum specimens for the presence of antibodies to all known rickettsiac—parasitic microorganisms intermediate in size between viruses and bacteria. No rise in antibody level had yet been discerned for any rickettsia. McDade himself was following a quite different and much more esoteric experimental route involving embryonated eggs and guinea pigs. Using legionnaire lung tissue specimens, he was attempting to isolate the specific rickettsia that caused Q fever, *Coxiella burnetii*. McDade was Shepard's expert on the disease.

The thirty-six-year-old, his piercing blue eyes enlivening an otherwise serious face, was cast in the same classic scientific mold as his superior: totally dedicated, gentle and self-effacing, motivated professionally only by a desire to do his work well.

Before joining the CDC eleven months ago, McDade had been a research associate at the prestigious University of Maryland medical school for four years, had spent a year doing fieldwork in Ethiopia and three years in Egypt, and before that had also put in a three-year hitch as a U. S. Army captain at Fort Detrick around the time controversy raged about the base's role as keeper of the nation's CBW arsenal. Though he was known to only a few at the CDC, the consensus of opinion among them was that Joe McDade had found his natural métier in the agency.

When he had finished briefing Shepard, the two men agreed they could not expect anything definite to emerge from the tests already begun for at least a couple of weeks. In the meantime McDade would initiate further animal experiments in case those now under way were inconclusive.

Dicko felt keenly disappointed. He had come to know them all in the past few days. At regular times, morning and evening and some-

times late at night, they would appear in his living room; then Joyce
and he would stop whatever they were doing and listen. He now clearly
recognized their very different styles and the little tricks they used.
Bachman was short and sharp, cutting off questions with a sudden
clamping of the lips; he was usually surrounded by a coterie of strong-
faced silent men who never said anything. The health secretary was
like something out of a Mario Puzo novel. So, for that matter, was the
Italian from Philadelphia, Gaddi-something-or-other, who spoke in long
bursts as if trying to mow down his audience, and who didn't always
seem to agree with what Bachman had said. The Italian frequently
turned up with someone with a name like a dance at one of the ethnic
evenings the post regularly held: Polk. Then there had been that handsome young fellow, the one who had phoned him, who sounded and
looked just like Dr. Kildare: Thacker. And just once, briefly, the boss
himself. Even seated, Fraser had radiated authority and confidence.
What Dicko especially liked was that Fraser hadn't tried to snow him
or minimize what was involved.

There had been others who had made fleeting and barely lasting impressions, flickering across the TV screen in the corner of his living
room. But Fraser's appearance stuck in Dicko's mind. Afterward Dicko
had assured everybody: *That guy's going to get things done; he'll make
the shit hit the fan to get his own way.*

Fraser had not appeared on Dicko's screen for some days, but newscast after newscast, edition after edition of every paper he could lay his
hands on, Dicko was following the progress of the investigation. Seeing
and reading about the way EIS officers had fanned out across the state
reminded him of the promise Thacker had made on the morning of
Jimmy's funeral: *Somebody would be in touch.* Dicko had continued
to believe that at any moment the medical detectives would descend
upon Williamstown to seek his help in uncovering the truth.

Instead, he rumbled at Joyce, somebody had sent him *this.*

In his hand Dicko held a copy of Fraser's questionnaire. Together,
they read it through.

Just another piece of goddamn paper, growled Dicko.

But it must be important, reasoned Joyce, otherwise it wouldn't have
come by special delivery.

Just another way of wasting taxpayers' money.

Joyce didn't think so; anyway, filling in the form might not just help
the health authorities but also somehow bring the Williamstown people together again—make them come to their senses in time for the
Sesquicentennial, the town's 150th birthday celebrations, which were
planned to run for a week from August 22. The festivities had been in
preparation for months. Many townsfolk felt they were even more important than the nation's Bicentennial. Now the deaths of Jimmy and

J.B. had thrown a cloud over the entire affair. It wasn't hard for Dicko to find a source to blame.

The goddamn press, he growled: nobody could come to their senses while papers wrote the sort of things they did and television and radio continued to behave as they had.

Joyce sighed: there was a good deal of truth in what Dicko said. The media's interest in Williamstown continued unabated. The tiny town was typical of so many Pennsylvania communities caught up in the drama. But since it was such a tightly knit place, the tragedy of Williamstown's dead and stricken, with the attendant fears and rumors, had a poignant impact which the media was quick to exploit. One Sunday paper had mulled over the significance of the selection of readings for J.B.'s funeral from the Book of Job and their references to wormwood, gall, running sores, death—and mystery. Other papers had published some of the latest rumors sweeping the town.

Doris was supposed to have said the outbreak might be the work of Taiwanese getting back at America for not supporting their bid to stay in the Olympic Games.

That sounded too goddamn smart for Doris, Dicko growled at Joyce. He doubted Doris knew where Taiwan was.

She was smart enough to have held on to Jimmy, Joyce reminded him. And Jimmy was no dummy.

Yeah, but that was over with now. And how long before Doris found another man?

It wasn't only Doris who was saying wild things, said Joyce, anxious to divert him from such thoughts. Look at Virginia Anne: she was still going on about sabotage.

Jesus, said Dicko, smiling, allowances had to be made for Virginia Anne. She was spiritually beautiful but a little out of touch with the world. If she wanted to get her name in the papers by saying it was sabotage, that was okay with him.

Doris and Virginia Anne, he went on, drew too many of their values from television. Viewing was as much a part of their daily routine as brushing their teeth: from "Today" to "Tonight," with regular stopovers for Mike, Merv, and Walter on CBS who five nights a week said that was the way news was—they accepted it all. He watched, too, but he refused to become conditioned. He didn't want Cronkite or Carson to do his thinking for him. That was why he had been so cautious about all that was being said on TV about the investigation.

Joyce smiled, happy and relieved. Dicko was getting back in form, arguing for the sake of it and enjoying himself, just as he had always done. What had Father Simpson said? The whole process of death was a ritual in which pain almost always gave way to healing. Dicko was coming out of it quicker than even she had dared hope.

Fill out the form, she said, interrupting him: he had a duty, everybody had, to do anything possible to end what was happening in the town.

Goddamn press, growled Dicko again, stirring up things.

Yet they both knew that what was being reported was not only sensational, but also largely true. The town *was* in trauma, *was* gripped in a collective terror. Arthur Grubb, its mayor, had told one reporter the minute anybody took sick, they immediately assumed they had the disease. And stories in the press about Police Chief Seip's sick wife and son had not helped matters. But now that, at least, seemed to be over. Seip had recently driven to Harrisburg to see his son in the hospital and returned home in high excitement: the boy's fever had gone as suddenly as it appeared. Mrs. Seip wept tears of relief and joy—and within minutes her own fever broke. It was nerves, just nerves, which, she thought, had made her ill.

Understandable enough, rumbled Dicko, only he just wished the press hadn't gotten hold of it.

If it hadn't been the Seips, it would have been somebody else, argued Joyce. There were any number of other cases of fright. Had he heard of the doctor's secretary who went to a Little League baseball game to watch her son play? When she sat down next to some other mothers they quickly moved away. They didn't want to be near her. They knew her boss had been the doctor who had sent Jimmy to the hospital.

Dicko shook his head.

And a lot of people, continued Joyce, were thinking twice about making trips to Philadelphia. One woman had refused to let her husband go to a Phillies game; another neighbor, whose husband couldn't avoid attending a conference in the city, had packed him lunch—and made him solemnly swear not to eat or to drink a drop while in Philadelphia.

Williamstown had lost more than his two best friends, said Dicko, recognizing a new truth: the town had lost some of its innocence.

He saw further evidence of that when he later drove up Market Street. People waved quickly and then looked the other way, as though they wanted to avoid contact with him and were embarrassed by their own behavior. He had heard the same thing had happened to others who had been at the convention. No matter how politely it was being done, the legionnaires *were* being ostracized. In its wake the outbreak had stirred primeval forces long dormant in the Williams Valley.

Dicko reached the post. Ordinarily he would have expected the usual crowd at the bar, gossiping and drinking.

The club was deserted.

Grim-faced, looking more than ever like that marine raising the flag on Iwo Jima, Dicko went into his office. He cleared a space on his desk for the questionnaire, and read it through again: *What in hell was all this about?*

He began to telephone fellow commanders in the Nineteenth District. They had also received the form; they were filling it in and returning it. The general feeling was one of optimism. Here was proof something positive was being done. The form might help dispel the uncertainty and fear being felt in many communities throughout the state.

That fear was going to affect Hoak's chances, predicted one legionnaire.

Dicko remembered: the state adjutant was running for the office of national commander of the Legion. His involvement in the epidemic—among other things, Hoak was trying to visit every post with a sick or dead legionnaire—had virtually put an end to an electioneering campaign he had planned for six years. There was no way he would now have time to present his case in other states. The epidemic had chained him to Pennsylvania.

That, said Dicko flatly, was Hoak's problem. He had no strong feelings, one way or the other, about whether Hoak made national commander. He rolled the questionnaire into the battered post typewriter and, using two fingers and a thumb on the space bar, began to type in his replies.

Room number: 826–28.

No, dammit, that wasn't right. He fished around the desk top and found the bill for the Holiday Inn suite.

Tap-tap-tap: 822–24.

Jesus, he had better get the suite number right. He wouldn't want those medical detectives going to the wrong room to track down the mystery of the leak around the air-conditioning vent.

He looked at another question: How many hours did you spend in the Bellevue Stratford on Wednesday, 21st?

Tap-tap-tap: *?Aprx 1 hr.*

Was that right? Hell, he didn't know. Maybe it was more. He couldn't remember now. Not for sure.

He glared at the paper. What was the point of all this? How could he accurately answer *all* those questions? How could anybody *really* remember exactly where they had been and what they had done at any given moment during the convention?

How long had he spent in the Bellevue on Friday, 23rd?

He thought for a while. About forty minutes at that breakfast. Maybe another hour or so on the convention floor. Say two, to be on the safe side. Maybe ten minutes afterward in the hotel lobby. Make it safe. Tap: 3.

Then the same question came up in more detail. How long had he

spent in the hotel or on the sidewalk that July 23rd? There were blocks
of time to be filled in. He selected: 8 to 10 A.M., 10 A.M. to noon, 2
P.M. to 4 P.M. But that was more than three hours—that was *six* hours.
How would anybody square up the two answers? Oh, the extra three
hours must have been on the sidewalk. Yes, that was it.

Pausing from time to time to scratch his head, Dicko continued to
type in his responses, trying to remember what he, Jimmy, and J.B. had
done. It brought back many memories.

So, too, did the newspaper clipping J.B.'s mother was reading at
about the same time. It described J.B.'s funeral and had been sent to
her by a reporter from the Washington *Post*. The press, sighed Mrs.
Ralph, had really been so kind in honoring promises to mail their reports. She put the clipping with the others on her Italian marble table.

Virginia Anne poured her mother more coffee and they continued to
make small talk.

Every once in a while Mrs. Ralph would break off and stare at the
couch where J.B. had lain dying.

The couch's covering, thought Virginia Anne, hung loose, like an old
skin. It should go, at least from the room. But it was too soon to make
any such changes. She couldn't remember how many times recently she
had caught her mother staring around the room, at its soft pink walls
that J.B. had found so soothing, at the velvet chairs with gold-leafed
backs he had usually preferred to sit in rather than the French provin-
cial love seat, at the Chinese screen hiding the TV set which he'd
pulled away to watch a ball game, at the mahogany breakfront he'd
kept his papers in, at the two icons, of Jesus and the Virgin Mary,
he'd sometimes paused to admire, even at the rose-colored carpet he'd
walked on: Mrs. Ralph stared at them all, almost as if she expected
J.B. suddenly to appear in this familiar and now, to her, empty room.

At other times Mrs. Ralph had just sat and looked at photographs of
J.B., going silently from one to another, drawing something she never
shared with Virginia Anne from the succession of faded prints.

Then slowly, as the day passed, and once the pain at waking had
gone, and the shock of realization become accepted, Mrs. Ralph returned to the present and spoke of what might have killed her son.

Occasionally the shrill sound of the telephone would interrupt her
soliloquy. She would thank the callers for their condolences, but no,
there was nothing she wanted; Virginia Anne was a great help. They
would manage.

Then she would come back into this room and talk endlessly about
her dead son.

Perhaps they should speak to Carol, said Virginia Anne. What had
happened at the cemetery was over. It had been an aberration. Carol

had not been herself. And whatever her motive might have been, the boys *were* Ralphs. They were part of J.B. Did she understand?

Mrs. Ralph nodded. She understood. But would anybody else? Maybe she would talk to Dicko: he was sensible beyond his years. And he had loved J.B. almost as much as she did. She would call him— soon. But not today. Now she just wanted to be alone, recalling all those memories she had of J.B. No mother could have had a finer son; why had she let him marry Carol? She would go to her grave regretting that.

Mom, said Virginia Anne again, she really should call Carol. Maybe the boys could come this weekend?

Mrs. Ralph nodded absently. If Virginia Anne wanted to phone Carol, she could. But she musn't plead. There was no need for that. They had a blood right to see the boys, who were J.B.'s.

Virginia Anne went to the phone.

Dear Lord, thought Mrs. Ralph. I never dreamed it would hurt like this. Nobody knew how much it had cost her to turn away from the grave holding the folded flag and walk through the silent crowd. Some of the reporters had described her as the Iron Lady with a will of steel. They meant well. But they couldn't see into her heart. And nobody, not even her daughter, would ever know the extent of the pain she felt there.

Virginia Anne returned to the room, almost triumphant. Carol had agreed. The boys could come for the weekend. Her mother and she would be able to spoil them just like her mother had spoiled J.B.

Mrs. Ralph nodded. *Sure.* But she would never be able to spoil anybody quite like she had spoiled her son.

She doubted even Dicko would understand that.

In Dolan's Hole, Dicko came to the end of his questionnaire. The point of many of the questions still eluded him. But the frequent mention of the Bellevue Stratford made him ponder. He leaned back in his chair.

Jesus, he said to himself, that hotel with its snooty staff and airs and graces could be hiding a goddamn killer.

Graitcer tried again, sitting comfortably in the boardroom armchair, giving the aged bellhop a man-of-the-world smile, lobbing the question across the expanse of polished table.

"Are you really sure no prostitute came into the hotel during the Legion convention?"

It was not voyeurism that made the epidemiologist press the question; around the city health department there was a continuing thought that whatever had struck the legionnaires might somehow have been sexually transmitted. A change in the nation's sexual mores had ensured that, except for the common cold, venereal diseases afflicted more Americans than all other infectious illnesses combined. And there was that "super gonorrhea" in Maryland and California that was impervious to treatment by the standard means, penicillin; the new strain actually produced an enzyme capable of destroying the drug. The CDC had already issued a nationwide alert about the disease. As a matter of routine, Graitcer had been putting his question about prostitutes to any hotel employee he met.

The bellman looked uncertainly at Varr. The general manager stared icily across the table at Graitcer.

Varr found such questions offensive. He did not see the relevance of the presence, or otherwise, of prostitutes in the Bellevue. He thought it was another one of those red herrings which seemed to abound in the investigation. Much of what he had observed or learned about the activities of the medical detectives had not impressed him. There often seemed to be no pattern or purpose to their inquiries. They repeatedly asked the same questions. But it was the point of those questions that baffled Varr—to the stage where he had sometimes felt it necessary to intervene. Further, he believed he was justified in doing so because he had formed the impression many of his staff were either confused, bewildered, or resentful at the way they were being handled by some of the medical detectives. So far Graitcer had behaved with propriety. But now, in pushing the question about prostitutes, he was arousing Varr's wrath.

Graitcer continued to wait, remembering the advice the detective had given him: *When you sniff something, tough it out; you're in the driving seat, don't rush.*

Varr leaned forward, elbows on the table, fixing Graitcer with an angry look.

"I have five hundred staff here. They all have one thing in common, watchfulness. They'd spot a hooker."

"I'm not disputing that," said Graitcer, keeping his voice light and even. "I'm just asking a perfectly valid question."

"You've asked it of every one of the staff you've interviewed so far. And they've all told you the same thing—"

"Right. None of them have been sick. And none of them saw any hookers. I accept that. But I've still got to go on asking," said Graitcer equably.

"What is this . . . this obsession you have with hookers?" Varr was irritated now, rather than angry.

"Simply that a hooker could have transmitted the disease. Nothing else."

"In this place a hooker would be a marked person by the nature of her business."

"Mr. Varr, I am not thinking of the girls who parade up and down the sidewalk outside. I am sure you can keep that sort out. But what about the better class of hooker? The ones who might come in unnoticed and operate from inside the hotel?"

Varr considered. The question bothered him; it would bother any hotelier. Varr knew there was always the risk of a high-class prostitute booking into the Bellevue. But if that had happened, there was nothing he could now do. And he would strongly resist any request to hand over to Graitcer or his superiors the guest lists for the period covering the Legion convention; that would mean breaching what he believed was the almost sacred trust existing between hotelier and guest—that the latter's presence would never be revealed without permission. The best way to handle the increasingly delicate situation might be to give ground.

"There are hookers and there are hookers," he conceded. "There are the very expensive hookers who sort of fit in. The hundred-dollars-a-turn type. But that class of hooker *never* interferes with the running of the hotel."

Graitcer pounced. "So you might have had a high-class hooker here?"

"I didn't say that! Don't put words in my mouth, young man."

"I'm not," said Graitcer, his voice suddenly hard and flat. "I think we'll all get along a lot faster if we remember this is an investigation which has the full backing of the city administration. If you don't like my questions, maybe you would like to state your objections to Al Gaudiosi or even Mayor Rizzo!"

"I'm sorry," said Varr. "This is not easy. You must appreciate no one likes being asked these sorts of questions."

"Rest assured, nothing said here will go beyond the proper authorities," said Graitcer. He looked steadily at the bellman. "Okay, you didn't see any hookers." Graitcer drew a questionnaire toward him. "Have you been sick since July 1?"

The bellman shook his head.

"You sure?" Graitcer glanced at a pad. "I heard from one of the other bellmen you had flu."

"Just a touch."

"When was that?"

"After the Legion left."

Graitcer made a note.

"Were you off work?"

"No."

"Run a temperature?"

"Never checked. I just took some medicine."

"What sort?"

"Some capsules my wife had left over from her flu last spring. Tetra-something-or-other."

"Tetracycline?"

"Yeah. Sounds right."

"How many did you take?"

The bellman thought. "Maybe half a dozen."

Graitcer sighed. Another busted lead. It had been like that all day: as a backup to Goldberger's employee survey, a procession of hotel staff who worked in the lobby had come to the boardroom to be interviewed by Graitcer in the presence of either Varr or Chadwick. After several hours Graitcer had learned very little—except that, either through inclination or training or perhaps through being cowed by the presence of the hotel's two senior executives, the employees were unforthcoming. The dentist in Graitcer thought it was a bit like drawing teeth out of stone.

And yet, somewhere early on in this mammoth session of questions and guarded answers, something important had emerged. A front desk clerk had been the first to mention that the air-conditioning vent above the desk had been malfunctioning. He had not elucidated—perhaps because Chadwick's glare stopped him. Subsequently other employees had, when prompted, mentioned the faulty vent in vague, nonspecific terms.

"Were you aware of any problem with the vent?" Graitcer asked the bellman.

"The desk staff complained about it."

"Specifically, what did they complain of?"

"It didn't work properly."

"Yes?"

"It was clogged."

Varr interrupted. "That's normal, it can happen with vents."

Graitcer sighed. "Mr. Varr, will you please let the bellman answer."

"Like I said, it was clogged. No air came out. One of the maintenance men came last Friday and took down the unit for servicing."

"Where was the servicing done?"

"In the basement area," said Varr. "We're not the sort of establishment which does running repairs in public. We have a proper place for that."

"I'm sure." Graitcer continued to probe the bellman. "Can you remember how long it was clogged?"

The employee pondered. "A week. Two weeks. I'm not sure."

"Okay. So it was taken away and brought back."

"Right. And it now works fine."

Graitcer turned to Varr. "They probably cleaned it in some liquid. Do you know where that might be now?"

"Probably thrown away. There's no reason to keep such stuff."

"Well, it'll have to be followed up. I'll pass it on to Mr. Mallison."

"I can't see what this has to do with anything," protested Varr.

"Who knows?" Graitcer shrugged.

There was a knock on the door. The black homicide detective came into the boardroom, pausing to drop ash from his cigar into a cuspidor. He smiled pleasantly at Varr, nodded toward the bellman, and then addressed Graitcer.

"No problems?" He winked at Graitcer. "Otherwise we'll invite them down to headquarters."

"No problems. They've been very helpful."

"Just checking." The policeman took another draw on his cigar. "Anyway, I think we got ourselves a real lead."

"What sort of lead?"

"You might say I'm keeping it on ice for you." The policeman grinned.

Graitcer became excited. "You found the ice suppliers? The one the legionnaires got their ice from?"

"Sure have."

Minutes later Graitcer was being driven quickly across the city to the ABC Ice Company at Seventh and Washington. When the Bellevue's ice dispensers had run out—and for some reason the hotel had been unable to replenish them—many of the legionnaires bought ice in plastic bags from the ABC Company. The firm's manager explained to Graitcer that ABC sold ice that was, in fact, manufactured by another firm.

Graitcer phoned Sharrar and arranged for a health department sanitarian to meet him there; the sanitarian would judge whether proper care had been taken in the ice-making process.

The policeman was optimistic. "If this ice plant is suspect, we've got ourselves a hard lead. Phil, I can see them pinning a medal on you and your picture in the *Daily News:* 'Doc De-ices Bug Outbreak'!"

"I still want to talk to the Pigeon Lady," said Graitcer.

For days now the epidemiologist had been trying to locate the old crone who regularly fed the birds on Broad Street. But for some reason she had not been seen recently at any of her haunts. The thought had crossed his mind she might be ill, a victim of the disease George Mallison suspected—psittacosis. There was, mused Graitcer, a problem with this investigation: the outbreak fitted so many possible theories. But he had to find the Pigeon Lady so she could be crossed off his list.

"Phil, you continue to amaze me," said the policeman with heavy

irony. "First it's hookers. Now it's nuts. Maybe you should have studied psychiatry."

"The way you drive, I'd have you certified for a start," Graitcer responded, grinning.

An hour later, after thoroughly inspecting the ice-making plant, the
sanitarian said he had found nothing to suggest it was the source of the
infection. Even so, he would take samples of ice for further analysis.

The detective would not give up. Maybe the trouble was in the vehicles that had transported the ice to the hotel. The ice plant manager
explained that some of the legionnaires had struck a deal with a cab
driver to ferry the ice to the Bellevue. The detective asked to use the
phone. He soon traced the name and address of the cabby.

Shortly afterward he and Graitcer drove slowly along Tenth Street.

"There it is. A couple of blocks up."

Graitcer spotted the cab, parked outside a tenement building.

The detective parked behind it, peering at the cab's trunk.

"You think there's a body in there?" asked Graitcer.

"No. Maybe a leak."

The policeman climbed out of his car and walked slowly around the
taxi, finally crouching to look underneath. He straightened up and
wrote the license number in his notebook.

Graitcer thought: *It's just like working with Kojak.*

"Hey. Wassamatta? Whattya doin' with my cab?"

A fat, middle-aged man in an undershirt and trousers puffed up to
them.

"You Constantinos?"

"Yeah. Who're you?"

The detective flashed his badge and casually displayed his shoulder
holster.

"I wanna ask you some questions. You run ice for the legionnaires?"

"Wassamatta widdat?"

"You got a license to haul ice?"

"I need a license?"

The policeman smiled. "No. But don't get smart. Show us where
you carried the ice."

"In the trunk."

"Open it."

"Wha' for ?"

"Open the trunk—or I'll bust it open."

Constantinos opened the trunk.

Graitcer and the detective peered inside. The detective straightened
and faced the cab driver. "I'm going to have to take this trunk apart."

"You can't do that. I need da cab for my living. Wassamatta with
you? You can't stop a guy makin' a living."

"Listen, fella. People might have died from that ice you carried. You know what that could make you?" The policeman made a cutting motion across his throat. "Savvy?"

Constantinos winced. "I ain't done nothin' wrong. You gotta believe me."

"We just want to check your car," said Graitcer placatingly.

The detective made a decision. "Constantinos, get in your cab and drive to headquarters. You know where it is. I'll be right behind you. And don't get cute. The lab guys can run tests—"

"But, mister, I gotta be on the road in an hour. I gotta wife, five kids. Whattya doin' to me?"

"Constantinos—get in that car and drive. Otherwise I'm arresting you for resisting an officer in his lawful inquiries. Now *move!*"

Within an hour police department forensic science technicians had begun to disassemble the trunk—watched by an ashen-faced Constantinos, a fascinated Graitcer, and an impassive detective who had growled just once, "You're looking for icewater," and then lapsed into silence, chewing on his cigar.

No water was found.

The technicians reassembled the trunk.

The detective shrugged and told Constantinos he was free to leave. As they watched the taxi drive away, the policeman turned to Graitcer.

"You got any ideas—apart from your Pigeon Lady?"

Graitcer shook his head.

15

Concentration

It was, Fraser agreed with Bob Craven, totally terrifying. He continued to read the photocopied pages of the classified U. S. Army manual Craven had brought with him from Pittsburgh.

Craven's anonymous telephone caller had been as good as his word: two days after the man's alarming call, which Craven had followed up all the way to the Pentagon, excerpts from the secret manual arrived on his desk in Pittsburgh. When Fraser ordered him to join the others in Harrisburg, Craven had brought the photocopies with him.

To a strong pacifist like Fraser, the papers were entirely abhorrent with their coldly calculated estimates of kill ratios and megadeath predictions. The photocopies also indicated the Pentagon duty officer might have been telling less than the truth when he said the Army was "out of the CBW game."

Craven was right, thought Fraser, the symptoms produced by the particular chemical agent referred to in the papers did indeed mimic some of those seen in the epidemic. But there were significant differences: the incubation period of legionnaires' disease was longer and the course of the illness different. While unable to exclude other CBW agents, Fraser was certain the lethal disease described in the photocopies was not the one he was investigating.

He pushed aside the papers, aware of, but still not responding to, the speculative looks of the two older men seated near his desk. He knew they were taking a keen interest in the decisions he was making.

Fraser concentrated on Craven, listening raptly as the epidemiologist gave a graphic account of his work in Pittsburgh. Right to the very end, Fraser was pleased to hear, Craven had stayed on top of a number of running strands, including checking on the condition of the Keystone Cadets, the marching band whose ranks had been decimated by what seemed to be the illness that had killed their bus driver, Andrew Hornack. The ten sick cadets were now all recovering.

Nevertheless, warned Craven, there was another unresolved problem in Pittsburgh: coroner Cyril Wecht was continuing to behave like "a rumbling volcano" over the way the investigation was being run. Wecht, explained Craven, liked his "daily injection of ink and air time," and in the course of his many public criticisms—the coroner matched Bachman or Gaudiosi in the amount of column inches specifically devoted to his caustic views—Wecht had, in Craven's view, "made some fairly preposterous statements."

Fraser abruptly told Craven to stop worrying about Wecht.

Craven reacted. From the moment he had stepped into the Harrisburg complex, he had been struck by its "boiler-plate" atmosphere. Tiredness and tension abounded. Fraser himself was at times "abrasive, very curt and difficult." Craven got the impression he was trying "to do too much himself, he didn't delegate things as much as he should." Perhaps that could account for the presence of the two watchful men who had just arrived from Atlanta.

When Craven had finished his report on the winding up of the CDC involvement in Pittsburgh, Fraser assigned him to work on the line list with Thacker and Tsai.

Craven could barely contain his disappointment. He had hoped for something more exciting—possibly even a chance to go where "the real action" was: Philadelphia. Being restricted to line list work was barely appealing; he enjoyed "being out in the field rather than taking information down by phone and working with that."

Looking around the War Room, Craven's mind began to cast about for ways of diversifying his duties. He quickly learned nobody in Harrisburg was acting as central keeper of information on what researchers outside the CDC were doing about the possibility of a toxin's having caused the outbreak. Craven recognized that, since the origin of the epidemic remained unknown, in effect a huge, nationwide competition had been thrown open. Scientists of every standing and many disciplines were eager to join the race to be first to announce a solution. Nowhere was that race keener than among the specialists looking at toxins. And Craven soon discovered one of the most distinguished of these was Dr. F. William Sunderman, Jr.—the same Sunderman who had previously passed to the FBI the anonymous letter he had received stating the legionnaires had been poisoned. Now Sunderman was himself actively investigating that very possibility. In his impressively equipped laboratory at the University of Connecticut, urged on by his father, an eminent fellow scientist in Philadelphia, Sunderman was conducting tests to try to ascertain whether the victims had died as a result of poisoning by nickel carbonyl—a clear, colorless liquid that is relatively easily transformed into a lethal gas. Sunderman was particularly intrigued by how closely the symptoms of nickel carbonyl poisoning paralleled those of legionnaires' disease. It was not a perfect match—the longer incubation period and higher fever of the disease did not fit the pattern of the poison—but it nevertheless looked a most promising lead. Craven, as competitive as the next EIS officer, decided to run with it.

Fraser immediately agreed to let him act as coordinator of all research into the possibility of a toxin's being the culprit. He had sensed Craven's frustration: for all his studied casualness, Craven had not fooled Fraser—who privately shared his desire to be in Philadelphia. Fraser wanted to move his team and himself as fast as possible to the center of the city, to converge the search on the most suspect area.

Bachman, he guessed, would resist such a move. Taking the team out of his immediate orbit would inevitably take some of the limelight away from the health secretary. It was a tricky situation. That was why Fraser was now glad of the presence of the two men who had been quietly watching him at work during this Tuesday morning of August 10.

One of them was the director of the Bureau of Epidemiology at the CDC and Fraser's boss, the man he had telephoned religiously every morning around two o'clock to discuss developments. Well used to assessing the pressures on his field officers, the bureau director had become increasingly concerned by the exhaustion and edginess Fraser displayed in those nocturnal calls. At the end of their conversation early on Sunday morning, he ordered Fraser to have a night off, to relax and take out as many members of the team as possible for dinner. They had eaten a Chinese meal, which ended with the traditional fortune cookies, and there was a lively discussion as to whether some of the advice on the slogans baked into the cookies might be applied to the investigation. Afterward, in spite of what his chief had suggested, Fraser went back to work. This almost compulsive inner-driving force of Fraser's had, among other things, decided the bureau director to come to Harrisburg. He had brought with him another senior CDC officer, a specialist in influenza. They were both anxious, as Fraser's superior expressed it, "to get a better feel of what the situation was, seeing Philadelphia, seeing the hotel, just to get a feel for it."

Having observed the Harrisburg operation for some hours, the bureau director concluded that "the quality of the investigation" could not be bettered and that Fraser was "well in command, knew what was going on, what everybody was doing"—but was "frustrated" because Bachman wanted to keep the CDC team in Harrisburg.

Having listened to Fraser's arguments for moving to Philadelphia, the bureau director made a decision. He asked Fraser to introduce him to Bachman.

Bachman was going over his brief for that morning's press conference when the men came into his office. The health secretary was growing increasingly angry with the sniping of the Rizzo administration, but he was determined not to "get into a pissing contest with a skunk," or to be upset by the scathing attacks of the *Daily News*: he thought the Philadelphia-based newspaper was out to hatchet him. Bachman was careful to keep such thoughts from his visitors.

Nevertheless, the bureau director could see that the harassed health secretary was under "tremendous pressures," and wanted the help of the CDC at a time when the "going was really sticky."

It was not an unfamiliar situation to the CDC man. After Fraser had completed his introductions and left, he set about handling it.

Five minutes later he was back at Fraser's desk. There had been no "arm twisting." But Fraser was now free to move his team "forthwith" to Philadelphia.

Fraser immediately began to give orders to wind down the War Room. Then he telephoned Sharrar and explained what was happening. He told him he wanted a War Room prepared at 500 South Broad Street along similar lines to the one in Harrisburg. He suggested they use the large room on the ground floor of the building. He wanted wall boards and easels for the line lists, adequate secretarial help, at least ten telephones installed—Fraser reeled off a lengthy list of requirements.

Sharrar asked: Where did he want the computer terminal?

Fraser snapped: He didn't care where it went. There were more important things to settle.

What about the detectives?

Fraser knew they were already conducting a critically important telephone survey of hotel guests who had been in Philadelphia between July 6 and August 7, and who had stayed at one of the four hotels the legionnaires used. His decision whether he would have to order the Bellevue closed—or any of the other hotels—depended largely on the results of this survey. Fraser told Sharrar he did not want to disturb the detectives until they had finished this work. Sharrar should reserve space in the room so the detectives could move in as soon as the hotel survey was done.

Anything else?

Fraser hesitated: Was something wrong?

There was silence.

Then Sharrar spoke. He was exhausted. He was going to take a brief vacation to be with Karen in the last stages of her pregnancy. He'd booked this time off months ago.

Fraser told him not to worry. It was fine.

There was one other thing, said Sharrar. Goldberger had just quit the investigation. He hadn't been happy for some time. He would be gone before Fraser got to Philadelphia.

Fraser said he wasn't surprised. He told Sharrar to thank Goldberger for his work, and ended the call.

Shortly afterward Fraser was sent for by Bachman.

Whatever the health secretary might privately have felt about the outcome of his brief encounter with Fraser's chief, he was now his usual ebullient self, rocking back and forth in his padded chair and firing a fusillade of questions at Fraser.

Was it just another press scare—or could there be a connection between the present epidemic and what had happened in Philadelphia almost exactly two years ago?

In September 1974 the national Odd Fellows convention had been hit by a mysterious outbreak that killed three persons and hospitalized nineteen others. The newspapers had now begun to speculate whether the two outbreaks were linked. The fifteen hundred Odd Fellows, like the legionnaires, had used the Bellevue Stratford as their convention headquarters.

Fraser explained to Bachman that it would be impossible to prove conclusively whether the two were connected until the agent for legionnaires' disease was known. But it did seem a remarkable coincidence.

What about that other connection the press were still playing up, persisted Bachman, the pneumonia-like outbreak at St. Elizabeth's Hospital in southwest Washington? A smart reporter on the Washington *Post* had noted the death rate then—fourteen out of some eighty known cases—was about the same as in the current epidemic. Was that significant?

Fraser said the statistic by itself proved nothing.

Bachman would not let go: he needed more than that for his morning press conference. Since they didn't yet know what the disease was, perhaps Fraser might tell him exactly what it *wasn't*?

Fraser left Bachman briefly and returned with a list. Within forty-eight hours of the first specimens arriving in Atlanta, laboratory tests had eliminated typhoid, tularemia, lymphocytic choriomeningitis, the Lassa and Marburg viruses, pertussis, plague—

Some of the press were still flirting with that one, interrupted Bachman.

Some of the press also promoted flying saucers—because it helped their circulations.

Bachman grinned and motioned for Fraser to continue.

After five days the lab tests had ruled out swine flu and other influenzas, streptococci, staphylococci, meningococci, pneumococci, *Salmonella, Shigella, Histoplasma*, blastomycosis, cryptococci, brucellae, and coccidioidomycosis.

Tests were now being run to confirm or exclude the presence of *Mycoplasma*, spiroplasma, Q fever, adenoviruses, respiratory syncytial virus, herpes virus, mumps and measles viruses, enteric viruses, *Thermoactinomyces*, leptospira, coronaviruses, tin, thallium, beryllium, chromium, paraquat, pesticides, herbicides, and flame retardants. Still further tests were scheduled for arsenic, mercury, ethylene glycol, cadmium, *Candida*, toxoplasmas, *Ascaris*, and *Entamoeba*.

Bachman whistled, impressed: that was one hell of a checklist. Fraser should have it ready when he took him along to the morning press conference.

Fraser tried to beg off. Couldn't Parkin continue to handle the media? He had a great deal to do in the next few hours.

Bachman was terse. He wanted Fraser there.

Fraser thought: *Politics again; it's just astonishing the way administrators like Bachman can put on a show when the occasion demands.*

He also sensed that this time there was no way out.

As usual, a large crowd of reporters, cameramen, and TV technicians assembled for the conference. There was a ripple of excitement when Fraser entered the room.

Bachman confirmed there had been no new cases reported overnight. The latest figures stood at 27 dead and 128 still sick. Some of them were in critical condition. He did not expect further outbreaks, though the situation was being closely monitored. There had not been and he did not expect to see any signs of secondary spread. He then introduced Fraser.

Immediately a *Daily News* reporter was on his feet, hurling a barrage of questions at Fraser. What had caused the outbreak? What was the source? Were there ten thousand people at the convention, as the Legion claimed? Or twenty-five hundred, as hotel registrations seemed to show? How many had not stayed in the four hotels under suspicion—

Fraser stopped the reporter in mid-gallop, knowing he must take immediate control or he would be swamped in a sea of questions.

The issues the *News* man had raised, he replied, were among hundreds the investigating epidemiologists had already asked themselves.

With what answers?

Fraser smiled. Lots of thoughts had gone through his head, but his job was to generate a firm hypothesis and then test it.

Lawrence Altman of the New York *Times*, himself a former EIS officer, raised the possibility of a link with the Odd Fellows outbreak.

Fraser was as frank as he had been with Bachman: It *was* going to be hard to pin down any connection; as yet he wasn't even certain a disease was responsible for the earlier outbreak.

Altman held up a copy of the questionnaire that had been sent to all Legion posts. Several of the twenty-three questions focused on events of Friday, July 23, when the legionnaires had paraded along Broad Street "in humid, smoggy, seventy-three-degree, showery weather." Why so many questions for this Friday?

Altman's sharp as a tack, thought Fraser, beginning to enjoy the probing.

He explained he was considering whether a geographical factor could be involved: "all kinds of things" were on the sidewalk in front of the Bellevue; there were "grates on the sidewalks, trees, a subway entrance, and a median strip in the road—each of which could be the source of a toxic substance that could make people sick who stood near it for a long period of time while watching the parade, but leave others unaffected if they were just passing by or waiting for a bus."

There was silence as the reporters digested the implication of what he had said.

Would Fraser elaborate, asked Stuart Auerbach of the Washington *Post*.

Fraser explained that the degree of sickness and how quickly it appeared were probably related to the amount of exposure—which could explain the varying incubation period of from two to ten days.

Auerbach raised a related matter. As it had been a hot and rainy afternoon before the parade, could that have caused a chemical reaction with agents generally found in the area, so creating some poisonous substance?

It was, conceded Fraser, not only a good question but a real possibility.

The concern in the room grew.

But so far lab tests had failed to show *anything* that could have caused the outbreak.

The reporters slumped back in their seats.

A *National Enquirer* reporter took up the questioning. Was Fraser able totally to rule out chemicals?

Fraser considered. He would not, at this stage, rule out chemicals.

Did that mean a chemical could be the agent?

Fraser sighed: he wished it was as simple as that. He suspected many of the reporters had only a rudimentary knowledge of science—and almost certainly no real idea of how difficult it was for him to be positive about anything. He decided to play safe. He was "leaning more toward a chemical than I was before because so much of the microbiology seems unlikely."

How *far* was he leaning? The question came from one of the team of *Wall Street Journal* reporters covering the story.

Fraser explained he was seriously considering toxins as a source.

Poisons, demanded the *National Enquirer* reporter, was that what he meant?

Fraser agreed he was anxious to establish whether somehow poisons had been introduced into the legionnaires' air, water, or food.

Why was it taking so long?

Fraser kept his temper: The tests to establish the veracity of this were time-consuming, the possibilities numerous, and the results so far negative.

What had been tested for?

Fraser repeated the list he had given Bachman.

Hell, yelled a reporter, what was there left?

On that imponderable note the press conference ended.

Returning to the War Room, Bachman warmly congratulated Fraser on his performance. More than ever, continued the health secretary, he was going to miss having him around.

Fraser sensed the older man's mood. For Bachman the cut and thrust of the hunt was all but over. When Fraser and the CDC team moved to Philadelphia, the main media attention would go with them.

Bachman would be able to catch up with his vacation, suggested Fraser.

The Health Secretary brightened: He would start making plans at once to go sailing. In a week's time he could be at sea, he added, while Fraser could be swimming for his life in the whirlpools of the Rizzo administration. Look sharp, young fellow, repeated Bachman, there were more sharks around Philadelphia City Hall than off the Maine coast.

Fraser promised to be careful.

Bachman had a final piece of advice: Watch out for the *Daily News.* Its people would swarm all over Fraser and his team like bees around a honeypot. And—Bachman grinned—he would not be on hand to ward them off.

Then, with a gruff admonition to solve this goddamn thing and a quick handshake, Bachman was gone.

Parkin had no advice to give. Instead he told Fraser that their time together had been one of the most exhilarating in his career. He was engagingly frank: Before Fraser arrived he looked upon the CDC as a bunch of hotshots who would leave him behind to pick up the pieces. Parkin no longer thought that. He had learned a good deal working so close to such a professional team.

It was the nearest Fraser came to blushing.

Having said good-bye to Parkin, he plunged into the task of moving to Philadelphia. The mood among his EIS officers, he saw with quiet satisfaction, was bullish. Whatever the difficulties ahead, they were homing in on the place where the enemy had struck. So far close to $250,000 had been spent in tracking that enemy to his lair in downtown Philadelphia. And while his actual identity was as much of a mystery as ever, he was probably still there, somewhere, waiting for them to flush him out.

Watching Tsai packing his special sample-carrying box, Craven assembling his files and the other EIS officers all the paraphernalia they must take with them, Fraser felt quiet pride. In a relatively short time, from scratch, they had been molded into a well-knit team.

Thacker interrupted such thoughts with a question: Where would they be staying in Philadelphia?

Fraser told him: The Bellevue Stratford.

A small adjustment, a mere touch from well-manicured fingers, and a minute portion of J.B.'s lung tissue came into greater magnification. The scientist looking down the microscope worked at the CDC, in the highly restricted Toxicology Branch, which was part of the Clinical Chemistry Division, in itself a part of the Bureau of Laboratories.

The CDC was structured like an army, she had thought when she first came to work here. Nowadays the analogy seemed particularly apt: like the brigades, corps, companies, and platoons within a huge army fighting to be first to capture some strategic target, so the many CDC laboratories involved in the hunt—from bureaus down through divisions and branches—were all competing to be the first to crack the case. This in turn led to internal competition for the limited number of samples available. From a toxicological viewpoint, the scientist poring over that sliver of J.B.'s lung was not entirely happy with the size and quality of the specimens her lab had received. Nevertheless, a good number of tests had been successfully performed. All proved negative. With no real expectancy of a change in that pattern, the toxicologist continued to study the sample.

Some eight miles away, other laboratory staff in the main CDC complex were also pursuing analyses performed under the most stringent safety precautions the agency had known.

Nobody, unless directly concerned, was allowed into a laboratory looking for the agent of legionnaires' disease. Each lab door carried a bold biohazard warning sign. Engineers continually balanced each lab's ventilation system to provide directional airflow from the corridor. Inside the labs, all staff were masked, gowned, and gloved. All their work was done in biological safety cabinets. All their protective clothing was autoclaved before they left. All waste was burned.

Throughout the maze of laboratories, researchers considered to be at the top of their professions were conducting a wide range of meticulous, ongoing experiments. There was no panic, no outward signs of urgency; even the rawest lab technician knew nothing could—or should —hasten or change the scientific procedures under way.

Slowly, often infinitely so, the process of detection unfolded.

Virologists, preparing nutrient broths on which they hoped viruses would grow, used ingredients that often sounded as though they had been culled from some biological cookbook—double-concentration vitamins, fetal bovine serum, Hank's balanced salt solution, and Eagle's basal medium. To this they added penicillin and streptomycin; the antibiotics were there to exclude bacteria from confusing the tests. Viruses were untouched by such drugs. Yet despite experiments involving cell cultures, eggs, and animals, as yet no viral agent had been isolated.

In the laboratories of the Viral Pathology Branch, scientists conducting electron microscope studies of legionnaires' lung tissue were so far seeing only what they expected to see: "the sort of bacteria that pile up in the lungs of people who die of pneumonia."

In the laboratories of the Division of Bacteriology, which was working mainly with white mice, the results were equally inconclusive. The division's director reported to Sencer, "From what we have done, there are no bacterial pathogens that we are able to demonstrate; if there's that sort there, it's one we don't know anything about."

In the laboratories of the Bureau of Epidemiology—charged with serving EIS officers such as Fraser in the field—nothing specific had been found, but tests were continuing on the material being regularly received from George Mallison.

In yet other CDC laboratories, tissue samples were being analyzed for abnormal concentrations of more than thirty metallic elements by using the very latest techniques: neutron activation, atomic absorption spectrophotometry, electron- and proton-induced X-ray fluorescence. Organic toxic substances were being looked for by high-pressure liquid chromatography, gas chromatography, and mass spectroscopy.

And in the Antimicrobics Investigations Section, experiments were in preparation to establish the most efficient antibiotic for fighting the disease. Among the twenty-two drugs chosen to be tested was the one used on Maria Reeves—erythromycin.

Collectively, it was an antiseptic world where men and women spoke easily about branched-chain amino acids and double bonds, where technicians compared the difference in retention times between methyl ester peaks and methyl ester standards. Above all, it was a world where there were no shortcuts and where precision was everything.

So far, a great deal had been learned about what the disease's alien agent was *not*. But its true identity remained as unknown as ever.

That situation, admitted the usually stoic Joe McDade, accentuated the "sense of curiosity" that normally motivated him. He was spending almost all of this Tuesday in the highly restricted hot lab of Building 7, continuing with his attempts to isolate the rickettsia which caused Q fever and which it was thought might have killed the legionnaires.

Dressed from top to toe in disposable garments, the chunky microbiologist turned to the last legionnaire lung tissue specimen he would deal with this day: J.B.'s.

Standing before a biological safety cabinet, McDade carefully ground up the thumbnail-sized tissue with a sterile mortar and pestle, using Alundum as an abrasive. He next suspended the ground-up tissue in a saline solution.

He then selected a 25-gauge hypodermic needle and carefully drew off some of the tissue suspension into a syringe.

McDade turned to the first of the four adult male guinea pigs he had just brought to the hot lab from the Animal Building. All were of the same age and weight, 600 grams (about 21 ounces). He gently picked up the animal, holding it so that the abdomen was exposed. He injected precisely 1 milliliter of the suspension into the abdominal cavity. Stroking the guinea pig, he replaced it in its cage. McDade then repeated the procedure with the other three animals. Previously he had similarly inoculated four guinea pigs with lung tissue from bus driver Andrew Hornack, and yet another four guinea pigs with tissue from the oldest legionnaire who had died, eighty-two-year-old Abe Ruben.

Now, with twelve guinea pigs inoculated, for the moment there was nothing more to be done.

McDade left the windowless isolation room and walked down a corridor past other laboratories where specimens were fed in by conveyor belt and scientists placed their hands through portholes fitted with long rubber gloves that extended into the rooms.

Before he could leave the building, McDade had to undress, pass through ultraviolet light, and shower.

Behind him an orderly gathered up his discarded garments. They would be autoclaved and incinerated.

It was early morning when McDade came out of Building 7 and mounted his bicycle for the two-mile ride home. There he would relax with his wife and children before going jogging, to complete what for him had been just another relatively "routine day at the lab."

Quit pushing, said Anna Taggart tersely.

The photographer apologized. The two reporters continued to bombard her with questions as the elevator descended to the lobby.

Was it true that room occupancy had fallen significantly since the Eucharistic Congress ended? Did she know the FBI was running checks on Puerto Rican and non-American employees? Had she heard the hotel was now the prime suspect in the whole investigation? What was it like working in a place that could be responsible for so many deaths?

Anna studiously ignored all the questions. Only her clenched fists betrayed her mounting fury at such outrageous suggestions.

The hotel security man standing beside her pleaded with the newsmen: Look, fellas, the lady doesn't want to talk. She can't talk. None of us can. It's a hotel rule. No talking to the press.

The reporters smiled at each other triumphantly. Had the staff been gagged? Was this part of a deliberate cover-up? Were the rumors after all true?

Anna glanced sharply at the security man. It was all his fault.

The man stared miserably at the elevator door, wishing he had stopped the newsmen when they first entered the hotel. Now he could hardly wait for the cage to reach the lobby and end this wretched journey from the eighteenth floor.

The reporters continued to question Anna. Was it true a medical detective had been searching the hotel for several days? Where was he now? Had she seen what he'd been collecting? What did he look like?

Anna gritted her teeth. So that's who the tall, gangling man was, the one whom both Mr. Varr and Mr. Chadwick called respectfully "Mr. Mallison." She smiled to herself: she *had* been right; he *was* a detective —though she couldn't be certain where a *medical* detective fitted into the police hierarchy.

The security man spoke again: Listen, fellas, anything you want to know you must get from Mr. Chadwick.

The reporters laughed derisively. It would be easier to get a Mafia boss to speak than persuade the hotelier to comment.

Anna glared again at the security man. If he had been doing his job properly he would not now be acting like a nervous sheepdog shepherding the three newsmen down from the Oak Room, where they had been caught searching for Mallison.

She knew where he was: up on the roof, watching the pigeons.

What sort of a job was that—watching birds making droppings and wandering around picking up all sorts of unconnected items? He must be crazy, she thought, spending hours out on the roof.

But she would never tell the reporters where he was. She would tell them *nothing*.

The elevator reached the lobby. Anna opened the cage.

The photographer backed out first, raising his camera, focusing on Anna.

She moved swiftly toward him, speaking at last: If he dared take her picture, let alone publish it, it would be the last thing he would do.

The fury in the voice of the petite chief elevator operator was strong enough to make the photographer quickly lower his camera.

Anna had one last piece of advice for the crestfallen newsmen: Stay away from the hotel. Let honest people get on with their living.

She watched them walk across the lobby and out into Broad Street.

The music of the string trio playing in the Stratford Garden dining room drifted across to Anna. It did little to lift her spirits. The reporters had been right: the hotel *was* being hit. Dozens of rooms were unoccupied; just as that darned local newspaper said, fear was stalking the Bellevue.

She walked quickly past the entrance to the Stratford Garden. The restaurant, with its high ceiling and soothing colors, renowned for its impeccable service and gourmet food, was almost empty. She continued to walk around the lobby, her experienced eye assimilating the signs. At reception a couple of room clerks were gossiping. Behind the cashier's grille a woman was reading a newspaper. A page was taking his time emptying the ashtrays scattered around the lobby. At his desk, the duty assistant manager stared broodingly at the bell captain's post, where half a dozen bellhops were marooned for lack of business. Small indications—but significant.

Anna moved past the wood-paneled Hunt Room. It was almost empty at an hour when the cocktail bar was normally crowded.

Those darned reporters, she thought again angrily: the hotel was reeling under what they were writing and now even the staff was becoming demoralized. Why didn't management fight back? Go to the media—hold daily press conferences, adopt an aggressive attitude? Instead Mr. Chadwick had sent another reminder that no one was to talk to the press. That, mused Anna, was playing into their hands. If nobody challenged what they wrote, they would go on asking even more impossible questions and publishing even more lies. She would dearly love to speak her mind.

She returned to stand before her elevator, still fuming at the way she had been questioned. What did those reporters really know, or care, about what it was like to be under suspicion, to know that jobs, futures, lives could be in jeopardy? Working at the Bellevue was like being part of a family. Reporters wouldn't understand that. All they cared about was getting a story.

Anna felt a lump in her throat; she bit the inside of her lip to hold back the tears.

Suddenly there was a flurry of activity by the Broad Street entrance. The doorman held open the door and the bell captain led a team of men toward the entrance.

So that's *them*, thought Anna grimly, staring at the group coming into the lobby.

Fraser and his superior were first, handing their suitcases to bellmen while looking inquisitively around the lobby.

Strange, seeing such a lovely hotel so empty, said Fraser's companion as he led the ten-strong CDC team toward the front desk.

Ted Tsai politely refused a bellman who wanted to carry his special specimen case.

Craven and Thacker ambled across the lobby, pausing at the newsstand, glancing into the cocktail bar and restaurant, nodding appreciatively at the ornate surroundings.

It sure beat hamburgers in Pittsburgh, Craven joked.

Or a motel in Harrisburg, added Thacker.

The bureau director and Fraser reached the front desk. One of the room clerks pushed a registration pad forward.

Fraser spoke: The CDC party was prebooked.

His words had an immediate effect.

Both room clerks looked up at the guests, smiling welcomes. The assistant manager came forward, solicitous respect in his voice. The bell captain and his team hovered around, beaming, saying it was nice to have them all stay at the Bellevue. The clerks shuffled reservation and room slips.

The EIS officers began to crowd around the registration desk. None of the CDC group noticed two men in formal dress standing on the marble staircase.

Should they meet them now? Varr asked Chadwick.

No, murmured the hotelier, let them check in. Time enough in the morning. The two men turned and walked back up the staircase.

Clerks were calling out names. Dr. Fraser and his chief were allocated the Delaware Suite on the third floor.

The bell captain stepped forward to lead them to the elevator.

Dr. Craven—311.

A bellboy picked up the key to a large single room overlooking Broad Street.

Dr. Thacker and Dr. Tsai—408.

The two had decided to share and had been given a spacious corner room that overlooked both Broad and Walnut streets.

Walking toward the elevator, Tsai confided to Thacker that in spite of all its trappings and grandeur the Bellevue still gave him a spooky feeling.

Tsai would likely have been even more concerned had he known the reason they were staying in the hotel. Fraser was using them all—himself included—as human guinea pigs. If any of the team became ill, it would strongly suggest that the unknown killer was still somewhere in the building.

Al Gaudiosi growled into the telephone: *How many?* Automatically he reached for a yellow legal pad; nowadays he soon filled one after another with scrawled notes about the epidemic.

Polk repeated the figure: Thirty-two. The acting health commissioner added: Some of them have checked into the Bellevue.

Gaudiosi scribbled the figure on the pad. He settled back in his chair, one elegantly shod foot resting on an open desk drawer, the other tapping impatiently on the carpet, trying to keep pace with his thoughts.

Thirty-two CDC officers in the city was startling enough; that a number of them were actually staying at the Bellevue was potentially explosive. Gaudiosi's well-developed gut instinct told him their presence in the hotel was no coincidence.

He barked into the phone: That way they could monitor the Bellevue around the clock. Right?

Polk remained confident. His people had combed the place. Nothing.

Gaudiosi repeated: *Nothing?* Nobody found *nothing?* How come? There was something wrong with every building. Small things, maybe, but something wrong. Everybody knew that. That was the way of things.

But, Al, nothing serious had surfaced at the Bellevue. A few minor faults. Nothing to get excited about. . . .

Gaudiosi wasn't really listening. His gut signaled potential trouble: *somewhere in all this a time bomb is ticking.*

Still cradling the phone, he stood up, loosened his shirt collar, and looked out over the city, staring at the downtown section. He couldn't pick out the Bellevue in the fusion of lights. He didn't have to—just as he knew he didn't need a map to see that if the hotel was threatened it could have serious repercussions for the entire area. In many ways the Bellevue was the hub around which so much of center-city Philadelphia revolved. Its presence dominated the business and shopping districts; its massive, craggy grayness gave substance to an area of new skyscrapers and blocks of uniformly unexceptional shops, broken here and there by the raw emptiness of asphalt parking lots. Without the Bellevue, the aspect would be even more dismal. The hotel, as Gaudiosi had told out-of-town reporters, was one of Philadelphia's great assets—the epitome of that impossible-to-define Philadelphia Taste. It bore, like a thumbprint, the impress of playing host to generations of old Philadelphian families. It was in the same category as the Free Library, the Franklin Institute, and the Museum of Art. They, and many other venerated institutions in the vicinity of the Bellevue, would be grievously hurt if anything happened to the hotel.

The Bellevue was a magnet that attracted people and business to the entire downtown section.

To Al Gaudiosi the situation was agonizing. From the start of the investigation he had insisted there must be no fudging, no cover-ups, no granting of exemptions or favors. In rigidly enforcing that rule, he had, in turn, been brusque, rude, and abrasive—some even said cruel—in his decision-making. Yet even his enemies had often not only shown grudging respect for the iron control he kept on the flow of information out of City Hall on the epidemic, but also come to accept every fact he released as gilt-edged truth.

Late on this Tuesday night, Gaudiosi knew that no matter what the consequences, he would not begin to lie now—not even to save the Bellevue. On the other hand, he would take every legitimate step to protect the hotel.

He slouched back in his chair and began rapidly to question Polk.

Who knew the CDC were staying at the hotel?

Polk guessed: Nobody—yet.

Gaudiosi scribbled a reminder: Call Chadwick.

He barked again into the phone: Was Fraser still in charge of the Feds?

Yes.

Would he want to talk to the media?

Polk's answer was unequivocal. No. He had avoided the press while in Harrisburg. He'd told Sharrar he'd do the same here—

Gaudiosi interrupted: Was it true Sharrar was going on vacation?

Polk began to explain.

Gaudiosi growled: Everybody was tired. He returned to Fraser. What else did Polk know about him?

He could be prickly—as Bachman had discovered.

Gaudiosi laughed. At least Bachman was out of his hair. How was Fraser going to operate?

Polk explained. Fraser controlled the CDC team. It meant he was effectively running the investigation.

Gaudiosi bristled. Didn't Polk have any say?

Consultation—yes. Control—no. The CDC people were a self-contained unit. Polk groped for a graphic comparison: a bit like the Green Berets in a normal army command; the EIS team was highly trained and highly individualistic. Polk had a question: Would Gaudiosi like to meet Fraser?

Again, Gaudiosi's instinct prevailed. No, anything he wanted to know from Fraser, or vice versa, would be passed through Polk. That way lines couldn't get crossed. The arrangement also gave Gaudiosi an advantage should he require one: he could keep Fraser at a distance while swiftly reaching him anytime he wished.

After he had finished talking to Polk, Gaudiosi sat quietly and thought. The presence of the EIS officers in the hotel could be handled in two ways. The media could again be told that whatever had caused the outbreak was no longer a threat. He could argue, with considerable force, that the very presence of the medical detectives as guests in the hotel was additional proof of this. He believed not even the most dedicated investigator would deliberately expose himself to possible death. Yes: there was a persuasive case to be argued that the mysterious killer had gone and that the city should put the dreadful affair behind it and resume the serious business of celebrating the Bicentennial.

Yet Gaudiosi hesitated. The sheer number of EIS officers now in the city clearly suggested that they were searching for something they thought was still there—that possibly the killer could be lurking, replenishing itself, preparing to strike again. Perhaps, developing Polk's analogy about the Green Berets, he should look upon the CDC team as a commando unit about to smoke out the enemy. Yet that tactic could well damage the Bellevue. Already some press reports seemed strongly to suggest that the hotel was somehow implicated in the epidemic. If it became known that EIS officers were now actually living in the Bellevue, it would not only focus further unwelcome attention on the hotel—the newspaperman in Gaudiosi told him it would be too good an angle to pass up—but could considerably contribute to its difficulties.

He called Chadwick and said the presence of his CDC guests was not to be publicized.

Gaudiosi continued to brood.

Even from the little he had gleaned from Polk, Fraser sounded formidable. And in his press interviews he came across as strong-minded and determined; during his appearance on the "Today" show, he had shown himself to be completely in command. It would be sensible, then, not only to keep him at a distance but also to give him a free hand. And if things worked out well—if the agent was identified and a suitable medicament produced to combat it—there would still be a possibility of apportioning credit, of ensuring that a degree of luster rubbed off on what even Gaudiosi recognized was the tarnished image of the Rizzo administration.

The mayor's position as head of one of the most powerful cities in the nation daily became more insecure. With Gaudiosi's blessing, Frank Rizzo had just gone on vacation, in part to prepare himself for the recall hearing result due next month. In an almost unprecedented move, a large portion of the electorate planned to oust the controversial mayor from office before his term ended. Inevitably Gaudiosi, being so closely associated with Rizzo, had come under attack. Over his handling of information on the epidemic the media was especially caviling. The *Daily News* accused him of news management. And *Philadelphia Magazine*—a vociferous antiestablishment monthly—was about to publish a wounding diatribe guaranteed to fan the criticism.

The personal attacks, as such, did not unduly bother Gaudiosi: he was thick-skinned enough to shrug them off. The reports angered him only because they portrayed what he felt was an unfair picture of how the epidemic could best be handled; he was controlling the information flow to try to ensure responsible reporting. And he doubted any of the hundreds of reporters covering the story had any idea of the tremendous effort he had made. There were, he knew, few other people in Philadelphia who could have worked harder—or achieved more. And yet, for all his expansive and outgoing manner, he was reluctant to project himself. By nature he was not a braggart.

Given the chance, Frank Rizzo might have behaved differently. But nowadays Rizzo was a figurehead; a common belief was that Gaudiosi had deliberately placed the mayor on the back burner—"out of sight, out of mind."

If that was so, Gaudiosi still maintained the closest contact with Rizzo; they spoke as often as twenty times a day on the telephone.

And as always, when Gaudiosi reported the arrival of the EIS officers at the Bellevue, the mayor immediately agreed with his chief lieutenant's decision: their presence as guests should not be revealed to the press.

Gaudiosi looked out again over the city and for a moment visualized a scenario in which the downtown area became a wilderness, devoid of tourists, a place to be totally avoided. The prospect was even more scary than having Frank Rizzo booted out of office.

And more than ever Gaudiosi was determined to do everything in his power to ensure that neither of those circumstances occurred.

George Mallison casually tacked himself on to the cleaning party making its way toward the Bellevue kitchen and coffee. It was barely dawn and, as Mallison had planned, there were few people about to notice him. In his coveralls and stout boots he looked like one of the hotel's engineers. The cleaners didn't give him a second glance.

Reaching the kitchen, he paused to watch the early shift at work; it was a reflex action, to check against memory whether anything different was happening at this time of day than had happened during his previous walks through the area. He spotted nothing unusual.

One of the woman cleaners was listening attentively to a kitchen hand animatedly describing something; the man was continually gesturing to make his point in between carrying trays of eggs to the breakfast cooks. Caught up by his story, the woman went with him to a storeroom. Both of them were momentarily out of sight. When they emerged, the cleaner bid her companion farewell and walked out of the kitchen past Mallison.

Even the worldly-wise sanitary engineer—seldom if every surprised by anything—would undoubtedly have been astonished to know that, suspended on a hook between her legs, the woman carried a plastic-wrapped chunk of prime cut.

Mallison walked from the kitchen, heading for the subbasement.

The cavernous area at this early hour of Wednesday, August 11, was deserted, the wine cellar locked, and the laundry in darkness. He picked his way past the clutter of laundry baskets and empty wine cases. From the dimly lit engine room came the steady hum of machinery. Days before, Mallison had inspected the facility and the adjoining area containing the hotel's main circuits and fuses and had found nothing untoward except for the leaking air-conditioning chiller unit. He passed the incinerator, glimpsing through the doorway its solitary guardian patiently sifting the refuse for retrievables.

Mallison reached a gloomy space beside the incinerator and paused to get his bearings. He swung his flashlight slowly along the wall until the beam rested on a set of iron steps anchored to the wall. He let the light travel up the rungs. The trapdoor set in the ceiling hardly looked big enough for even his spare frame.

He patted a coverall pocket, checking that his smoke pencil was securely clipped. From another pocket he fished out a pair of gloves and put them on. Then, gripping the flashlight in his right hand, he began to climb the ladder, carefully testing each rung to make sure it would bear his weight. Close to the ceiling he reached up with his left hand. The trap creaked upward, sending a shower of fine debris down on his head. Craning his neck, Mallison directed the beam into the stale-smelling hole. The light bounced off the metal walls and ceiling of the air duct.

Mallison was about to pursue his theory that droppings from sick pigeons might have been carried by the flow of air through the hotel's ventilation units. It was conceivable the droppings could have come into the building through the fresh-air intakes set in the hotel's side walls. But if so, how had they been distributed from there?

He had already made a study of potential routes, establishing that there were some ventilating units receiving fresh air through sunken window wells, others from air shafts running from the basement up to the seventeenth floor. Ventilating units on the upper floors—excluding the loft where he had found that faulty cross-connection with the hosepipe—brought in fresh air through louvered grilles in the side of the building. The grilles were sufficiently fine to prevent birds from entering the ventilation system but not, of course, their droppings or dust. Some of the grilles faced onto internal light wells and others onto the street. He had been interested to see there were light wells adjoining the ceiling of the ballroom—where the Legion's formal sessions had been held—and around the rooftop Oak Room and Rose Garden, where the conventioneers had held their Go-Getter's Breakfast.

Mallison also studied the various types of air-conditioner units used in the hotel. Some were self-contained and mounted into windows, such as those serving the bedrooms on the sixteenth floor. A single large unit served the basement beauty shop, as did another the Viennese Room off the lobby. These packaged units had been checked, and samples of dust taken from them. And then there was the ventilation unit located above the reception desk, which served that area only. Unlike other ventilation units in the hotel, this particular vent provided only recycled air, without any fresh air content whatsoever. Graitcer had been quick to spot the possible significance of its malfunctioning. But in a way that raised more questions than answers. At some stage almost every guest in the hotel came to the front desk, yet not every guest had been taken ill. Again, while a few of the staff working in the vicinity of the unit had complained of headaches, none of them developed symptoms that fitted the case definition for legionnaires' disease. And because the unit had recently been cleaned, there was now no real way of establishing whether it was really implicated in the outbreak. Mallison planned to inspect the unit later this morning, but he doubted he would learn much. It was tantalizing to think that if he had known about it a few days before, he might well have discovered something important. His only hope now—and one he didn't rate highly—was that since the unit had been cleaned five days ago, fresh deposits of dust might have accumulated in its mechanism that could provide a clue.

Mallison had also learned that 25 percent of the air throughout the Bellevue was supposed to be in a constant process of removal by exhaust fans and through a number of other outlets from the hotel. Because of the stack effect in tall buildings, air also tended to move upward through stairwells and elevator shafts—a phenomenon Fraser had been aware of when formulating his Elevator Theory—to be exhausted at the upper levels. All this exhausted air was of course replaced by fresh air, drawn in mainly through intakes into the ventilation system. And it was by this means that small particles of sick pigeon droppings could have entered, spreading the psittacosis Mallison believed might have caused the outbreak.

What he was about to do was not only dirty work but dangerous into the bargain. He was going to begin to explore the ducts along which such infected air could have traveled.

He reached up and placed the flashlight on the floor of the duct. In its beam he could see twenty feet along the square-walled tunnel before it reached a T junction.

Mallison eased himself up, moving slowly, anxious not to disturb the thick layer of dust on the floor. When his head touched the roof, he paused, his feet still on the ladder, his body half into the duct. He scooped some of the dust into a small plastic envelope, which he sealed with wire and stowed in a coverall pocket.

He bent forward, pulling himself slowly up into the duct, pushing the torch ahead of him, the noise echoing in the confined space.

Mallison was now kneeling on his elbows and knees, very much like a combat soldier about to crawl into the unknown. The bulk of his body blocked out the light from the trapdoor behind him. His shoulders rubbed against the metal walls. The air smelled unpleasant.

He began to move forward. He breathed slowly, lifting his head to inhale and exhale so as not to scatter the dust under his elbows and knees.

He quickly established the best way to move. He pushed the flashlight forward with his right hand a foot or so. He brought his left hand and knee forward in one move. Then he completed the maneuver by bringing his right knee level, leaning forward from his hips to gain additional stability.

In this manner he reached the T junction. He paused, fishing for his smoke pencil. He held it at arm's length before him. He pressed the switch. A tiny whiff of smoke puffed into the air. In the light he watched it slowly eddy and dissipate. It was enough to indicate the direction of air flow in the duct. He turned the corner and crawled in that direction for a few feet. It was time to collect another sample. He scooped dust into a fresh envelope, sealed it, and pocketed it. Analysis would determine how long the dust had been in the duct; judging from experience, Mallison thought it might have been there almost from the time the duct had been installed over twenty years before.

He crawled a few more feet and stopped. Tracks. There was no doubt at all that the faint zigzagging lines were tracks. Moving with infinite care, he turned on one side, supporting himself on an elbow to make himself comfortable while he studied the traces more closely. They were old and almost indiscernible. He lowered his head, staring at close range at the marks in the dust. They weren't pigeon tracks. He couldn't be certain, but they looked like rodent trails. Somewhere in this confined space could be rats. He scooped up a portion of the dust with the tracks; back in Atlanta laboratory tests would establish what animal had made the marks.

Mallison resumed his crawling position, his eyes straining ahead, pausing from time to time for any telltale scurrying sounds. A cornered rat in this enclosed area could be a formidable foe.

He reached a crossroads of four pipes. The dust here was different; it contained what looked suspiciously like rodent droppings. There was no doubt now: the channels were natural runs for the rats which, despite stringent precautions, still inhabited the building.

Mallison used his smoke pencil. The air flow was down the right-hand branch of this intersection. He moved forward into the new duct, then reversed slightly, bumping his body against the roof of the shaft in the process. He paused to look down the route he had just traveled. He could discern a faint glimmer at the T junction, reflected light from the trapdoor opening. He moved forward a few feet into the new duct and turned his head to glance behind between his elbow and body. Now there was nothing but darkness.

He stared ahead. The beam of light bounced back, half blinding him. He pinched shut his eyes for a few moments and then opened them. It helped to relieve the glare. He resumed crawling.

After a few more feet he paused to use his smoke pencil. The air current was stronger here. He guessed he might be near one of the shafts rising through the building.

His palms and knees hurt. And in spite of his care, the dust was hovering in a fine cloud around him.

Another junction. Another test puff of smoke. He had to crawl into a tunnel to his left, which seemed to be rising.

Suddenly he heard it: a strange swishing sound. He felt the hair on the nape of his neck rise. There it was again. *Swiiissshhh.* He froze, pulling the torch closer to him, wishing now he had brought some sort of weapon to defend himself. *Swiiissshhh.* He held his breath, trying to identify how far away the sound was. He breathed out slowly. About fifteen feet ahead was yet another junction. The sound appeared to be coming from one of the ducts branching off the intersection.

Mallison continued to crawl forward, moving warily, frequently stopping to hold his breath while he tried to determine what was causing the sound. He didn't know too much about rats, but this sound didn't match the rustling of rodents back in the Animal Building at the CDC. If it was a rat, it must be a large one.

He arrived at the junction. In turn he shone his torch down the ducts and on either side of the one he was in. There was nothing to see.

But the sound was much louder here. And now it was not just swishing but gurgling, intermingling, one sound on top of the other. He remained totally still, tracing in his mind how far he had crawled and what part of the hotel he had reached.

He smiled with relief. He was probably over the laundry. The noise he could hear was from the washing machines filling and spinning.

Mallison inched forward, trying to keep a rhythm between elbows and knees, concentrating hard to blot out the reverberating sound.

He pushed forward the torch—and his hand touched something furry and hard.

He quickly pulled back his hand, staring at the rat, dried out and withered by the poison that the hotel's rodent killers regularly put down.

Mallison moved on past the carcass.

Rats' teeth, that's what the old crone's pointed and discolored incisors reminded him of as she quacked like a duck.

Graitcer had finally found the Pigeon Lady in an alley close to the Bellevue. He continued to ignore the curious stares of passersby as he tried to find some way of making her talk.

"Have any of your pigeons been sick?"

"Quack-quack-quack!" The woman ruffled her rags.

"Quack—yes? Or quack—no?"

"Quack-quack-quack!"

"Okay. Have you seen any dead pigeons?"

The crone rolled her eyes.

"Where did you see them?"

She shook her head.

"You mean you didn't see them?"

She quacked several times.

"Would you like a drink? A coffee maybe?"

"Quack-quack-quack-quack!"

"Some bird seed . . . for your feathered friends?"

Another burst of quacking accompanied by a birdlike shaking of her head.

Graitcer thought: *She's as crazy as a loon; Philadelphia's famous Pigeon Lady isn't that at all—she's a Duck Lady!*

"Do you have enough food for your birds?"

"Quack-quack!" The crone patted her bags of moldering bread.

"Can I see?"

"Quack." She pulled the bags closer to her.

"Where did you get the bread?"

She quacked several times.

"Where's that?"

"Quack! Quack! Quack!"

The woman sounded irritated.

Graitcer tried again. "Can you tell me, in words, where you got the bread?"

"Quack."

"That means yes—"

"Quack."

"—or no?"

"Quack."

"Have you always quacked?"

"Quack."

"Why?"

"Quack-quack-quack!"

Graitcer shook his head, defeated. He had run another lead to ground—and like so many others, it had finally proven fruitless.

He smiled at the crone. "Lady, you just quacked yourself out of our investigation."

She quacked happily on as he left her.

16

Realization

The bedroom curtains were drawn back, for this was high summer and Doris liked to sleep with the window open. She watched the light pale from gray-blackness to a milky white which became flushed with the pink and gold that were the harbingers of another fine day. The sun, she knew, would continue to wither the flowers and fade the inscriptions on the wreaths.

And, she reflected, it was not only Jimmy and J.B. who had died so suddenly: almost overnight, the entire town had changed. Those who had gone to the convention, or who had relatives who went, found themselves isolated. She had almost gotten used to the way people moved away from her in the stores and on the streets. She kept reminding herself they were frightened, that it was all so understandable.

Doris looked at the calendar on the wall opposite the bed: Friday, August 13—the start of the ninth day since Jimmy had been put in the ground.

Normally the day and date would have fanned her superstitions about bad luck. Instead, she felt surprisingly optimistic, as if she were awakening from a long sleep and something had told her life still had much to offer.

She thought: *The sun will rise over his grave, warming the earth.*

Doris lay quietly, listening to the dawn chorus of birds and watching the sky change and deepen.

Other thoughts returned, stronger than they had been the last time: *Jimmy is dead, I am alive. He's gone forever. I feel my life is only beginning, even though in years it's probably half over. Jimmy would*

want me to go on living, not to forget him, but also not to live with no
purpose.

She watched the sun creep over the horizon. The light grew more intense, picking out the grain and patterns on the old, familiar furniture.

Doris continued to think: *Jimmy is dead—that part of my life is dead. I must not waste the time ahead. He would not want that. I must plan a proper future. The kids need me. That's what he would have wanted.*

With every passing moment, she felt better, stronger, and more certain.

The sun was climbing; it was going to be a perfect day. Through the wall she heard the children awakening and talking to each other.

Doris kicked back the sheet and trod barefoot across the faded carpet. Jimmy had always said they must get a new one—

She stopped: she must quit thinking like that. The decisions now were hers alone to make. She looked at the carpet. It would stand a lot more wear. Its replacement would have to wait. There were more important things.

Doris could hear the children whispering and laughing at the same time. She thought: *We're all coming out of a tunnel; we're in the light, alone, but together.*

She opened the wardrobe and began systematically to take out Jimmy's clothes, folding them neatly in a pile on the bed. They'd go toward paying the bills that had accumulated.

Doris had also planned to sell Jimmy's car, but Dicko stepped in. It was the first time he had spoken to her since the funeral. His voice on the phone had been cold and formal. The car was not hers to sell. That's all he had said; not a word about how she was making out, how the kids were, what her plans might be. It was as if, with Jimmy dead, she was no longer of any importance to Dicko.

Even now, as she folded the last of Jimmy's things, her anger at Dicko's attitude gave Doris a hollow pain in her stomach. It was, she thought sadly, so typical of him just to think of the car. Sweet Jesus, he can have the car. She would manage.

The bedroom door burst open and the children stood there, staring at the pile of clothes.

Charlie, the oldest, broke the silence. "Mom, what are you going to do with them?"

"Sell them to help us."

"Mommy, won't Jimmy need them when he meets Jesus?" asked little Trina.

"No, hon, Jimmy's got all he needs."

"Mom, will you get enough to buy me a pair of sneakers?" asked Tommy.

"I'll get you all sneakers," she promised. "Now go and get dressed."

The phone rang. She looked at her watch. Who could it be at this early hour?

Doris picked up the receiver. It was Virginia Anne. She had been adding up the bill for Jimmy's funeral. It came to $1,800. Could Doris send over a check?

"Eighteen hundred dollars. But that's a fortune."

Not really, said Virginia Anne sharply, not for the best funeral the Ralphs could lay on.

"Virginia Anne. Right now I don't have eighteen dollars to spare. You're going to have to wait."

Mrs. Ralph came on the line. She was firm. Doris must pay the bill.

"I haven't the money. I'm trying to sort things out but it's going to take time."

What about insurance?

"I've no idea."

Doris ended further discussion by putting down the phone. She thought: *The Ralphs must be getting over their loss to be out chasing money at such an early hour.*

She was still worrying about the call when later that morning there was a knock at the door. A stranger stood there. He showed her an ID card; the man was from the Department of Defense. He explained he was looking for a key that Jimmy must have brought home with him.

Doris was incredulous. "You've come all this way for a key?"

The man smiled. Did she know where it was?

"No. But you can have a look."

While he searched, she tried to question him further. What was so important about a key? What had Jimmy used it for? And anyway, what exactly had been Jimmy's job at Fort Indiantown Gap? Was it something to do with the CIA—

Had Jimmy told her that? The man looked at Doris carefully.

"Well, he sort of hinted. Said his work was top-secret."

The man said nothing.

"You from the CIA, too?"

He shook his head.

"Then what do you do?"

He looked for lost keys. The man turned away to search a kitchen cupboard. Soon afterward he found the key and left as mysteriously as he had arrived.

His visit made the lasting impression on Doris that somehow the key was not only connected with Jimmy's secret work but could also be linked with his death. Maybe Virginia Anne was right about her sabotage theory. Doris wished suddenly she had not put down the phone on Mrs. Ralph. It might have been helpful to ask her daughter some questions. No chance of that now.

With tender, almost loving care, Joe McDade used his gloved right hand to insert the thermometer into the rectum of a guinea pig that had been inoculated with lung tissue from J.B. Even though he was completely masked and gowned, McDade took infinite care in how he handled the animal; its watery eyes, ruffled fur, and signs of increasing prostration clearly indicated it was dying.

Since inoculating the twelve animals, the microbiologist had carefully observed and taken the temperature of each at regular intervals. Now, three days after injection, some of them were showing signs of being acutely ill, especially those inoculated with tissue from J.B. and Hornack.

McDade withdrew the thermometer. The mercury stood at 41 degrees Celsius—106 degrees Fahrenheit. The guinea pig's high fever had remained constant since its onset two days ago; the animal could not survive more than a few hours.

He took the animal to a small, totally sealed cabinet and placed it inside. Within minutes it was dead, painlessly killed by carbon dioxide vapor pumped into the cabinet. He waited for the gas to clear and then took out the animal.

McDade placed it on a dissection table inside the lab's biological safety cabinet, where he would be protected by the all-important flow of sterilized air. He swabbed the guinea pig's stomach with surgical spirit. Then he dipped first a pair of forceps and then scissors in an ethanol solution and passed each instrument through a flame. He used them both to open the animal.

He then repeated the process with a second set of identical forceps and scissors before using them to remove the animal's spleen, liver, and lungs.

McDade used the scissors to snip off a small sliver of each organ from which he would later prepare slides to be examined under the microscope. He then placed the remainder of the spleen in a sterile mortar, adding a little Alundum to act as an abrasive. He ground up the spleen and diluted it in a phosphate-buffered saline solution to form a 10 percent tissue suspension. McDade did the same with the animal's liver and lungs, keeping the three 10 percent tissue suspensions in separate vials. Afterward, in an attempt to grow artificially whatever organism had caused the guinea pigs to become sick, a measured amount of each of these suspensions would be inoculated into various bacteriologic mediums.

But now McDade prepared to inoculate chicken eggs with the tissue suspensions in the hope that within a few days the organism would grow inside them. He first measured out 1 milliliter of each of the three suspensions into separate test tubes. The unused suspensions would be flash-frozen and stored at minus 70 degrees Celsius for possible future use.

The microbiologist had already placed in the lab's biological cabinet a dozen embryonated hens' eggs. Each egg was between six and seven days old. Since other CDC labs had effectively ruled out a bacterium as the agent causing legionnaires' disease, he was anxious that no bacteria should be present to confuse the results of his work. The guinea pig just sacrificed should have acted as a biological filter, successfully destroying most harmful bacteria while at the same time succumbing to the rickettsiae. As an additional precaution against a bacterial reaction's confusing his findings, the eggs contained penicillin and streptomycin, which should preclude any remaining possibility of a bacterial contaminant.

McDade carefully inspected, or candled, each egg to confirm it was healthy. He would inoculate four with lung tissue suspension, four with liver suspension, and the remainder with spleen suspension. He numbered the eggs with a soft lead pencil and then turned to the spleen suspension in the test tube. He transferred 1 milliliter to another test tube containing 9 milliliters of saline solution, to dilute the 10 percent spleen suspension down to a 1 percent suspension. He would do the same later with the liver and lung suspensions.

The microbiologist reached for a 6-milliliter syringe fitted with a 20-gauge, 1½-inch needle. He completely filled the syringe with the 1 percent solution. Next he covered the needle with a safety shield and cautiously placed the syringe on the work surface.

He returned to the eggs, selecting them in the sequence they had been numbered. He held the first in his left hand and disinfected its top with an ethanol solution. He waited for the disinfectant to dry. He picked up an egg punch and immersed it in a 70 percent solution of alcohol, and then passed the instrument through a flame. Satisfied it was sterile, he used the punch to puncture the top of the egg.

McDade picked up the syringe and inserted the needle completely inside the egg. He depressed the plunger to inoculate precisely one half milliliter of the guinea pig's spleen suspension. Finally he sealed the egg with Duco cement and placed it in an incubator.

He then began to repeat the painstaking process with the second egg.

In his private suite on the Bellevue's eighth floor, Chadwick pushed aside his plate. The food had been perfectly prepared by Castelli. But,

Chadwick growled at his solitary luncheon companion, Harold Varr, he had little appetite.

Varr again murmured that Chadwick was putting himself under too much pressure.

Chadwick stared morosely across the dining table.

That they were here at all, thought Varr, was a pointer. Normally they took their meals in the Stratford Garden. Today, at Chadwick's suggestion, they were lunching in the suite so they could talk without being interrupted or overheard. Varr had arrived just as Pat Chadwick was leaving to attend one of her charity functions; in his wife's presence, her husband had been almost relaxed and carefree. As soon as she left, Chadwick's mood changed, and the anxiety that nowadays he found so hard to shake off returned, clouding his face. Momentarily Varr wondered whether Chadwick really thought he was fooling his wife. Pat was a shrewd observer. She must, he guessed, know the truth: her husband's lifetime's work was now under serious threat. And with that the threat to his health grew that much greater.

The Bellevue had become a huge research laboratory, a test-bed for doctors, scientists, engineers, and even police officers to work in—all under the additional scrutiny of scores of reporters, photographers, and TV crews.

Mallison, Varr thought bitterly, had been "the shout which launched the avalanche." Now other investigators, independent consultants brought in by the city, were checking the hotel's ventilation and air-conditioning systems, the kitchen, the fixtures and furnishings, the chemicals used by the maids and cleaning crews; even the pesticides employed to keep down vermin were being taken away for analysis.

Though the media had still not realized EIS officers were actually guests in the hotel—an irony that made Chadwick wince—Varr was unhappily aware of their presence in the building. And now there was a proposal to ask legionnaires who were recovering from their illness to return to the hotel and retrace their movements during the convention. The legionnaires would be accompanied by EIS officers. Philadelphia's deputy health commissioner had announced he wanted each epidemiologist "to look for whatever he thinks might be relevant; we want to know what bed a legionnaire slept in, where and when they went to the bathroom—everything in as much detail as possible."

Varr feared that this idea, once the press got hold of it, could be disastrous. Yet he knew to protest would be pointless. Many of the same activities were also being pursued at the other hotels where the legionnaires stayed. And only this morning, when he encountered Mallison clambering down out of a duct, the CDC specialist had explained one of their objectives was to collect comparable data. If, for example, a substance or microbe found in the Bellevue looked suspicious, it might be ruled out if tests showed the same agent was in hotels where no guest got sick. Varr had accompanied Mallison to the lobby, where the sanitary engineer had stood on a ladder and removed the grille over the air-conditioning vent above the registration desk. He then carefully scooped out black dust. Afterward he photographed the hole. It was all done in full view of reporters; what was even more upsetting for Varr was the effect Mallison's actions had on the lobby staff. He had heard a bellman say, "If it's up there, we're dead."

Once more Varr had realized there was little he could do. To bar the media would be to invite a retaliatory blitzkrieg which might not only totally demoralize the staff but empty the hotel of guests. He felt he must continue to set an example to the other employees by displaying steadfast resolve. His own immediate, and still unspoken, concern was how Chadwick would continue to cope.

Increasingly, Varr felt an almost overwhelming sense of sadness for the older man. In virtually everything he said or did, Chadwick indicated that the hotel was for him a way of life which he had inherited at its peak and which seemed to be slipping from his grasp.

It had been partly Chadwick's old-fashioned attitude that had attracted Varr to join him in the first place. They made a perfect team: Chadwick the genial host, Varr the capable administrator. Now the even-handed partnership was disrupted. Chadwick frequently had to attend board meetings of Bankers Security, the Bellevue's owners, to help try and decide how best to meet the worsening situation. He was also sticking to his policy of almost never talking to the press.

The behavior of most of the reporters, Varr knew, continued to upset his superior. He had once lost sufficient control of himself to describe them as "a plague of locusts, hammering questions down the phone, trampling through the public rooms, snapping photographs and still more questions as if they were in at a kill."

Varr could understand such anger. But he believed the fight should be carried back to the media. He had his own ideas how that could be done. And knowing what was going on in the hotel even at this moment, he believed more than ever that the time for action was overdue.

Since early this morning two senior engineers had been conducting, on behalf of Philadelphia's water and health departments, a cross-connection survey. It arose partially from Mallison's discovery of the makeshift hosepipe arrangement in the loft. Varr regarded the outcome of the survey—basically intended to establish whether contaminants *might* somehow enter the hotel's supply of drinking water—to be a foregone conclusion. He was willing to bet there was not a hotel in the city, probably in the whole country, of a similar age to the Bellevue, where some cross-connection faults could not be found.

And sure enough, within a short time of the inspectors' starting their checks in the basement area, one of them noticed in the laundry that the starch blender had an unprotected potable water inlet at the bottom. Given very unusual circumstances, impure water *might* backflow into the hotel's drinking water system. Nearby, the bleach crocks were seen to be fed with potable water from submerged hoses, providing the same potential for back-feeding. And so it had gone on: one small fault after another noted in the inspectors' books.

When he heard about these discoveries, Varr regarded them as no more serious than the sort of faults that must almost inevitably occur in the somewhat antiquated plumbing systems of older hotels; in no way could these infractions be seriously considered a major health hazard: the remote possibility of a small amount of soapy water flowing the wrong way hardly constituted a real risk. And the hotel's systems had successfully passed the previous regular inspections. Nothing had changed. Why all the fuss now? Nobody was saying such faults should be ignored, only that they should be placed in perspective. To talk of them as "violations" was, in Varr's view, preposterous—it was also just the sort of emotive word the press could leap upon. They did: the nineteen separate "violations" unearthed after a great deal of diligent peering and poking this morning would bring a further crop of what Varr firmly believed were misleading headlines; additionally, the media would make almost no mention at all that similar faults were found in the five other Philadelphia hotels examined about the same time.

Though he feared the cross-connection survey could only bring trouble, Varr, over luncheon, kept such disconsolate thoughts from Chadwick. Instead he began to paint an optimistic picture. Business in the restaurants and bars had started to improve—

Without warning Chadwick pounded the table. "My God! Don't you see? We're having to dance to their tune! Any two-bit reporter can walk in here and ask the most God-awful questions and then write what they like!"

It was the opening Varr needed. But first he had to clear the ground.

"We have lawyers."

Chadwick reacted sourly. "So we sue. It'll take months, maybe years, to bring the case to court. By then it could be over for us."

Varr began to speak. While it was true the hotel was caught up in a publicity treadmill that threatened to drown them all, there was a way out—

"How?"

"Advertise. Locally, then across the nation. In every major newspaper."

Chadwick smiled bleakly. "Harry, you know what that would cost. A couple million. Maybe more. I doubt even Bankers Security has that sort of money available."

Varr, appraisingly, looked at Chadwick. He must not be allowed to lapse into defeat. If they could not afford to advertise widely, they must do the next best thing: get the Bellevue the sort of editorial coverage that would negate the unfavorable publicity it was receiving.

"Bill, we've got to hire the best PR firm in town."

"That sounds like a vote of no confidence in me."

Varr shook his head quickly. "Anything but." He wished now he hadn't put it so baldly; Chadwick prided himself on being the best publicist the hotel had. "Bill, they'd follow up your contacts, your ideas. Give us their ideas. Produce a campaign to save the hotel."

For a moment Chadwick's expression changed and Varr wondered whether he had still gone too far.

"You really think it has come to that?"

Varr knew there was no turning back. "Yes. This is the biggest fight you've had. You need all the help going."

"Tell me."

While Chadwick listened, Varr developed his arguments: a professional publicist could act as a buffer against the media; he could prepare and arrange for the publication of proper rebuttal stories; he could remind the nation that one of its most venerable hostelries was endangered; he could recruit famous people who had stayed at the hotel to lend their support or even their presence; he could arrange events in the hotel that would draw favorable press comment; he might even produce some sort of function where the elite of Philadelphia society would come to bestow a special accolade on what had traditionally been its first choice of hotel.

When Varr finally finished, Chadwick remained deep in thought for a few moments.

Then he banged the table again, this time in excitement. "Dammit, Harry, you're right. We *are* going to fight—all the way!"

The noise was like a shock wave, hitting Fraser as soon as he stepped back into the Philadelphia Health Department War Room after a quick lunch. The large, windowless, featureless room on the ground floor of 500 South Broad Street was filled with a babble of voices, ringing telephones, and clattering typewriters. It was remarkable, Fraser thought again, how much was being achieved in such bedlam.

All around him shirt-sleeved EIS officers were engaged in implementing decisions he had helped formulate in Atlanta a few days ago. Making a lightning round trip to the CDC, Fraser had attended a couple of important meetings, snatched enough time to pick up a suitcase of fresh clothes from home, and then flown back to Philadelphia.

The first meeting had been with a panel of toxicologists who spent a great deal of time eruditely eliminating any number of possible causes while complaining about the size of specimens they were getting. Sunderman had already announced that his first tests for nickel carbonyl poisoning were inconclusive; the distinguished scientist inferred that this could be because the samples he received were contaminated: post-mortem surgical instruments and basins often contained nickel, trace amounts of which could rub off onto specimens and be picked up by the extraordinarily sensitive instruments he used in his nickel carbonyl research. Sunderman had asked that in the future "plastic surgical instruments" be utilized when obtaining his samples. He had gone on to explain to his bemused audience that the utensils provided for airline passengers were ideal for this purpose. The upshot was that Eastern Airlines was contacted "for information about its dining utensils." It caused panic among the airline executives, who feared the airline was about to be implicated in the epidemic. When the real reason emerged and the corporate agitation ceased, Eastern gladly supplied sets of its plastic utensils to be used at autopsies.

The second meeting Fraser attended had been to review the results of all the questionnaire and other surveys conducted so far. It had been a daunting task, with statisticians and departmental heads on hand to offer advice and opinions, which were often contradictory. But Fraser was pleased to hear that analysis in Atlanta had confirmed what the Philadelphia detectives' four-hotel survey had found: although the outbreak appeared concentrated among legionnaires and guests at the Bellevue during the convention, there was a distinct falloff in cases afterward. Additionally, the telephone survey of Bellevue guests showed that those who checked in after the legionnaires left ran a much lower risk of becoming ill. Until he carefully studied these findings, Fraser was uncertain whether he should order the Bellevue closed. Now it was clear he need not. He was much relieved.

Even so, all the data—particularly the information culled from the 3,683 responses to the legionnaire census that had been sent to Atlanta for analysis—led Fraser and his colleagues to conclude that the source for the outbreak was indeed the Bellevue, although a new and disconcerting factor had emerged.

Computer analysis revealed that a number of victims who seemed to have legionnaires' disease—whose clinical symptoms of high fever and cough or lesser fever and X-ray evidence of pneumonia satisfied the case criteria—were in actual fact *not* legionnaires, had *not* attended the convention, and, most important, had *not* set foot inside the Bellevue. But they *had* been in Philadelphia around the time of the convention, and they *had* at one time or another walked along Broad Street within a block of the Bellevue.

As a result of this analysis, Fraser decided to categorize these victims as cases of Broad Street pneumonia. At the same time, the original case definition was revised; the clinical symptoms remained as before, but an important epidemiological rider was added. To qualify as an "official" case of legionnaires' disease, a victim now had to be either "an American Legion conventioneer" or someone who had "entered the Bellevue Stratford after July first."

As a matter of routine, Fraser passed on this revision to the city health department and to Parkin in Harrisburg. Within hours the new criteria formed the basis for one of the press releases Bachman's office continued to issue.

It caused immediate confusion in the minds of the media and the public. One result of the change was to reduce the number of "official" deaths from legionnaires' disease by three. Although not explained, those three deaths were simply transferred to the new category of Broad Street pneumonia. But to the baffled public it now appeared that, somehow, three persons who had been dead no longer were—at least not "officially," whatever that meant. Among those now classified as having died from Broad Street pneumonia was the bus driver, Andrew Hornack.

Fraser did not consider it his job to explain the finer points of epidemiology to the media. And certainly this afternoon his mind was far removed from the headlines that followed reports of the altered case criteria.

Looking around the overcrowded and stuffy War Room, he could draw considerable satisfaction from the way everything was working. The EIS team he had brought down from Harrisburg slotted in perfectly with those who had been here from the start; there was not only cooperation but genuine camaraderie among them. He had even grown used to the sight of the shirt-sleeved detectives occupying one corner of the room—known as the Precinct—hunched over their telephones and oblivious of the stares their shoulder holsters drew.

Fraser paused to have a word with Tsai. Had any new cases surfaced from the Eucharistic Congress?

Tsai shook his head. There were still just the two, a nun and a priest.

Fraser showed his relief. The news that victims had now been found among the million or so persons who attended the Congress had fueled media speculation for the past few days. Tsai was one of several EIS officers checking whether any more fitted the new case criteria.

Something caught Fraser's attention at the far side of the room. A stranger was talking to the operator manning the computer terminal; the man was jotting down the operator's responses in a notebook.

Fraser turned to one of the local health department workers: Who had let that reporter in?

The man didn't know. But that was no ordinary reporter. That was a correspondent from the New York *Times* who had worked on Watergate.

Fraser couldn't help smiling; the *Times*, like the Washington *Post*, continued to bask in the wake of the Nixon scandals.

There was no way he could bar the press from this room. The appearance of the reporter was merely another reminder of the delicate and often diffuse demarcation lines that existed within the investigation. The mood still prevailed in some quarters that the CDC were "invited guests" whose presence, while welcome, must also be subjugated to the local bureaucracy. Everybody higher up the bureaucratic ladder was very pleasant, and nobody actually raised the issue in so many words, but at times the overall effect was clear enough: the CDC team was not going to get all its own way.

Keeping a wary eye on the reporter, Fraser turned to Craven. What progress was he making in listing the Broad Street pneumonias?

Craven shuffled his papers. There were now thirty cases and two deaths. Doubtless more would be listed as the results of fresh surveys came in. Apart from the fact they had not been in the Bellevue, the Broad Street cases seemed virtually identical to those classified as victims of legionnaires' disease.

Fraser nodded, perplexed. Perhaps they were "just background," not really related to the disease being investigated. As yet he couldn't be sure. He walked to his desk at one end of the War Room. It afforded him the minimum of privacy to contemplate what more he should or could do before he made one of the most difficult decisions of all: when to withdraw his team and return to Atlanta. There, supported by all the scientific backup needed and away from the high-pressure atmosphere of his work in the field, he could quietly review the huge amount of information still awaiting analysis.

The timing of the move was crucial. To keep an increasingly tired EIS team in Philadelphia—many of them had yet to have a proper night's sleep since leaving home—could be counterproductive: mistakes could arise, leads chased to no purpose. Yet to pull out before every possible avenue had been explored would be equally unthinkable and could only increase the criticism being directed at the CDC for its not having isolated the agent that caused the outbreak.

It was a balancing act that required a high degree of medical acumen mixed with political sensitivity.

Fraser was still trying to find a way across this tightrope when a tall, straight-backed, well-dressed stranger was brought to his desk. The man introduced himself as an attorney for Bankers Security.

Fraser looked at him blankly.

"My clients own the Bellevue Stratford Hotel. Can we talk some-where more private?"

"Okay." Fraser led the way out of the War Room to a nearby office. He indicated a chair. "Please sit down. Now—how can I help you?"

"Your new case definition. My clients object to it."

"Why?"

"I must advise you of the grave financial consequences the definition may cause, to the detriment of my clients' business. Their hotel has been directly linked with this particular outbreak and investigation. I urge you to remove the name Bellevue Stratford from your definition so that we can all avoid a potential multimillion-dollar lawsuit."

Fraser stared at the lawyer. There was no doubt: the man was seri-ous. He had also been courteous—and specific. Fraser would answer in the same vein.

"Our case definition was chosen for scientific purposes. It is serving those purposes. If it needs to be changed for scientific purposes, it will be. But as long as it is serving those purposes I do not anticipate chang-ing the definition."

"That is your considered position?"

"Yes. But let me add one thing. I am sorry about any negative effect the outbreak may be having on the financial status of the hotel. I cer-tainly do not want to contribute to that problem. But my primary re-sponsibility is to see that the scientific investigation is carried out as efficiently as possible."

The lawyer rose and bade Fraser a polite farewell.

Though he had been careful to hide the fact, the visit had shaken Fraser. In all his experience he had never before met a legal threat over a case definition. He called his superior in Atlanta. The bureau director listened carefully, then pronounced, "If you're *right*, then you'll be sup-ported by the federal government."

Fraser put down the phone and thought that didn't sound very sup-portive. He decided the best thing he could do was dismiss the attor-ney's visit from his mind and concentrate on what needed to be done before he and his team left the city.

McDade had to agree with his superior, Dr. Charles Shepard: the test results so far simply didn't make sense.

Not one of the eggs McDade had inoculated four days ago showed any sign of becoming ill, let alone dying. Surely whatever had killed the legionnaires, and which presumably had made the guinea pigs mori-bund, should also have killed the embryonated chicken eggs. Nor had McDade seen anything significant in the microscopic slides of the guinea pig tissue he had spent so many hours examining. Nor had any of the artificial culture mediums proved suitable as a base for enhancing the growth of any unusual organism that might have been in the guinea pigs' tissues.

There was something wrong.

Although none of the animals inoculated with lung tissue from the elderly legionnaire, Abe Ruben, had become sick, three of the four inoculated with J.B.'s lung tissue had developed high fevers and become moribund, as had three of those inoculated with Hornack's tissue. McDade had sacrificed two of the guinea pigs inoculated with J.B.'s lung tissue and one of Hornack's. From each of these three guinea pigs he had removed the spleen, liver, and lungs, prepared microscopic slides, and inoculated tissue suspensions into various bacteriologic mediums and also into the eggs.

It all, seemingly, had no effect.

Throughout the CDC other scientists, conducting quite different experiments, were equally unsuccessful in their attempts to isolate the agent. A few, much to Shepard's chagrin, suggested that McDade's guinea pigs became sick as a result of "some kind of common contaminant" or even that "all guinea pigs get fevers." Shepard knew animals in his labs didn't normally develop fevers without very good reason: he felt confident they hadn't become ill because of any contamination unwittingly introduced during the tests.

Shepard and McDade concluded it was much too soon to give up the search. Perhaps, given more time and different culture mediums, the organism could finally be grown. Perhaps the eggs just needed a little longer before they, too, showed signs of infection. And perhaps there was something in those guinea pig tissue slides that McDade had so far failed to spot. The microbiologist returned to his microscope and began again to peer at the first of them.

Fraser sat on the edge of a desk in the center of the War Room, informally addressing the assembled workers.

As far as the CDC was concerned, the epidemiological investigation in Pennsylvania had run its course. In the past weeks, they had done everything possible to collect all the evidence needed. Their task had been to cast as wide a net as possible, to try and capture anything that looked of interest or suspicious. They had done so brilliantly; a great deal had been learned, but much remained to be discovered. Now the focus of the investigation must again shift, this time to Atlanta. The hunt was far from over.

Epidemiologically, the Bellevue had been implicated. And hundreds of separate samples had been taken from the hotel; some would need lengthy testing in the CDC laboratories to determine their culpability or otherwise.

The ad hoc test Fraser had himself devised—exposing himself and a number of EIS officers to any hazard lurking in the hotel—had failed. None of them had been taken ill.

But every one of the victims or their families or friends had been interviewed. Literally thousands of others had answered questionnaires containing hundreds of questions. Much of this information remained in an unorganized state and required the most careful evaluation; it would best be done by a much smaller team, which Fraser would lead, working closely with the laboratory scientists still engaged in the hunt.

The field investigation, Fraser had to acknowledge, had often been performed against a background of confusion and sometimes even recriminations. Physicians treating desperately ill patients were frantic, floundering from diagnosis to diagnosis. A variety of treatments had been tried. There were reports of a doctor who had prescribed intravenous penicillin because he couldn't think of anything else to do; of another who began treatment with intramuscular penicillin and oxygen, added streptomycin, switched to ampicillin and gentamycin, and then brought in steroids as a last hope. His patient died. But in one case there was said to have been a marked improvement after a doctor prescribed only aspirin.

Until the CDC laboratories made a final determination, Fraser would remain unwilling to indicate a drug of choice. And, as everyone in the War Room was aware, the lunatic calls continued. There was hardly a person present who had not received one. The calls were further evidence, if any was needed, that they had dealt with a phenomenon which had probably never before occurred in the world and for which there were almost no guidelines.

Yet in spite of everything their work in Pennsylvania was virtually finished. There was now no practical or useful purpose served by Fraser and the EIS team's remaining in the city. The local health department and their colleagues in Harrisburg could cope with the day-to-day residue of the investigation. And if necessary, Fraser could always return to Philadelphia.

He now had one final job to perform. Moving among the workers, Fraser distributed his personal going-away gift to each of them. He had spent a lot of time trying to find something appropriate. In the end he settled on distributing the souvenir kits legionnaires had been able to purchase when they arrived at the convention. Many of the veterans had quickly discarded the ragbag of souvenir items. But to the medical detectives they would remain proud possessions—a reminder that they had been part of an event unique in the annals of epidemiology.

At about the time Fraser was preparing to leave Philadelphia, another, quite different, investigator arrived in the city. Ray Cole was the chief investigator for the Congressional Subcommittee on Consumer

Protection and Finance, a body chaired by the peripatetic congressman John M. Murphy. Cole was in town to try to uncover evidence and find participants for hearings Murphy planned to hold into how the entire medical investigation into legionnaires' disease had been conducted. Cole was ready, indeed eager, to listen to anybody who had any information that would show, in particular, that the CDC had been either negligent or inept. If things developed as Cole hoped, Murphy's subcommittee would be in a position, in effect, to put the CDC—and Fraser—on public trial.

17

Resolution

Now that she was here, Doris didn't know why she had come to the dell. It all seemed such a long time ago she had sat here with Jimmy. It was late summer now and the birds had grown fat and moved slowly in the woods; she had almost forgotten how noisy they could get, rustling in the undergrowth, snapping dry twigs, startling her. Yet she doubted there was any other person up here in the woods. They would all be down in the town, celebrating its 150th birthday.

All week the bunting had gone up, flags had been unfurled, colored lights strung across the streets. The beauty parlors and barbershops had done record business. There was a carnival mood in the air that her mother said reminded her of Victory Against Japan Day in 1945. And everywhere Doris turned nowadays, she encountered people determined to have a good time.

Perhaps that was why she had come to the dell. Though she had learned to smile and laugh again, and told those who commented on the matter that Jimmy would not have wanted her to go on grieving forever, she still felt a certain deadness inside her. Doris wondered whether, however cheerful she forced herself to be, the feeling would ever go away.

She looked around her. The first sign of seasonal change was there; a few leaves had drifted onto the floor of the dell. In no time at all, just a few more weeks at the most, the leaves would fall thick and fast to form a crunchy carpet and the trees would appear to move closer to the town spread out below.

Doris sat hugging her knees, feeling the cool of the earth penetrating her skin. She stared down at Williamstown, thinking: *Five weeks, and this is the first time I have been back here. I thought it would hurt, but it doesn't. There's nothing here to show this was our place, that this is where he proposed, and before Father Simpson made us promise, this is where we liked to come and cuddle and be close. Jimmy called it loving in nature. And sometimes when he'd quarreled with Dicko or J.B., we'd come here and I'd soothe his anger and pain.*

Coming here now, she suddenly realized, had been a form of exorcism, severing another link that could interfere with her new life, which was steadily taking on a meaning and purpose of its own. She had accepted a job at Fort Indiantown Gap, working as a waitress in the base cafeteria. It meant an early start and late home; then it was time to feed the children and get them off to bed. On Sundays there was barely time to go to mass and listen to the rolling homilies of Father Simpson before she had to hurry back, prepare brunch, clean up, and get ready for the week ahead. It was a hard, demanding routine that allowed her little time to dwell on the past.

Sometimes she'd watch the news: the mysterious outbreak was still commanding attention, but nowadays nobody ignored her. Those primeval fears which had so suddenly surfaced in the town had just as quickly dropped out of sight. Yet Doris had seen them and would not easily forget that behind all the friendly greetings, the have-a-nice-day-see-you-in-church-say-hello-to-the-kids pleasantries, there lurked something else. Something evil.

On this Saturday afternoon, August 21, she found herself with time unexpectedly on her hands. The children had gone off early in the morning to watch the opening day of Williamstown's Sesquicentennial celebrations. Impulsively Doris had dressed in a light summer dress, one that showed off her deep suntan and enhanced the golden sheen of her legs. She attracted a lot of admiring looks as she walked out of the town and up the winding road that the coal miners once trudged. Thirty years had passed since the last black-faced collier had made the return journey from the pithead. She'd never understood why the mine closed; everybody knew there was more coal and methane gas below the ground than had ever been brought up. She was certain that, with the energy crisis worsening, it would only be a matter of time before the mine reopened.

From far below she heard cheering. The demonstration by the fire company was over. Doris rose to her feet and began to meander back down the road, thinking hard. In the past month she had managed to put aside $100 for the lawyer she had engaged to try to make sense of the complicated legal tangle Jimmy's death had left: there were his will, his insurance policy, the bequests he made to the children. When he was alive and they had spoken of these things, it sounded so simple.

Now it seemed so messy. To make matters worse, creditors were pressing from all sides. Mrs. Ralph was the most demanding, to the point
where she was threatening to take legal action. It was one more pressure to bear. Doris found the best way to cope was to plunge herself
into unremitting work that left no time to think about the consequences of not meeting all the demands.

Coming into the town, she came to a decision: never again would
she visit the dell. The place only kindled pointless memories. Doris
began to think of more mundane matters as she became lost in the
crowd lining Market Street to watch the parade of fire trucks.

The sight of the Hahn Custom Pumper leading the parade reminded
Mrs. Ralph of the part J.B. had played in raising money to pay for the
town's new fire engines and firehouse; through his efforts, Williamstown could now boast of having one of the finest private fire services
in the state.

It was only now he was gone, sighed Mrs. Ralph, that people were
coming to realize just how much J.B. had done for them. She had
impressed this upon her two grandsons when they had stayed with her;
they must never forget, whatever their mother said, that their father
had been a wonderful person. That was why she was a little disappointed with the otherwise splendid Sesquicentennial Book the town's
History Committee had produced. As it was, the Ralph Funeral Home
had to be content with an entry between Billy Adams' Shoe Repair
Shop and John Trotman's Coal and Ice Company. Mrs. Ralph would
not wish anybody to think her snobbish, but she really would have
thought a little more could have been made about J.B.'s many contri-
butions to the town, especially since Virginia Anne was on the History
Committee.

Virginia Anne patiently explained that if her mother read the anniversary book carefully, she would see there were other—and flattering—
references to J.B.

It wasn't the same, insisted her mother. The references were spread
out. They didn't have impact.

Her daughter smiled, relieved. In a way her mother's reaction was
healthy, a sign she was coming out of her grief, that in wanting recognition for J.B. she was coming to terms with his death.

Virginia Anne pointed to the growing pile of newspapers and magazines from all over the country that had written about her brother and
his funeral. She was certain nobody alive in Williamstown today had
received such universal publicity. And, in death, J.B. had made the
town as famous as it had briefly become on that day Jack Dempsey
visited.

Mark her words, Virginia Anne urged, J.B. in the end would be
remembered long after the world had forgotten Dempsey's visit, or the

visits of other celebrities who from time to time found their way into the valley, John L. Lewis and the Harmonicats among them.

The moment the fire trucks were safely rolling down Market, Dicko plunged back into his office to check the final preparations for the crowning of the Queen of the Sesquicentennial later in the day. Like almost anything else of importance, the ceremony would take place in the post, which would also host in the coming week a Micky Finn Night, a Splash Party, a Tommy Dorsey Night, a German Night, a Veterans' Breakfast, and a Turkey Dinner.

It was, he had conceded to Joyce, marvelous the way the town had recovered from the trauma of July. The Seip family and all the others who had been taken ill were fit again. The press had departed, the TV no longer featured shots of Williamstown, the radio had ceased to broadcast stories of a community in torment.

None of this slackening of media interest had diminished Dicko's own burning interest in the progress of the medical hunt. His collection of clips would not have disgraced a newspaper library. He probably also knew more about the endless twists and turns of the investigation than did a lot of reporters.

And now a Russian newspaper—of all things, he had growled on hearing the news, it had to be a Commie one—had given credence to those fears which Dicko did not like to contemplate: that his fellow legionnaires who had died or were still sick were the victims of out-of-control experiments with chemical and biological weapons.

Jesus, he didn't want to believe *that*. And yet here was this god-dammed Commie newspaper claiming that during the last few years the CIA had tested 139 fast-acting substances on what the paper called unsuspecting Americans.

One thirty-nine: how the hell did they know *that?* That didn't sound like a figure anybody could invent, did it?

And look what else the paper said: There were secret CIA places all over Pennsylvania making poisons.

No, *that* had to be crap. How the hell did anybody keep a poison factory *secret?* It was all horseshit. It *had* to be.

But was it? He couldn't help remembering what J.B. once said: that the CIA had tried to suborn Pennsylvania mushroom growers to produce noxious fungi. And never mind what that jerk-off Commie paper published, elements of the U.S. media were beginning to explore a question the *Daily News* stated in its usual razzmatazz style: "Is it possible some mutilated germs or bizarre poisons created in the Pentagon's super-secret labs during the last few decades could have been stolen? Lost? Misplaced? Duplicated?" In the case of legionnaires' disease, flatly stated the Philadelphia newspaper, "the CBW theory seems to be the one that COULD fit."

Jesus, Dicko thought with feeling, what sort of world was Williamstown celebrating?

Fraser pushed aside another pile of reports, saying, grinning, to Tsai that after weeks away from his desk the CDC seemed more than ever a bureaucratic paradise of circulating files and documents.

Tsai smiled. "And memos. Some of them work wonders."

"You mean my bicycle memo?"

"It's the talk of the place. You scored a memorable victory."

Fraser grinned again. When he returned to the CDC this Monday morning, August 23, among all the correspondence claiming his attention were two items that both pleased and intrigued him. The first was a memo from Security saying a special area had been set aside where he could now safely store his treasured bicycle. The second was a note stating that two army officers would be visiting the center this morning. No reason was given for the visit. Fraser didn't need one: the CBW specter that had haunted him in Pennsylvania was about to resurface. Well, when the time came, he'd handle it. But right now he wanted to concentrate on briefing Tsai.

After a great deal of thought, Fraser had chosen Tsai to spearhead the next phase of the investigation: the ongoing analysis of the massive amount of information the team had gathered in the field. While Thacker had returned to Washington, D.C., and Graitcer and Craven had resumed their vigil for swine flu, and all the other EIS officers were back at their original posts, Fraser and Tsai would continue the formidable task of interpreting the results of the numerous questionnaires that had formed the unexciting but essential backbone of the entire investigation. As before, computers would be used to help tabulate the data. But in the end it could be the sharp eye of either Tsai or Fraser, attuned to relate what they saw on the printouts to what they had witnessed in Pennsylvania, that might spot some deeply buried but crucial detail amid the myriad of facts and figures the computers produced.

With all his other duties—for now that he was back at the CDC, he must again assume full responsibility for the daily running of his Special Pathogens Branch—Fraser knew he could not handle the analysis alone.

Tsai, apart from being a member of Fraser's own unit, had been the obvious choice: with his infinite patience, highly developed power of reasoning, and great physical stamina, he was the best possible person to pick his way through and draw conclusions from the reams of information that would confront him.

"Where shall I begin?"

"Might as well start at the end—the Case Control Survey we completed just before leaving Philly. It hasn't been studied at all yet."

Tsai made a note. The replies of 147 legionnaires who had remained well after the convention were compared in this survey to 113 who became ill. Among the questions asked was one which puzzled many an interviewee: Were you close enough to touch any pigeons in the area of the Bellevue Stratford? Fraser had to admit the question might have been phrased better.

"After you've done that, I think we should go back on the Legion Census. We got well over three and a half thousand responses. There's bound to be a lot of good material in there waiting to be dug out."

Tsai looked thoughtful. "It's going to take time to summarize the demographic results. And I want to review all the hospital charts."

"You'll get them. As well as everything that comes up from testing in the labs," promised Fraser.

"How high a priority do you want to give the survey Goldberger and Graitcer did of the Bellevue employees?"

Fraser considered. "Only that air-conditioner man fits the criteria. But I'm interested in the lobby personnel. We need to relate them to that question about the time legionnaires spent in the lobby."

"Okay. What about the Hospitality Room Survey?"

The three-page questionnaire was meant to establish whether there had been an increased risk associated with visiting rooms where free drinks, food, and cigarettes were dispensed.

"We got a good response, considering. The trouble is, people don't often really remember. But they want to be helpful. So they try and say *something,* instead of leaving a blank. We have to allow for that. Better cross-check the replies with those we got in the Legion Census and the Epidemiological Survey."

"Okay."

Both knew it would require weeks of intense concentration to correlate and spot patterns within the mass of statistical data. Tsai would work in the office adjoining Fraser's, spending long hours at a stretch poring over the statistics, while Fraser concerned himself largely with another critically important aspect of the investigation: keeping track of the laboratory work to find the agent. It would require fine judgment on his part when to sit back and curb his own impatience and when gently to chivvy, to offer advice and encouragement. The lab scientists could be tetchy; Fraser knew he would have to exercise even more diplomacy than he had at times displayed in Pennsylvania.

In the meantime there was the more immediate problem of how to handle the visit of the two CBW specialists.

The senior army officers had traveled to Atlanta partly as a result of

Fraser's original request that the Department of Defense be contacted. Both officers were scientists knowledgeable about the toxic effects of chemical and biological agents.

Fraser had only the vaguest idea of what went on nowadays in Fort Detrick, despite some of the lurid tales reporters in Pennsylvania had hinted at. When the possibility of sabotage or a noxious substance being involved had surfaced early in the investigation, the fort's name had cropped up and refused to go away. The Truck Theory—the scary scenario that an army truck loaded with lethal germs had found its way into Philadelphia—revolved around its traveling either to or from the military base. Then there was the rumor that had persisted in the city that other equally deadly germs had vanished from the fort. And there had been all those hints that some demented worker at the fort had got hold of a canister of something lethal. And the army manual Craven received: it, too, had referred to Fort Detrick. Literally every theory about CBW in the end included some reference to the mysterious establishment that, it was now only just emerging, *had been*, in the fifties and sixties, the hope of the Special Operations Division, the Army's biological research unit producing germ weapons for the CIA's use. In the early fifties the cold war was at its height and the CIA had been engaged in far-ranging schemes to liberate Eastern Europe by any means: Stalin lived, Joe McCarthy raged; it was a foreboding era suited for the introduction of consciousness-altering technology. Officially, behavioral experiments were now back in their box. Fort Detrick, officially, was nowadays only concerned with monitoring Soviet and Chinese CBW developments and not with the production of new weapons for the United States. But many people believed that American researchers were still, by the very nature of their monitoring work, making advances in the field.

To try to establish whether there was the remotest possibility a secret noxious substance had been responsible for the outbreak, a handful of the CDC's most senior scientists, including Fraser, assembled in a large office to meet their military visitors. The CDC men hoped for an informal and open exchange of information; they were all willing to answer any question and assumed the two officers would, in turn, be equally forthcoming.

The military men sat, ramrod straight, facing the sports-jacketed, baggy-trousered doctors and researchers.

There was a momentary awkward silence while the two sides eyed each other.

The leader of the CDC delegation, a distinguished scientist, asked, pleasantly enough, how the visitors would like to conduct the meeting.

The taller of the two men, a crew-cut officer with a smile that never reached his eyes, reminded the CDC team what his terms of reference were.

"We are here to listen to everything you have to say."

Instinctively Fraser throught: *This is going to be a waste of time.*

The senior CDC scientist explained that the agency was not just interested in "the possible involvement of a chemical warfare agent but also members of families of that type of compound. . . ."

Fraser continued to stare at the two officers: *They're cool all right, not by the bat of an eyelid do they show what they're thinking.*

". . . The agency is concerned to know whether what we are seeing is similar to what might be expected from some of the material you might be working with."

There was silence in the room when the CDC scientist ended his presentation.

The tall officer finally responded. "I can only repeat what you have already been told. We have no reports of anything missing. There is no possibility the Army is in any way involved in what you are looking for."

Another scientist spoke. "How can we be certain the agent involved in our outbreak is not at least related to what your people might be working with?"

"Do you know what the agent is?"

"No."

"Then how can we tell whether it might be associated with something we might, or might not, be involved in?"

Fraser thought: *This can go on forever.*

He became aware that the younger officer was looking toward him "Dr. Fraser, perhaps you would be good enough to run down the clinical and symptomatic aspects of your outbreak."

Fraser did.

The first officer reacted. "I know of no match for that pattern of illness. I am willing to refer this back to persons with the basic expertise."

His companion added, "We'll be surprised if we know of any agent you haven't thought of already."

"Maybe we should explore that," suggested a CDC doctor.

"That would serve no useful purpose."

The taller officer repeated, "We're here to listen. If you have any further information, we'll gladly take it back and have our experts evaluate it."

Fraser tried. "Could we talk directly to your people?"

"We will contact the CDC if we have anything to communicate."

Fraser gave up, taking no further part in a meeting that lingered on, with the two officers frequently hedging, ducking, and sometimes even flatly refusing to answer questions. But at the conclusion—a vague promise to hold further discussions "on neutral ground" should the need arise—Fraser was satisfied that whatever was going on within the highly restricted confines of Fort Detrick, there was now no possibility a CBW agent could have triggered the epidemic.

It hurt so much she wanted to scream—this all-pervasive mood of flatness that touched everybody and everything in the lobby. It was an almost physical thing; the lackluster dullness settled on her skin and clung to her hair. Anna Taggart closed her eyes, trying to remember how it had been when Marlene Dietrich, King Hussein of Jordan, President Eisenhower, and John F. Kennedy had walked toward the special elevator always reserved for notables—Elevator 4—smiling, and sometimes shaking her hand. Heck, her hand had been wrung by more famous people than almost anybody's on the staff. Now, *there* was something for that publicity fellow who was always running around nowadays trying to think up new ways of promoting the hotel.

Anna opened her eyes. She would mention it to him. He certainly didn't seem to be having much luck so far. The hotel was still being publicly drubbed. The lobby on this Friday morning, September 3, was like a faded photograph. With it almost empty of people, the genteel, old-fashioned shabbiness of the place, the wear and tear Anna had always found so homey, now seemed to belong to a bygone age. The colors were suddenly more faded under the dimmed lights of the chandeliers, and even the carpet across which some of the most famous feet in the world had trod looked drab and sad.

The image of a faded photo stayed with her, embracing the lobby staff. There was a lifeless, sepia look, for instance, about Tony Delia, the bell captain who had carried bags for fifty-three years; in these past weeks he had seemed to grow more stooped and desolate. The same defeated air clung to his aged, red-jacketed bellmen. And it was there, too, in the usually smiling face of Jimmy Callos, the headwaiter in the Hunt Room for more decades than Anna cared to remember. Callos now looked like a "man who had stared into the future and wished he hadn't."

Anna knew she had no need to look farther than the front desk to see the reason for this gloom. There wasn't a guest in sight. Slowly and remorselessly the Bellevue was being starved to death. Some of the cashiers put the hotel's losses at over $5,000 a day. Nobody, Anna guessed, really knew the true figure; Mr. Chadwick and Mr. Varr would be sure to keep that sort of information under careful lock and key. But she didn't need facts and figures to tell her the hotel was badly hurt. She thought: *We're like the* Titanic, *holed, but the bridge*

*is more concerned with pretending to the crew that any day now the
hole will be fixed and we'll go sailing on.*

Each morning when she came to work, the signs were a little more
ominous. When she passed through the basement area, the laundry
was that much less busy, the kitchen that much more slack. And the
slightest thing made everybody nervous.

The news that a dead pigeon had been found in the water tower on
the roof had spread like wildfire. What was so bad about one dead
bird, Anna thought angrily; it wasn't as though the bird had been
found anywhere near the drinking water. And again, there had been all
that brouhaha when yet another inspection team had suddenly spotted
that the hotel incinerator was being improperly operated. There had
been endless discussions about the significance of the discovery; as far
as Anna could make out, all it meant was that the furnace afterburner
had not been used to reduce the amount of smoke belching out of the
rooftop chimney. The oversight had been corrected, but for days afterward men had stood and stared solemnly at the smoke coming out of
the stack. Anna thought the whole thing was footling, just another example of how jittery everybody was becoming.

And as she had so often remembered her own mother's reminding
her, there was that very Irish saying about bad news bringing more bad
news. She had heard one of the "chain gang"—a member of the corps
of free-lance waiters who were called in to help with large banquets
and other functions—complaining he would starve if he had to rely on
the Bellevue for a living. And she'd overheard the credit manager telling the senior housekeeper he feared a lot of their hoped-for conventions might not now materialize.

The worst thing for Anna was just having to stand before her elevator, striving to numb her mind to such thoughts, trying to turn the
pages of memory, to conjure up a past rich in glitter and spectacle.

Time and again something would jerk her back to the reality of the
present. There would be the sight of a grim-faced Mr. Varr walking
quickly across the lobby, anxious, so it seemed to Anna, to avoid having
contact with anybody. Or one of the permanent guests in the hotel—
mainly fabulously wealthy widows—would emerge from her suite and
act as if nothing had changed. In a way, thought Anna, they were
being as escapist as she was. And as these elderly and imperious guests
made their way across the lobby, they were surrounded by a silence
which, too often, was rudely shattered by the whirr of a film camera or
the voice of a reporter.

Anna had come not only to loathe but actually to despise the media.
All this, she thought bitterly, staring around the almost deserted lobby,
is their doing. The Bulletin, *the* Inquirer, *and especially the* News, *and
those other out-of-town rags—they've all played their part. The radio*

reporters too, prowling around, using their microphones to pick up the slightest indiscretion. Creeps, that's what they are. No, not creeps, vultures. *Yes, that's what they are*—vultures.

Suddenly a burst of artificial light bounced off the glass doors of the Broad Street entrance.

Anna squinted: *My God, there they are again. Holy Mary, Mother of Jesus, this has got to stop! And I'm going to stop it!*

Her fury mounting by the stride, Anna strode across the lobby toward the TV crew and its reporter declaiming into the camera.

". . . There are many who say the Bellevue was doomed in any event. That it is part of the old world. Beautiful but obsolete. That what happened here in these past seven weeks has only hastened the inevitable. As yet no answer has been found to what killed twenty-nine legionnaires and hospitalized one hundred and fifty more, except that somehow this building—"

Anna launched herself at the reporter. "Put down your horn!"

The startled reporter lowered the microphone.

Anna rounded on the TV crew. "Get off our doorstep, you squirts!" She gestured toward the reporter. "And take this bimbo with you!"

The camera team backed off as Anna continued to rail at the luckless reporter. "You bimbo! You poor, pathetic bimbo! You dare to stand here and talk of a fine lady like this hotel. A punk like you has no right to even be in the same street!"

"Look, lady, you're wrecking my story—"

"I'll wreck more than that if you don't clear off!"

"Lady, please—"

"Listen, you squirt. I'm Irish, see. Fighting Irish! And the Irish don't fight on the left side or on the right side. They go right down the middle! Now beat it before I send you all into the middle of nowhere!"

The crew continued to back away, filming Anna as she advanced on them.

"Okay, you punks. You want a story. I'll give you a story. When you come here and criticize the Bellevue, you are criticizing my home. And nobody does that. Nobody!"

She motioned toward the hotel. "What you have done to this place is an outrage." Anna turned back and faced the camera. "The Bellevue has been blackballed from here to the end of the world. It's been crucified because of this disease, and there's no such disease in this place! If a disease was around, some of us would have taken it in some shape or form. We dealt with the legionnaires directly. The doorman, the bellman, the elevator girls, the maids. None of us is sick."

Anna paused for breath. "I stand there at the elevators and watch you people and I tell you I'd rather be cleaning offices than seeing you!"

She turned to the dazed reporter. "Don't twist my words around or I'll personally punch you in the mouth!"

Before the reporter could respond, Anna had turned and marched back into the hotel to resume her post at the elevators. She felt happier than she had for weeks.

Fraser and Tsai pored over the computer printouts that covered all of Tsai's desk and overflowed onto the floor of his office. In the past two weeks they had done a considerable amount of analysis. Among other things, it allowed them to conclude that advanced age, smoking, and underlying illness were all factors that increased the risk of dying from legionnaires' disease.

Perhaps most significant of all, Fraser was becoming persuaded that whatever agent had caused the epidemic was airborne-transmitted, and that not only was the Bellevue implicated, but the agent's most likely habitat was the rooftop water tower that fed the hotel's air-conditioning system. The data also suggested it was entirely possible the agent emerged into the Bellevue through the vent above the registration desk; lobby employees might well have become immune to its effect over a period of years.

Epidemiologically speaking, the computer results were helping to prove that Fraser's investigation had been a success. Initially, clues had been spread over an entire state, yet he had managed to trace the source of the outbreak to a single building in one of the largest cities in the nation. That had been his task, and he had done it in almost textbook manner. And now, just as the textbooks demanded, he must wait for the labs actually to confirm what kind of agent he had cornered within the confines of the hotel. Few outsiders, he suspected, would fully understand such an esoteric difference. That was one more reason why he was reluctant to talk to the media.

Tsai ran a hand over his weary eyes. "Anything new from the labs?"

"No. Nothing from bacteriology or toxicology."

"What about Dr. Shepard? It still looks to me like it could be Q fever."

"Or maybe a new rickettsia. I keep pestering Shepard. He and McDade are looking into it. But so far nothing."

"That's tough, especially with these hearings."

Fraser grimaced. "They sound more like a trial—with us in the dock."

Congressman John Murphy had just announced that his subcommittee would hold two days of public hearings in Philadelphia, "to examine the handling of the medical investigation." The news had brought a further splash of headlines criticizing the CDC.

Fraser turned away from the printouts. "Ted, Sencer wants me to put together our evidence for Murphy. I won't be able to be here as much as I'd hoped. And I'll need your help."

Tsai smiled. "Sure. We'll manage. You just get the best case together to stop Murphy."

Fraser looked pensive. "I think it's going to be pretty unpleasant. From what I've heard, hearings aren't meant to be fair."

On that sobering note, he left Tsai and returned to his own office to begin preparing an explanation and defense of the CDC's involvement in the investigation. Fraser was now cast, willy-nilly, as the champion of the agency, the strategist who would help formulate the crucial statements for Sencer to deliver at the hearings. Fraser knew he must ensure that his arguments were not only uncluttered yet scientifically sound, but also unassailable by the garrulous congressman and his subcommittee. When the time came, he could expect a hostile reception. He had never before been involved in such an inquiry. Typically, once he had accepted what lay in store, Fraser began to relish the challenge of meeting Murphy head on.

Chadwick slowly put down the telephone and stared at Varr.

"The President won't stay with us. Somebody close to Ford must have passed the word we're bad news."

"What about Carter?"

"The governor's staying at the Ben Franklin."

Carter and Ford were due in the city shortly for the first of their televised preelection debates. For weeks Chadwick had nurtured and worked on a dream of having both the President and his rival staying at the Bellevue. Instead they had opted for the Ben Franklin. When Ford heard that Carter was booked in there, he had, however, canceled his reservation. Chadwick had tried, again, to get the President to come to the Bellevue. Ford had preferred to stay in a private home.

"Maybe we can persuade Carter to move here, to our Presidential Suite. Sell it to his people as a sort of lucky omen."

"I tried. The Carter people won't budge. Now their man's so far ahead in the polls, they're doing no favors. The best I could get was a maybe the governor will stop by if he has the time. That's still more than Ford will do."

Varr thought: *It's the worst blow yet.* He'd banked on his connections and the reputation of the Bellevue as host to every President and candidate who visited the city. Now two no's.

Varr tried to be encouraging. "There's still the ball. That'll get a lot of good coverage. The PR people are pulling out all the stops."

In a week's time the hotel would stage the glittering centerpiece of its fight for survival, the Save the Bellevue ball, the creation of its PR consultants and the climax of their forceful publicity campaign to get all Philadelphia's "movers and shakers" to come to the hotel. Thousands of "I Love the Bellevue" buttons had been given out, countless news releases had bombarded the media: announcing that the hotel had retained its own epidemiologist, that state governor Milton Shapp had dined in the Stratford Garden, that some one hundred leading local businessmen and tourist and convention officials had met at the hotel to "restore confidence in the safety of the city," that an eminent local professor of occupational medicine had said the outbreak was "largely peculiar to the legionnaires, probably brought by them to the hotel," and that it had "left with them," that Bellevue employees had donned colonial costumes and, led by a fife and drum corps, paraded to Independence Hall to demonstrate their support for the hotel, that a "Friends of the Bellevue" committee had been formed. The committee was sponsoring the black-tie gala.

In publicity terms, it was a brave effort, achieved in spite of Chadwick's insistence that he would continue to give the media as little hard information as possible. Perhaps as a result, a great deal of what the PR firm hoped to achieve had fallen by the wayside.

Varr could well understand Chadwick's dilemma. The media, for whatever reasons—and *perhaps* Chadwick was not entirely blameless—had sunk their collective teeth into the Bellevue. Reporters were hammering away at one basic theme: How was the hotel doing with room occupancy? Even the greenest newsman knew that tied to that was the question of how long the hotel could stay open.

And, Varr recognized, Chadwick would not, *could not*, admit the dire truth. To do so would be publicly to sound the death knell of the Bellevue. But the fact was that on average just over 10 percent of the hotel's 750 rooms were occupied. Losses, in this last week of September, were running at a staggering $10,000 a day.

"That ball could be too late," said Chadwick morosely.

For once Varr could find no answer to cheer up the unhappy hotelier.

Fifty-seven days after what she later admitted "transformed my professional life," Dr. Sheila Moriber Katz suddenly became ill. In a matter of hours on Thursday, September 30, the tall, blond, determined young pathologist developed a splitting headache, chills that racked her body, and a temperature that climbed to 104 degrees.

By coincidence, that same Thursday the CDC announced the national immunization program would begin the next day, when the first swine flu shot would be given in a circus tent at a state fair in Indiana.

Dr. Katz doubted she had swine flu. She thought it could be something even deadlier, stemming from what she had been doing during the past fifty-seven days.

By the end of that Thursday, a number of alarmed people knew that Dr. Katz was prostrate in the bedroom of her home in a fashionable Philadelphia suburb.

On hearing the news, Sharrar arranged for blood and throat swabs to be taken from Dr. Katz. They were speedily sent for analysis to both the state laboratories and the CDC.

Though she was careful not to say so, for that would be both unscientific and not at all in keeping with her reputation as a careful researcher at the Hahnemann Medical College and Hospital, the thought had struck Dr. Katz that she might be stricken with legionnaires' disease—which she could possibly have caught from the specimens she had been examining since August 4. They included those Goldberger had rushed to her, as well as samples from other legionnaires.

Perhaps typically, even in her sick state she saw the situation as an opportunity rare for any pathologist, the chance to study the progress of a disease as it swept through her own body.

Subsequently, as soon as she could get out of bed, she started collecting further samples of her blood and sputum for analysis in her laboratory.

In the meantime, neither the state laboratories nor the CDC could determine which virus, if any, had caused her complaint. Treating herself with tetracycline, Dr. Katz made a swift and total recovery from an illness whose symptoms she would admit in one of her many press interviews were "very nonspecific; they were identical to legionnaires' disease, but they were also identical to viral pneumonia."

Whatever had caused it, the incident only furthered her determination to be the first to "crack" the legionnaires mystery.

Like everybody else, Dr. Katz had her own theory: a form of psittacosis.

For hours at a time she would sit in a darkened room in her laboratory focusing her electron microscope, seeking that one vital clue which continued to elude some of the best brains in the scientific world.

One day she moved the green luminescent viewing field of her microscope, and just as Fraser had enthused over his Elevator Theory—which he had subsequently discarded—so, too, did Dr. Katz give vent to her feelings: "There! That's it!"

Even retelling that moment later to an *Inquirer* reporter, she remembered how at the time her voice had betrayed awe. Visible in the green glow were mycoplasma-like, pebble-shaped forms. The shapes that so entranced her were, she believed, the organisms causing legionnaires' disease.

Later—in spite of a visit to the CDC that would perhaps have left other scientists crestfallen by the total lack of acceptance for her claims

—the unstoppable Dr. Katz burst into print in a prestigious scientific journal. Challenge and criticism were heaped on her paper.

In the end, professional colleagues would believe Dr. Katz had been close, but not close enough, to discovering the causative agent of legionnaires' disease.

Joe McDade found his hopes of reaching an answer diminishing with each day that passed.

The final results of tests run on blood samples from 164 ill legionnaires had just been received. They showed no sign of antibodies to the rickettsia causing Q fever. Neither had the tissue suspensions from the dead guinea pigs been successfully cultured on any of the media that were judged to be suitable. Nor had the inoculation of the eggs produced any result. After six weeks' research, all McDade's sophisticated attempts to isolate a rickettsia had failed.

He decided to have one more look at the slides made from the guinea pigs that had been injected with lung tissue from the dead legionnaires. Peering down his microscope at one slide after another, he still could see nothing of import. He picked up and scrutinized a slide marked E-76-21, J.B.'s. Afterward he put the slide back with the others and closed the box lid firmly.

As far as Joe McDade was concerned, his search for the agent that caused legionnaires' disease had come to an end.

Moving from station to station—tasting, checking, hurrying, and sometimes scolding—executive chef Frank Castelli dredged up from the memory of his days in wartime England a Churchillian clarion cry that he proceeded to improvise with equally telling effect: *Though the Bellevue will live for a hundred more years, people will say this was our finest hour!*

All day Castelli had steadily built toward the controlled panic that was erupting all around the Bellevue's kitchen on the night of Thursday, October 7, as the final preparations began for serving the one thousand guests at the "I Love the Bellevue" charity gala.

The maître d'hôtel appeared, almost magically, at Castelli's elbow. "The first ones are going in."

Castelli glanced at the kitchen clock: 8 P.M. "We'll begin serving at eight-twenty as planned. Start getting your waiters up to the soup station."

"Right."

As swiftly as he had materialized, the headwaiter vanished back to the Grand Ballroom.

The sous-chef, Castelli's right hand in the tightly planned operation, sensed rather than heard what was about to happen. He walked to the rows of caldrons holding a hundred gallons of the hotel's famous consommé Bellevue and began to supervise the loading of soup tureens.

Castelli moved to the bank of ovens in the center of the kitchen. An entire team of chefs and assistants had, for the past hour, been preparing the main course: broiled filet of beef. He addressed the senior chef.

"Be ready to start carving at nine o'clock," ordered Castelli. "You're going to have to move faster than usual. They're dancing in between courses."

"I don't care if they do a striptease—as long as we can work like this every night!"

Castelli grinned and moved to the vegetable station. Three side dishes would complement the beef: tomatoes stuffed with spinach puree and topped by grilled cheese, jumbo asparagus Polonaise, and baked potatoes. Several of the team at the station—like many of the other kitchen staff and most of the waiters—wore "I Love the Bellevue" buttons.

The executive chef had never known morale in his kitchen to be higher. Cautious by nature, he was slowly coming to believe the recent past was a nightmare that would soon be over. It was a belief reinforced by members of the hired public relations firm, one or two of whom had dropped by the kitchen during the early evening and left with the promise that this could be the start of a new life for the hotel. Already, as Castelli knew, the room occupancy rate had taken a turn for the better. It was now hovering around 20 percent. Following a successful ball tonight, the publicists believed, it might not be long before the entire hotel was operating at a healthy profit once more. The prospect brought a gleam to the executive chef's eyes, marking a determination to make this a memorable occasion. The smile on his face as he watched the final preparation of the vegetables was a mixture of energy and contentment.

"Chef, this is even better than the night Ford came," yelled a cook.

"You sound like a Democrat," Castelli shouted back, happy. "Sure it's better. Ford and his people didn't eat."

A couple of weeks ago the President had briefly addressed two thousand supporters in the Bellevue at the end of his televised debate with Carter. Apart from light snacks, there had been no demands upon the kitchen, though the bar service had reported a near-record night. Many of the staff believed that Ford, out of sympathy and respect for Chadwick, had gone against his advisers and insisted on making the quick last-minute visit to the hotel. Carter, on the other hand, in spite of his promise, had not put in an appearance.

Castelli stole another look at the wall clock: 8:10 P.M.

Dodging fellow waiters, a dining room captain was hustling across the kitchen floor.

"The mayor's arrived. So has Gaudiosi. They're in the Burgundy Room, being received by Chadwick."

"Where's Varr?"

"With the other VIP's. Moving them into the ballroom."

"Good."

Castelli dismissed the captain and turned his attention to the continuing intricate process of serving a six-course banquet to a thousand guests who had paid fifty dollars a head to eat it.

In the lobby, her hair coiffeured at her own expense specially for the occasion, Anna Taggart continued to bob her head at the rich and famous who passed her on the way to the cocktail reception in the Burgundy Room.

Mayor Frank Rizzo, just cleared of the recall threat by a Pennsylvania Supreme Court ruling, had grabbed her hand in both of his and fervently promised, in the hearing of a group of reporters, that she need have no fears; he personally wished to assure her the Bellevue's future was safe.

As he stalked away, she had thought: *For a man who's still got a load of problems, he sure knows how to put on a front.*

Singer James Darren—the featured cabaret spot—had winked at her; disc jockey Jerry Blavat had given her a thumbs-up sign and Channel 6 sportscaster Joe Pellegrino a boxer's salute. Even the overseas guests had said encouragingly that this night surely marked the dawn of a new era in the long life of the hotel.

Only the watchful presence of the reporters and photographers, for once allowed to roam the lobby without hindrance, reminded Anna of the true purpose of the occasion: it was window dressing, to try and make folk come in and buy again.

In the Burgundy Room, Chadwick was expertly moving the stars of the Philadelphia Phillies baseball team into the ballroom. Inside, Varr seated his VIP's near a twelve-foot floral arrangement bearing the words "I Love the Bellevue" picked out in red and white carnations.

Then, as waiters moved in swift succession bearing the consommé Bellevue among the tables, Varr slipped away to check the number of signatures on a giant greeting card in the ballroom foyer.

At a quick glance he could see that the cream of Philadelphia society had pledged their support for the hotel: the Adamses and the Astleys, the Belingers, Bookbinders, and Buntings, the Kellys and Kimballs, the Wilsons and Youngs. And there, too, were the scrawls of Al Gaudiosi and Frank Rizzo. Satisfied, Varr joined his wife at the table they shared with the Bookbinders.

Music and conversation blended, rose, and fell; people started to dance. There was applause and laughter. The second-course Caesar salad was served. There was more dancing.

In the kitchen, Castelli glanced at the clock: 8:55. Busboys were returning with piles of used salad plates.

The "chain gang"—free-lance waiters—assembled around the meat station.

At precisely nine o'clock, Castelli gave the order to start carving the main course.

With balletlike precision, meat was transferred to a plate, fresh mushroom sauce added, stuffed tomato, jumbo asparagus spears, baked potato, and finally a protective hot cover banged on the top. It took seconds. Eight plates to a tray. Then, fully loaded, the waiters returned to the ballroom.

There the musical mood had changed. A rock band was on stage, bringing still more dancers onto the floor. As the main course was served, the smooth strings of the orchestra took over, gently wafting people back to their seats.

At his table Chadwick recalled for his guests some of the momentous past occasions the ballroom had known. Yet, he had to admit to his listeners, he could not remember a more exciting start to an evening than this.

In the now almost deserted lobby—the reporters had gone to their table in the ballroom—Anna Taggart pondered: *It is indeed a wonderful show, but these are mostly local folk with their own beds to go home to; how will this help fill our empty rooms?*

At nine-thirty, Castelli moved upstairs to the large subsidiary kitchen just off the Grand Ballroom. There two lines of waiters were assembled. He began to inspect them, every inch a general reviewing his troops.

So far everything had gone off exactly right. Now it was time for the dessert.

Castelli had created Bellevue ice cream cake, decorated with whipped cream and chopped nuts, covered with warm vanilla cognac sauce.

It would be served with full ceremony.

The executive chef reached the head of his forces. He turned and looked back. Each waiter stood stiffly to attention, holding aloft in his right hand a silver tray containing portions of the confection.

Castelli turned toward the service doors leading into the Grand Ballroom. Through a gap in the door he saw the lights in the ballroom dim. A roll of drums began to build from the band stage.

Once more Castelli turned and checked the line of waiters. The pastry chef and his assistants were moving among them, distributing sparklers.

The service doors suddenly swung open.

A searchlight, operated from high in the ballroom, swung down, its beam cutting across the packed tables to pick out Castelli standing beaming in the doorway.

A wave of applause was lost in the crescendo of drums.

Then Castelli stepped back into the kitchen, nodding as he did so.

The pastry chef's team began to light the sparklers each waiter held.

The band swung into "What a Wonderful World" and the procession of sparkler-twirling waiters, marching in step, entered the darkened ballroom.

The applause grew into a standing ovation.

The kitchen door closed and Castelli, sweat running down his cheeks, a triumphant smile on his face, repeated: *In a hundred years they will still say this was our finest hour!*

Fraser had decided that one of the most effective ways he could prepare for the congressional hearings was to pose a series of questions that Murphy and his subcommittee members might ask, and then to formulate answers to them in well-reasoned detail.

During the past weeks, while Fraser prepared the CDC's defense, it was becoming ever more obvious that he would be appearing at what, to all intents and purposes, *was* going to be a trial, in which Murphy and his colleagues would act as prosecutor, judge, and jury. Clear evidence that a witch-hunt was in progress had surfaced on October 27, when Murphy circulated a "confidential investigative report" to his subcommittee. Conveniently, a copy marked "secret-classified" had fallen into the hands of columnist Jack Anderson of the Washington *Post*. In a major article, Anderson featured Murphy's prehearing's conclusion that the CDC investigation was a "fiasco."

Murphy had gone on to pour crude invective on Fraser and his team, stating: "Some governmental experts, who are highly regarded among themselves, are not nearly so well regarded by others who by reputation and assignment to reputable medical facilities are the possessors of impeccable credentials."

In large part, the responsibility for preparing a rebuttal fell on Fraser. And even before the Murphy report got into the press, there was a mounting furor in the media against the CDC, much of it dating from October 11, when another of the agency's scourges, Cyril Wecht, reemerged to announce that only hours after receiving their swine flu jabs, three people in Pittsburgh had died. The CDC-backed immunization campaign had been immediately suspended in nine states. There were more deaths. But as no connection with the vaccine could be proved, the program was now again in progress. Even so, the frightened public were shunning the shots, and confidence in the CDC had been severely eroded. Against this background, Fraser knew he confronted a far tougher task than he had originally supposed.

His wife, Barbara, had given him a highly useful legal maxim: let the facts speak for themselves; hyperbole is for those with a dubious case.

If that was so, her husband mused grimly, then Murphy should face certain defeat. Fraser suspected, though, that real life did not always follow the faultless logic of legal maxims. And matters, in some ways, would not be made easier, he realized, by yet another twist in the drama.

On November 10 the Bellevue Stratford had announced it would be closing its doors in just over a week, on November 18. In an emotional statement Chadwick said the hotel "found it impossible any longer to withstand the economic impact of the worldwide, adverse publicity which has been associated with the legionnaires' disease, even though no investigative agency found any link whatsoever to hotel operations."

Fraser felt for Chadwick; in recent weeks he had returned to the hotel—once, ironically, to address a symposium on the outbreak—and had come to know and respect the hotelier as a person who, for all his crustiness, passionately cared for the Bellevue. Yet what Chadwick had told the press, Fraser feared, was not strictly true.

In question 26 of the defense he was constructing, Fraser posed the question: *Was the headquarters hotel implicated? If so, how?*

Fraser had answered it fully and fairly. Legionnaires who stayed at the hotel had a significantly greater rate of disease than delegates who stayed elsewhere. In addition, illness among all delegates was correlated to time spent in the lobby.

To be absolutely scrupulous, he had also added a further note: "We have not proved that exposure occurred in the hotel, nor have we detected anything in the hotel that caused the outbreak."

Anticipating that this might be seized upon as further "evidence" that he had "mismanaged" the investigation, Fraser next dealt with a follow-up question: *Why do you think the lobby might be the place of spread?*

Again, he had answered as honestly as he could: "There were nineteen cases who were in the hotel for one day only. Those cases were carefully interviewed and the time spent in the lobby was the only place in common with all cases. In addition, the need for changing the lobby air-conditioner filter on August sixth is suggestive of an airborne outbreak. Our special survey of delegate cases and well controls showed that delegate cases spent significantly more time in the lobby than delegate wells."

He then posed and answered a third vital question: *If the lobby is the place of spread, why were none of the employees affected?* "The lobby personnel may be immune. An alternative explanation comes from the fact that the average age of lobby employees is more than ten years younger than that of the cases. The illness is known to affect older age groups more than younger and this may be responsible. In addition, the overall rate of illness in delegates who resided at the headquarters hotel was 9 percent. If we assume that employees might show the same low attack rate, with most spared, then we might not see any illness among them since the number of employees in the lobby was small, about thirty-six full-time employees."

It was now Wednesday, November 17. There were just six days to go before Fraser would return, yet again, to Philadelphia, with CDC director David Sencer and Joseph Boutwell, deputy director of the Bureau of Laboratories, to face Murphy.

For the moment, though, attention in Philadelphia was focusing on the last hours of the Bellevue Stratford—the hotel some commentators were implying had been "murdered" by a combination of a mysterious bug and CDC bungling.

Emerging from the Broad Street subway into the cold morning air of Thursday, November 18, Frank Castelli knew he was breaking a lifetime's rule. He was going to be late for work. He did not care. In a few hours he would be out of work.

Ahead of him he saw TV and radio crews entering the Bellevue. There seemed to be dozens of technicians and reporters going through the Broad Street entrance.

At the corner of Walnut and Broad he paused, as he had done every morning, to give the hotel a long, lingering look. There was still an air of defiance about the Bellevue, the way its windows gleamed and the brass around its entrance shone. But the pigeons, which some said had contributed to its downfall, seemed to be fewer on the ground. Perhaps, mused Castelli, as animals ran just before an earthquake, so the birds had flown, knowing that their roost for seventy-two years was now doomed. And soon, he suspected, the half-mad old crone—the Pigeon Lady of Broad Street—cooing and quacking to what birds remained, would scatter her moldy bread elsewhere.

The executive chef watched her for a moment, thinking: *She's lucky. She's in a world of her own. She doesn't know what's about to happen to the lives of the five hundred people working in that building.*

The realization that the Bellevue was closing at the end of this day was made all that much harder for Castelli to accept because after the gala ball he had clung to the forlorn hope there was going to be a genuine renaissance; time and an injection of capital, he had kept telling himself, would see the hotel through the crisis. He had argued with colleagues that the hotel's owners would ride out the storm, that they were wealthy enough to protect their flagship investment whatever the cost, that one day legionnaires' disease would fade from the headlines.

Then suddenly, with the speed of a guillotine, it was all over. Just eight days to pack up and close down. It was a bitter pill to swallow.

Close to tears, Castelli passed through the staff entrance. There were few greetings exchanged this morning, and he knew the reason: *It's like a funeral—everybody looks the other way because you can't believe an old friend is dead.*

He changed into his freshly starched whites, donned his chef's hat. For a moment he stared at himself in the locker room mirror. The misery in his eyes stared back at him. Suddenly he thought: *This is no way to behave.*

Bracing his shoulders, he marched briskly into the kitchen.

The duty crew was going through the motions of preparing the lunches.

Castelli addressed them in a commanding voice. "We've got plenty of work to do before the day is over. Let's get on with it."

Today, in its dying hours, the hotel restaurants were booked solid. Fifteen hundred lunches and eight hundred dinners were to be served.

Up in the lobby, Anna Taggart seemed to be engulfed by newsmen. Since her rout of the TV crew, she had become something of a celebrity, with reporters frequently seeking her views on the hotel's future. She had resisted all their blandishments, hoping against hope there would be a reprieve. But then Chadwick had announced the hotel was to close.

Anna had felt both angry and upset. It was enough for a sharp-eyed reporter to pounce. Unable any longer to keep her feelings secret, Anna had spoken frankly and, for the first time, critically of her employers.

It was as though a floodgate had burst. Other staff who had studiously avoided the press were now speaking freely and posing for photographs.

And the few remaining guests, who normally would have shown the media the door, now welcomed in newsmen.

If the press, too, had to have its finest hour, then this was undoubtedly it, when everybody spoke and delivered the sort of quotable statements reporters dreamed of.

One journalist from the Los Angeles *Times* found his way to Suite 1226 to speak to Mrs. Eva Weiland, a sprightly ninety-three-year-old, and her daughter, Kathryn, aged sixty-four; they had just obtained a court order requiring that "full services" be supplied to their spacious apartment even after the hotel closed. The Weilands had spent the past twenty-five years in the Bellevue, two of its twenty permanent guests. Most of those planned to leave before the end of the day, but the Weilands would fight on. It would be weeks before the legal wrangling was settled and they moved to another hotel. Kathryn Weiland solemnly explained to the agog *Times* man that what especially upset her was the effect the closure was having on her poodle, Gigi. The poodle, who got her teeth brushed twice a day, had gone off her food and taken to her bed.

As noon approached, the TV and radio crews added to the almost impossible congestion in the lobby as hundreds of people began arriving for lunch: the *Inquirer* Book and Author Luncheon filled the ballroom and its balcony with eight hundred guests, the Greater Philadelphia Community Development Corporation hosted a gathering in the Viennese Room, and the Burgundy Room was filled with the alumni of Temple Law School.

At one o'clock the crowd in the lobby paused to watch a symbolic spectacle. A workman clambered up an aluminum ladder to remove the state flags hanging over the registration desk.

The afternoon passed with the permanent guests—the doughty Weilands apart—checking out. By six o'clock the Weilands were the only occupants on the upper floors.

At eight o'clock Mayor Rizzo arrived in the lobby and made his way slowly through the crowd, shaking hands, signing autographs, and posing for pictures.

At nine-thirty, the lights in the ballroom dimmed: the last charity function the Bellevue Stratford would hold was over.

In the kitchen a grim-faced Castelli waited, eyes on the wall clock. At ten o'clock the last table in the Stratford Garden was served.

"Okay, that's it," sighed Castelli. He ordered the cooking appliances shut down.

He addressed the night crew for the last time. Choking back his own emotion, Castelli said, "Part of Philadelphia has just died."

He would remain for another hour. Then, when the kitchen was secured, he would leave, a lonely figure walking slowly through the subterranean corridors and out into the cold night air. He was departing the Bellevue with his reputation intact—but a personal mystery unsolved. He still did not know how all that meat had been so systematically stolen from his kitchen. Somehow it no longer mattered.

In the Hunt Room scores of people stood and mournfully sang the only song suitable: "Auld Lang Syne."

Chadwick and Varr were closeted on the Executive Floor, dealing with the mass of paperwork the actual closure entailed. They said little to each other. Varr thought: *What do you say to someone who has just seen part of himself die?*

In the lobby, as the gilded clock above the registration desk struck midnight, Anna Taggart told a reporter, "It wasn't just 29 legionnaires who died and another 151 who became sick. This thing has killed 500 of us, and the finest hotel in the land."

She watched, ashen-faced, biting her lip, oblivious to the tears streaming down her face, as security men barred and chained the Walnut Street entrance and posted a notice on the door.

THE BELLEVUE STRATFORD IS CLOSED

Other security men were shepherding the last of the people out of the Hunt Room.

At exactly 12:55 A.M. on the morning of Friday, November 19, Chadwick and Varr emerged into the lobby and announced the staff must now leave.

Waiters, bellmen, pages, and clerks departed. Finally Anna was left alone with the two executives.

They exchanged silent handshakes. Escorted by the two men, the tiny elevator operator walked toward the Broad Street door. There, drying her tears, she faced her former employers.

"All my life has been a series of ups and downs. This is just another down. But there will be an up. You betcha!"

Then she turned and walked for the last time through the splendid main doors of the Bellevue Stratford.

A reporter noted that the William Green Federal Building at Sixth and Arch in Philadelphia, looked, on the morning of Tuesday, November 23, monolithic and uninhabited, a modern monument to the facelessness of government. It would make a good line for the story he had been asked to write for *Philadelphia Magazine* about what his colleagues had dubbed, in the handy shorthand of daily journalism, the Murphy hearings.

They were being held in Room 3306–10, a large meeting room on the third floor of the building.

At one end of the room was an alcove. It was brightly lit by rectangular overhead lights and the powerful spots set up by TV technicians. In the alcove was a long table covered with microphones and ashtrays.

Seated at the center of the table was Congressman Murphy. Flanking him were his trusted investigator Ray Cole, Pennsylvania congressman Robert Nix, New Jersey congressman Matthew Rinaldo, and Pennsylvania senator Richard Schweiker. There were also the counsel for the subcommittee, and various aides who came and went.

The panel faced a small table at which the witnesses sat while giving evidence. It, too, was festooned with microphones.

Behind that table were rows of cheap imitation-leather and chrome chairs, arranged in neat lines. The reporters, witnesses, and public sat there.

Above and behind the panel, alone and lost on a yellow wall, noted the *Philadelphia* reporter, was a smaller-than-life framed photograph of President Gerald Ford. The side walls of the room were white, broken

in the center by vertical orange bands, the kind of happy color archi-
tects prescribed for anonymous government buildings or low-income
housing projects. The TV cameras were to the right; to the left was a
drooping American flag.

Shortly after 10 A.M., Murphy delivered an opening statement
tailored for the noon news shows: "This has been called the epidemic
of the century"; "we have not found the answer"; "we do not know the
cause of the disease—if it was a disease." And, of course, the carefully
placed smear: "CDC's apparent failure to consider all possible causes
from the very beginning, no matter what their expectations led them to
believe, is questionable."

The stage had been set. But first Congressman Rinaldo had to float
his brief bid for media attention: "It is entirely possible that a terrorist
group or single fanatic might possess the technology to distribute a
deadly poison or bacteria among a large group. . . ."

The Sabotage/Terrorist Theory had just had new life breathed into
it—enough to sustain it in the years to come.

The first witness was Polk. He read his prepared statement. Afterward he answered questions. Nothing he said caused much of a stir.

Bachman, who had brought Parkin along in case he was needed, was
next.

Again, and as with all the major witnesses, Bachman's opening testi-
mony had been typed and photocopies distributed beforehand to the
panel.

This was standard procedure for all congressional subcommittees, allowing the panel to know what each witness would say, so that suitable
questions could be prepared in advance.

The *Philadelphia* reporter noted: "It is all very cozy, and one might
wonder why the whole thing isn't done through the mail. But that
would steal the subcommittee's thunder. It must be public, it must get
publicity, it must be important because it *looks* important."

After lunch, legionnaire George Chiavetta, accompanied by his attorney, testified about the man in the bright blue suit he had seen in the
Bellevue's lobby all those months ago.

Nobody was very interested.

Everybody was waiting for the CDC team to appear at the witness
table.

In the end it was the next morning, Wednesday, November 24, that
Fraser, Sencer, and Boutwell were motioned to their seats.

Sencer read aloud from the meticulous brief Fraser had helped to
prepare. He concluded with a sentiment that patently reflected both
his and Fraser's honesty and compassion.

"Whether [the] causative agent is a microbiological entity of as yet
undescribed characteristics or an environmental chemical, our best

scientific capabilities have been unable to determine. However disappointing this may be, particularly for those persons afflicted by the disease and for their families and friends and for the hundreds of persons who labored exhaustively to uncover the cause, we must admit that there are diseases and conditions of ill health with which we are not familiar and which, as yet, we are unable fully to understand. This is not so much an admission of human failure as a recognition of how medical and biological science and knowledge evolve."

When Sencer sat down, Murphy looked at Fraser. Did he have any comments?

Fraser said he had none.

Murphy repeated and received the same response from Boutwell.

For a moment there was silence in the room. Then, in the measured tones that had made so many witnesses quail down the years, Murphy launched himself into his harangue. Fixing the CDC director with his eyes, he stated: "Doctor, at the outset you said that 'contemporary science is not infallible.' Of course there is no group that is probably more aware of the fallibility of people of science and Government than the panel in which we serve. . . ."

It was the opening shot in a sustained attack on the CDC. The more Fraser, Sencer, and Boutwell tried to apply reason, the more the panel heaped scorn and doubt on their answers.

It was wonderful copy for the reporters. But it did little to further the image of impartiality of congressional subcommittees.

Bruised but unbowed, in spite of the savagery of the subcommittee's attack, Fraser returned to his office in Atlanta to complete the draft of his EPI-2—the end-of-investigation report. It was a coolly reasoned and comprehensive recital of everything which had epidemiologically occurred since that morning, four months previously, when he had plunged into the maelstrom of the Harrisburg health department offices. The report contained no hint of the relentless battering he had received during almost the entire period of the mammoth inquiry.

Though he would never have said so, few others could have survived to recount the epidemiological triumph his EPI-2 contained. Many believed that by remaining resolute in the face of the unbelievable pressures, he had played the major role in stopping a public panic that might easily have caused a much greater tragedy. He had not been present when the deadly agent emerged so surreptitiously in the midst of the greatest birthday party a nation had held. Yet once on the scene, Fraser had very quickly shown that it had vanished as suddenly as it appeared. He could not prevent its possible return. But he *was* able to describe it: an infectious agent from a common source, probably airborne. It was up to those in the labs to isolate which particular agent it was.

When he had finished the EPI-2, Fraser sent the document in mid-December to all those scientists and doctors who had helped in the investigation. He wanted their comments and suggestions, critical or otherwise.

It was typical of the man.

On Monday, December 27, Joe McDade, for reasons that he would remain not exactly clear about, decided to interest himself again in the legionnaires' disease agent. He opened his box containing the slides from two victims. One of them was J.B.

After lengthy microscopic study of the slides, McDade saw what he had not seen in August—the presence of a new bacterium. It was the causative agent of legionnaires' disease which David Fraser had tracked so tenaciously, and whose effects he had described—without, until now, its actual presence having been confirmed in the laboratory.

CONTINUATION

Aftermath

Fraser listened intently as McDade explained in his soft drawl—which made some of the assembled news reporters strain forward and the TV recordists and radio reporters turn up the volume on their equipment— just what he had seen under his microscope.

It was Tuesday afternoon, January 18, 1977, and the media had been hurriedly summoned to the CDC to officially hear that, 147 days after the outbreak was brought to the attention of the agency, its agent had been discovered.

For days previously the CDC had been buzzing with the rumor that a breakthrough had been achieved. And indeed a handful of outsiders already knew the truth, Congressman John Murphy among them. Sencer, in what must have been a bittersweet moment, had personally telephoned the browbeating congressman to say that, after three weeks of intensive laboratory work following McDade's first sighting of the organism, he and Shepard were now confident they had isolated the agent. In reaching this conclusion, they had been materially helped by Fraser, who fed them essential epidemiological information as part of the careful checks and balances they had instituted to ensure there could be no question about the final result. Fraser had also supervised part of the scientific paper work associated with announcing the discovery. And his hand could also be detected in the careful review of events that Sencer used to open the press conference.

Anxious to avoid a publicity debacle, one that would only add to his other professional problems arising from what was now being roundly condemned as the swine flu disaster, Sencer had been careful to prevent the importance of the discovery from being dissipated by premature reporting. To outwit the medical Deep Throats lurking in the CDC, he had virtually sprung the conference on both the unsuspecting media and his staff.

Nevertheless, Auditorium B—where six months ago Tsai and

Graitcer sat learning the principles of epidemiology—was filled with the press and CDC staffers.

Sencer, flanked by Fraser, McDade, and Shepard, sat on the podium.

The director concluded his statement by announcing: "We are dealing with a very real phenomenon which has been present in the past but has never been recognized."

McDade then explained what he had seen through his microscope on that December morning two days after Christmas. It had appeared to him as a bright red cluster of tiny rods nestled inside the much larger purple blob that represented a single animal cell. Yet the rod-shaped organisms were not the rickettsiae he had been looking for but very unusual bacteria. He and Shepard had decided to rerun their tests, with one major change: they would exclude from the embryonated hens' eggs the bacteria-killing antibodies they had previously used. It made all the difference. The eggs died, fatally infected by the bacteria, which was now able to flourish and reproduce inside them. With this ready means of supply for the new bacterium, it had been studied further and characterized as "fastidious, gram-negative, rod-shaped, and a micron long."

For the next few minutes the quiet voice of McDade took the attentive news reporters on a journey of explanation into the subvisible world where this pathogenic organism had lived, reproduced, and died, its identity hidden, until now, from all human beings, perhaps from the beginning of time. Nobody would ever know how widely it had ravaged, how many it had annihilated, anonymously. There was still much to learn about the new microbe, but the world now knew what it looked like and something of how it fitted into the great family of disease bacteria.

It was described as "fastidious" because it could be cultured only on very specific artificial media and, even then, only very slowly; "gram-negative" meant the organism was stained red by the laboratory dye used to identify it; "rod-shaped" distinguished it from the spherical and spiral forms that bacteria also come in; and its length of a micron—one millionth of a meter, or 0.000039 of an inch—meant the bacterium was somewhat shorter than usual for such organisms.

Sera from thirty-three legionnaires who had been hospitalized and survived were tested for antibodies to the new agent. The great majority showed strong reactions, clearly indicating they had previously been infected by the organism. Similar results were found among cases of "Broad Street pneumonias," the category that had so concerned Fraser. Now that mystery, too, was solved: the cases were part of the same epidemic. The last missing piece of the legionnaires' disease puzzle was firmly in place.

Further, the prediction made by Fraser's superior all those months ago—that with the solution of the legionnaires' epidemic Fraser would also solve the outbreak at St. Elizabeth's Hospital in Washington—had come true. Stored blood from that outbreak contained antibodies to the new microbe. It was chilling confirmation that the bacteria which had killed or made ill 221 persons in Pennsylvania had also been at work eleven years earlier in the federal mental institution.

After the CDC press conference, interest in the story switched to Pennsylvania. There, Adjutant Hoak of the American Legion said that the news was "important to the whole country," and that though some Legion members had urged the disease should be given another name, he strongly disagreed. To do that, he argued, "would be a disservice to those who suffered and brought this to the attention of the medical profession and the general public."

William Chadwick lamented that the discovery "was too late—the hotel has closed and is on the market." Chadwick returned to manage the Ben Franklin. But he never quite recovered from the closing of the Bellevue. Almost three years after the Legion convention, in June 1979, Chadwick was taking a short vacation at Ocean City, New Jersey. He suddenly staggered and fell, dying on the sands of the heart attack his loyal deputy, Harold Varr, had always feared would claim him.

Varr and the other fortunate ones among the five hundred staff who worked at the Bellevue found employment in various Philadelphia hotels. They rarely talked about their experiences in the late summer and fall of 1976.

The Bellevue was eventually sold for $8.25 million to a local developer who, with a San Francisco–based hotel chain, spent a further $22 million in renovations. The first guest in the renamed Fairmont Hotel was Anna Taggart. She noted that not only were the elevators fully automatic but "the new place didn't have the style of the Bellevue."

The absence of that indefinable style perhaps contributed to a further change of management under which, by 1981, the hotel also reverted to its original name: the Bellevue Stratford.

Four years earlier, Dicko Dolan decided to commemorate the fiftieth anniversary of Post 239 by issuing matchbooks. They bore the legend:

J. B. Ralph
J. T. Dolan

In memory of our departed comrades.
Taken from our midst by the mysterious
and unsolved illness.

David Fraser would be the first to accept that some people will only believe what they want to believe, that no amount of scientific evidence will convince them otherwise.

But he could be satisfied he had done his job.

News of the discovery of the bacterium immediately traveled around the world. Scientists in research establishments in Europe and Australasia as well as in North America began attempts to duplicate the CDC results. Microbiologists at the state laboratory in Philadelphia were the first to succeed, isolating the bacillus from stored legionnaires' lung tissue.

The first serious epidemic to follow the Philadelphia outbreak began in Vermont in May 1977 and was apparently associated with the Medical Center Hospital at Burlington. There were seventeen deaths, giving a case-fatality ratio of some 25 percent. The bacterium, now named *Legionella pneumophila*, was reportedly found in water from the cooling tower of the hospital. Another epidemic apparently associated with a hospital broke out about the same time at the Wadsworth Veterans Administration Center in Los Angeles; later investigation would again point to the likely culpability of air-conditioning cooling towers.

In the late summer that year, the first recognized European outbreak occurred in Nottingham, England. Many of the patients were treated at the City Hospital. No common source was proved, but sera from six of the patients were sent to the CDC for analysis: five of them had antibody titers strongly suggesting legionnaires' disease. Two of the patients died. Other sporadic cases were soon discovered in Scotland and London.

The fear spread—fanned by a crop of scary headlines—that the deadly bug was more likely to stalk hospitals, that it chose its victims among those already weakened by other illness. There was more than a modicum of truth behind the fear. Hospital patients, especially elderly ones, are more vulnerable because their resistance has already been lowered. And cooling towers—an essential adjunct to the efficient running of any large modern institution—have been identified as a favorite abode of the bacterium. From those towers it has easy access to air-conditioning systems. And from those systems it is only a short journey for the bacteria to reach their final destination—the lungs of victims.

Again in 1977, the infection was suspected in scores of isolated cases in New York City and confirmed in a dozen instances. The city's health department was therefore not surprised when two further cases were reported in late August of 1978, but as further evidence accumulated, it became apparent New York was facing its first known major outbreak. The initial three victims had each worked on West Thirty-fifth Street, in the garment district. Epidemiological investigation focused on the area. Environmental samples were collected and sent to the CDC. Among them was water from the air-conditioner cooling tower atop Macy's. Just before Christmas—by which time the case count had reached thirty-eight and three people had died—*Legionella pneumophila* was reportedly isolated in the water. However, according to the New York *Times*, city health officials decided that in order to avoid "an unnecessary scare during the middle of the Christmas shopping season," the public was not to be informed of the discovery until January.

Just as hospitals and other large buildings such as department stores often have cooling towers on their roof, so, too, do hotels.

Perhaps the most widely publicized hotel associated with legionnaires' disease, other than the Bellevue Stratford, is the Rio Park in Benidorm, Spain. In 1973 three Scottish tourists died after vacationing there and thirty-five others became ill. Four years later, after *Legionella pneumophila* had been discovered, sera from three of the survivors were sent to the CDC. The sera were found to have significantly high titers, suggesting legionnaires' disease. Soon afterward, another Scottish vacationer who had recently stayed at the hotel died; *Legionella pneumophila* was seen in her lungs after autopsy. This deepened scientific suspicion that the 1973 outbreak had been caused by the legionnaires' disease bacterium. In September 1980 yet another spate of cases erupted among vacationers who had stayed at the hotel. One of them died. *Legionella pneumophila* was reportedly isolated from water in the hotel's shower heads; intensive research would reveal shower heads as another preferred niche of the bacterium.

Those outbreaks in Spain created a climate where even a suspicion of the bacterium's presence was enough to produce panic and commercial havoc. In March 1981 *Legionella pneumophila* was again believed to be in Benidorm; three more British tourists were reported as having been killed by it. Fear swept the resort; thousands of vacationers from Europe and the United States canceled their bookings to Spain. For Benidorm the seventh suspected visit in as many years by the dreaded bacillus threatened this time to claim the town itself: it faced ruin at the onset of the critical 1981 season, when fuel surcharges began seriously to cripple the tourist industry. The Spanish government acted swiftly. It sent a team to Benidorm which, after working around the clock for several days, confidently pronounced that legionnaires' disease was not responsible for the deaths. Not everyone was convinced. The bacterium has a hit-and-run record, an ability not only to erupt without warning but to disappear under cover of a confusing trail.

The disease has also been seen in France, Canada, Australia, Italy, South Africa, Sweden, Germany, Holland, and Portugal—in one form or another. For it is now known that *Legionella pneumophila* exists in at least four slightly differing serogroups causing either a long-incubation, potentially fatal infection or a short-incubation, nonfatal, self-limited illness. This further complicates diagnosis.

In the United States, throughout 1981 sporadic cases were reported. During the summer it was feared a major epidemic was about to begin in the area around Buffalo, New York, after sixteen people became ill with the disease. Three of them died. Later, experts concluded the cases only reflected the increased awareness of doctors to the illness. The suspicions of an alert physician are sometimes raised by a common sequence of events: the failure to recover from sputum or sera by conventional methods an organism known to be involved in pulmonary infection; the absence of response to antibiotics commonly used to treat pneumonia; the identification of an unusual epidemiological setting, such as a history of close contact with or exposure to the water of air-conditioner cooling towers; residence in an area where soil is being turned over during construction work; swimming in a creek or lake.

Though there have been isolated cases among children, the typical patient with legionnaires' disease is a middle-aged or elderly person. The first symptoms include malaise, muscular rheumatism, and headache, usually followed by a rapidly elevating fever associated with chills and a nonproductive cough. Three sets of additional symptoms may be seen: chest pain; diarrhea, abdominal pain, or vomiting; confusion or delirium. The patient's past medical history often includes cigarette smoking and, sometimes, chronic renal failure or immunosuppressive therapy, or both.

Unfortunately the physician caring for a patient with pneumonia before its cause is identified faces a difficult diagnostic dilemma. The final proof of the specific agent responsible often rests on specialized microbiological studies presently available only in research establishments and outside the scope of laboratories in even the best-equipped hospitals.

The currently available CDC data suggest that the drug of choice is erythromycin. In cases where this drug has been administered in time, patients with legionnaires' disease have shown a relatively low fatality rate.

Yet some people contend the bacterium's existence today signifies an eleventh-hour warning that there must be a change in the course of civilization, pointing out that this alien and dangerous thing survives because it is stronger than humans, able to adapt to a hostile environment, overcoming the most complex defense system ever developed—the one implanted in each human being at birth. Time and again the bacterium is able to enter and destroy a body.

It continues to kill—but with one significant difference. Today victims are subjected to the most intensive scientific study, part of the on-going process of investigating legionnaires' disease. Almost every month a little more is learned about the bacterium; there is a continuous flow of medical publications about these discoveries. And in an era of un-easy relations between East and West, this knowledge transcends polit-ical barriers. Information emerging from laboratories in the United States and Britain is swiftly transmitted to research institutes in the So-viet Union and China. Because legionnaires' disease has been called, not altogether fallaciously, "the disease of modern man"—with an im-plication that its presence, in part, is due to the sophisticated technol-ogy that provides for a more comfortable life-style of which air-condi-tioning and cooling systems are two main supports—mankind has mobilized its considerable arsenal to counterattack this denizen of the subvisible world.

The battle continues today. But there can be no doubt about the outcome. The human race will win this confrontation, just as it has emerged victorious from so many other battles it has waged with that world.

APPENDIXES

SPECIAL THANKS

Interviewees

Without the cooperation of those whose names follow, this book would not have been possible.

HSH Princess Grace of Monaco

Alotta, Robert
Aronson, Marvin

Bachman, Leonard
Balows, Albert
Beecham, James
Bennett, John
Berreth, Donald
Biddle, Edward
Bindie, Richard
Brachman, Philip
Bunting, John

Cairo, Patrick
Castelll, Frank
Chandler, Francis
Craven, Robert
Cresci, Frank

Dolan, Joyce
Dolan, Richard (Dicko)
Dowdle, Walter

Fellman, Nelson
Fetterhoff, Doris
Flynn, Joe
Flynn, Lorraine
Fraser, David

Gaudiosi, Albert
Gilbert, Harold
Goldberger, Mark
Graitcer, Philip

Greenfield, Bruce
Grubb, Arthur
Grubb, Ruth

Hattwick, Michael
Hoak, Edward
Hoover, Dale

Katz, Sheila Moriber
Kimbrough, Renate
Kleger, Bruce

Lattimer, Gary
Liddle, John
Lucey, Denis

McDade, Joseph
Mallison, George
Maniglia, Rosario
Matthews, Arthur
Murphy, Frederick
Murphy, John

Nash, Philip

Parkin, William
Polk, Lewis

Quaide, Carol (formerly Ralph)

Ralph, Mildred
Ralph, Virginia Anne
Reeves, Maria
Rosen, Morton
Runsdorf, H. Norman

Satz, Jay
Seip, Elaine
Seip, Robert
Sencer, David
Sharrar, Robert
Shepard, Charles
Sideman, Leonard
Smylie, Michael
Soricelli, David
Sunderman, F. William
Sunderman, F. William, Jr.

Taggart, Anna
Thacker, Stephen
Tsai, Theodore

Varr, Harold

Walsh, Joe

Research

Bessell-Browne, Elizabeth

Chardin, Barbara

Foley, Diane
Frutos, Eva
Furniss, Margaret

Greaves, Margaret

Haskell, Ann
Hendrie, Anne

Lawson, Alan

Myers, Patricia

Naccache, Ursula

Secretarial

Byrne, Tina

Clark, Barbara

ACKNOWLEDGMENTS

Individuals

Bartlett, Christopher
Blyth, Jeffrey
Boyle, Bob E.
Bregman, Denis
Bresson, Thomas
Brown, David
Buckley, Joseph

Cassens, David
Causse, Georges
Choisit, Paul
Cole, Roger

Dribben, Elizabeth
Dull, Bruce

Foege, William

Hitze, K. L.
Hooper, Betty

Johnson, Claude

Kelly, John
Keto, Yaeko
Knapp, Werner
Kondrates, Ramunas
Koornhof, H. J.

Lieben, Jan
Lacoste, Nadia
Lord, Katherine
Lorenzetti, Paul

McGough, Sheila
Macrae, Alistair
Maxwell, William
Mayon-White, Richard
Moberg, Anne
Mollaret, Henri
Morgan, John

Morrow, Charles
Murphy, Peter

Najera, Rafael
Neubaum, Charles

Perian, Carl
Pidcoe, Vern
Pio, A.
Polk, Phyllis

Reid, Daniel
Riley, William
Rosen, Morton
Ruckdeschel, Gotthardt

Spencer, Gil
Stille, Wolfgang

Wainerdi, Richard
Wallach, Arthur
Ward, Richard
Wecht, Cyril
Worsey, Gloria
Wratney, George
Wright, Lawrence

Organizations

Aer Lingus
American Legion, Department of
    Pennsylvania, Harrisburg
American Legion, Department of
    Pennsylvania, Williamstown

Carrier Corporation
Centers for Disease Control
Central Intelligence Agency

Daily News, Philadelphia
E. I. Du Pont de Nemours & Co.

Federal Bureau of Investigation
    (Washington, D.C., and
    Philadelphia)

Health Department, City of
    Philadelphia
Holy Spirit Hospital, Camp Hill,
    Pennsylvania

Pennsylvania Department of
    Health
Philadelphia *Inquirer*
Pottsville Hospital, Pennsylvania

U. S. Department of the Army

Reader's Digest

Smithsonian Institution, Public
    Health Collection, National
    Museum of History and
    Technology, Washington, D.C.
Spiro and Associates, Philadelphia

U. S. Environmental Protection
    Agency

Water Department, City of
    Philadelphia
Williamstown Historical
    Committee
World Health Organization,
    Geneva

Bibliography

The following is an abridged list of the written sources consulted.

Balows, Albert, and Fraser, David. "International Symposium on Legionnaires' Disease," *Annals of International Medicine*, Vol. 90, No. 4, American College of Physicians, Apr. 1979.

Burt, Nathaniel. *The Perennial Philadelphians*. Boston: Little, Brown, 1963.

Collier, Richard. *The Plague of the Spanish Lady*. New York: Atheneum, 1974.

Cordes, L. G., and Fraser, D. W. "Legionellosis," *Medical Clinics of North America*, Vol. 64, No. 3, May 1980.

Fraser, D. W.; Tsai, T. F.; et al. "Legionnaires' Disease: Description of an Epidemic of Pneumonia," *New England Journal of Medicine*, Vol. 297, 1977, pp. 1189–97.

Fuller, John G. *Fever: The Hunt for a New Killer Virus*. New York: Reader's Digest Press, 1974.

Jones, G. L., and Herbert, G. A., eds. "Legionnaires'": CDC Laboratory Manual. Atlanta: U. S. Dept. of Health, Education, and Welfare, 1978.

Kruif, Paul de. *Microbe Hunters*. New York: Harcourt, Brace, 1926.

McDade, J. E.; Shepard, C. C.; et al. "Legionnaires' Disease: Isolation of a Bacterium," *New England Journal of Medicine*, Vol. 297, 1977, pp. 1197–1203.

Moley, Raymond, Jr. *The American Legion Story*. New York: Duell, Sloan and Pearce, 1966.

Marks, John. *The Search for the Manchurian Candidate*. New York: Times Books, 1979.

Suspension of the Swine Flu Immunization Program, 1976. Hearing, U. S. Senate, 94th Congress, 2nd Session, Dec. 17, 1976, Committee on Labor and Public Welfare. Washington, D.C.: U. S. Government Printing Office, 1977.

Legionnaires' Disease. Hearings, U. S. House of Representatives, 94th Congress, 2nd Session, Nov. 23 and 24, 1976, Committee on Interstate and Foreign Commerce. Washington, D.C.: U. S. Government Printing Office, 1977.

Legionnaires' Disease, 1977. Hearing, U. S. Senate, 95th Congress, 1st Session, Nov. 9, 1977, Committee on Human Resources. Washington, D.C.: U. S. Government Printing Office, 1978.

Index

ABC Ice Company (Philadelphia), 267

Acute Communicable Disease Control Program (Philadelphia), 71

Adams, Billy, 170, 312

Adams, Joseph, xi, 97, 153, 223–24

Adams family, 327

Adenovirus, 275

Africa, 7, 29, 113

Air-conditioning units, xiv, 171, 174, 199–200, 344

  at Bellevue Stratford Hotel, 22–23, 24, 37, 41, 44, 50–51, 52, 61, 67, 68, 75, 80, 130, 162, 163, 174, 231–32, 233–34, 236–37, 239, 243, 321

  at Macy's (New York City), 345

Allentown, Pa., 181, 182

Altman, Lawrence, 275–76

Alundum, 280, 297

American Broadcasting Company (ABC), 172, 214–15

American Legion, 27, 39, 107, 127, 343

American Legion State Convention of 1976 (Philadelphia), 8, 10, 11, 13, 48–69, 80, 81, 94, 95, 97, 104, 105–6, 107, 110, 127, 133–34, 144, 156, 163, 174–75, 178, 181, 203, 245, 278, 289, 294, 303

  closing dance, 67

  fears of radical group attacks, 39–40, 48, 63, 67–68, 145

  police vigilance, 48–49

  Post Everlasting ceremony, 61

  prostitution at, 50–51, 55–56, 66, 68

  total number of legionnaires, 242

Women's Auxiliary, 54, 242

  See also Legionnaires' disease

AMP (electronics factory, Williamstown, Pa.), 170

Anderson, Jack, 329

Anemia, 70

Anthrax, 7, 144, 145, 240

Antimicrobics Investigations Section (Center for Disease Control), 279

Arizona, 7

Armstrong, Neil, xiv

Arsenic, 275

Ascaris, 275

Associated Press, 107, 158

Astley family, 327

Attica prison, xiv

Auerbach, Stuart, 276

Australia, xiii, 345–46

Autopsies, 90–94, 110–12, 115–16, 132, 136–37, 152, 174, 189, 222, 223, 225, 303

  cranial type, 92, 147

Aveni, Frank, 60

  death of, 78

A/Victoria influenza strain of 1975, 140

Avon Company, 122

Bachman, Dr. Leonard, xi, 104, 106–8, 109, 110, 112, 116–21, 124

  legionnaires' disease investigation, 126, 130, 131–35, 143, 152, 155–56, 157–60, 165–66, 175, 177, 205–7, 209, 215, 224, 237, 244–45, 258, 271, 272, 273, 274–76, 277, 285, 304

Murphy congressional hearings, 335

press briefings, 116–21, 143, 157,
     158, 165, 273
relationship with Fraser, 158–60,
     177, 178, 244–45, 274–75, 276,
     277
reputation for honesty, 116
Bacterial Diseases Division (Center
     for Disease Control), 4, 187
Bad Booze Theory, 135
Bankers Security Corporation, 36, 300,
     305
Bear's Den (bar, Williamstown, Pa.),
     170
Beecham, Dr. James, 76, 100, 102,
     104, 108
Belinger family, 327
Belles, Dr. Terry, 94
Bellevue Hospital (New York City),
     72
Bellevue Stratford Hotel
     (Philadelphia), 20–27, 71, 80,
     113–15, 130, 133, 138, 145, 154,
     162–63, 171, 174, 182–86, 217,
     225, 227, 229–37, 238, 241, 243,
     247, 252, 261–62, 263, 265, 268,
     274, 276, 278, 280–92, 298–302,
     303, 304, 305, 306, 309, 315,
     318–21, 325–29, 343
     air-conditioning system, 22–23, 24,
       37, 41, 44, 50–51, 52, 61, 67, 68,
       75, 80, 113, 162, 174, 231–32,
       233–34, 236–37, 239, 243, 321
     air ventilating system, 288–92
     arrival of EIS officers at, 283–87
     as asset of Philadelphia, 284
     basement service departments, 53,
       318
     Burgundy Room, 38, 66, 67, 327,
       333
     CDC investigating of, 186, 187–89,
       192–94, 231, 233–37, 239,
       247–48, 281, 287–92, 299–300
     charity gala, 325–29
     closing of, 330, 331–34, 343
     computer printout analysis of,
       321–22
     concessionaires, 38
     cutting back on expenses, 26
     "downstairs" (kitchen) operations,
       23–27, 182–86, 192–93, 287–88,
       318
     employee theft, 42–43, 49, 66, 333
     financial losses (post–Legion
       convention), 323

Grand Ballroom, 174, 328
     Hunt Room, 231, 282, 318, 333,
       334
     incinerator operations, 22, 23, 51,
       52
     laundry staff, 52–53, 318
     number of guest rooms, 21
     Oak Room, 235, 281, 289
     plumbing system, 300–1
     renamed, 343
     reputation of, 21, 37, 71
     rodent droppings, 22, 80, 291
     Rose Garden, 60, 61, 62, 235, 289
     Save the Bellevue attempts, 322–23,
       325–29
     security force, 49, 57, 67
     selling of, 343
     Stratford Garden restaurant, 38, 56,
       62, 65, 67, 231, 282, 299, 323,
       333
     telephone exchange system, 37, 50
     "upstairs" (management), 25–26,
       36–44
     Viennese Room, 333
     See also American Legion State
       Convention of 1976; International
       Eucharistic Congress
Benidorm, Spain, legionnaires' disease
     outbreak of 1981, 345
Benjamin Franklin Hotel
     (Philadelphia), 36, 192, 238, 322,
     343
Benny, Jack, 36
Beryllium, 275
B/Hong Kong influenza strain,
     140–41
Bicentennial of 1976, xiii–xiv, 10, 59,
     134, 138
Billy Adams' Shoe Repair Shop,
     (Williamstown, Pa.), 170, 312
Biological nuclear solvent (BNS), 221
Black Death, xiv, 144, 145
     See also Bubonic plague; Plague
Blastomycosis, 275
Blavat, Jerry, 327
Bloomsburg, Pa., 80, 136
BNS. See Biological nuclear solvent
Boldt, George C., 21
Bookbinder family, 327
Botulism, 144
Boutwell, Joseph, 331, 335, 336
Brennan, Ray, 60
     death of, 75

"Broad Street" pneumonia, 304, 305, 342
Brucella, 166, 275
Brucellosis, 144
Bubonic plague, 7, 22, 144
  See also Black Death; Plague
Buffalo, N.Y., legionnaires' disease outbreak of 1981, 346
Bunting family, 327
Bureau of Epidemiology (Center for Disease Control), 187, 272
Bureau of Laboratories (Center for Disease Control), 278, 331
Burgundy Room (Bellevue Stratford Hotel), 38, 66, 67, 327, 333
Buzzard, Dr. Harry, 95, 103, 104
Byerly, Louis, 60

Cadmium, 275
California, 7, 47, 138, 264
Callos, Jimmy, 318
Cambodia, xiv, 145
Canada, xiii, 345–46
Cancer, 47
Candida, 275
Cardinal's Committee on the Laity, 37
Carrier Corporation, 23, 231, 233
Carson, Johnny, 259
Carter, Jimmy, 20, 233, 252, 253, 322, 326
Case Control Survey, of CDC, 315
Castelli, Frank, 19–20, 22–27, 37, 39, 49, 52, 66, 162, 182–86, 188, 192, 193, 194, 233, 298, 325–26, 327, 328–29, 331–34
Catholic Philopatrian Literary Institute, 37
CBS. *See* Columbia Broadcasting System
CBW. *See* Chemical-biological warfare
Center for Disease Control (Atlanta), xi, xiv, 27, 72, 73, 75–77, 78, 96, 101, 102, 105, 109, 112–13, 116, 117, 119, 123–24, 126, 127, 128, 129, 132–33, 134, 137, 142, 147, 150, 151, 152, 157, 166, 167, 173, 179, 180, 182, 186, 187, 188, 199, 201, 202, 215, 222, 223, 226, 228, 236, 244, 247, 251–57, 264, 271, 272, 277, 278–80, 298, 300, 305, 306, 307, 308, 314–15, 322, 324, 329, 345, 346
Antimicrobics Investigations Section, 279
army interview, 316–18
Bacterial Diseases Division, 4, 187
Bellevue Stratford headquarters, 283–87, 299
Bureau of Epidemiology, 187, 272
Bureau of Laboratories, 278, 331
Clinical Chemistry Division, 278
Division of Bacteriology, 279
EIS course, 76–77
epidemiologic fieldwork, 6–7
headquarters, 254–55
"hot lab" (maximum-security laboratory), 29, 254–55, 280
Influenza Surveillance Center, 243–45
Lassa fever vaccine breakthrough, 29–30, 31
Leprosy and Rickettsia Branch, 256
monitoring programs, 5–6
number of employees, 6
pragmatic approach of, 31
research laboratories of, 278–80
Special Pathogens Branch, 4–5, 9, 30, 31, 47, 121, 125, 314
swine flu rift, 45–46
toxicology division at Chamblee, Ga., 255, 278
Virology Division, 140–42
  See also Epidemic Intelligence Service (EIS)
Central Intelligence Agency (CIA), 9, 35, 40, 134, 144–45, 154, 157, 158, 159, 168, 222, 235, 239–40, 296, 313, 316
LSD experiments, 145
mushroom experiments, 144–45
New York subway test, 146
Chadwick, William, xii, 26, 36–44, 51, 56, 65, 66–67, 113–15, 138, 143, 162–63, 183, 185, 186, 188, 192, 193, 194, 224, 229, 230, 231–32, 233, 245, 248, 266, 281, 282, 283, 285, 286, 298–302, 318, 322–23, 326, 327, 328, 330, 332, 343
background of, 36–37
ban on hotel employees talking to the press, 162
death of, 343
hotel booking policy, 38
optimism of, 43–44

Chadwick, Mrs. William (Pat), 36, 40, 299
Chamberlain, Charles, 97
Chamber of Commerce (Philadelphia), 224
Chambersburg, Pa., 103, 190, 191
Chambersburg Hospital, 80
Chemical-biological warfare (CBW), 144–47, 154, 175, 197, 198–99, 240, 257, 270, 313, 316, 318
Chiang Kai-shek, 28
Chiavetta, George, xii, 56–57, 63, 171, 252, 335
China, 28, 145, 347
Chinatown (Philadelphia), 61, 203–4
Cholera, 7, 253
Chromium, 166, 275
Church of the Sacred Heart of Jesus (Williamstown, Pa.), 9, 85, 169
CIA. See Central Intelligence Agency
City Hospital (Nottingham, England), 344
Civic Center (Philadelphia), 37
Clinical Chemistry Division (Center for Disease Control), 278
Closing dance (American Legion Convention), 67
Clover Club (Philadelphia), 21
Coccidioidomycosis, 275
Cole, Ray, 308–9, 334
Columbia Broadcasting System (CBS), 172, 214, 259
Columbia Presbyterian Medical Center (New York City), 29
Congressional Subcommittee on Consumer Protection and Finance, 308–9, 321
Contaminated Soda Theory, 135
Convention and Visitors Bureau (Philadelphia), 36
Coronaviruses, 275
Coxiella burnetii, 257
Cranial autopsy, 92, 147
Craven, Dr. Robert, xi, 76, 77, 104–6, 112–13, 314
  guinea pig exposure, 283, 307–8
  legionnaires' disease investigation, 121, 124, 127, 137, 151–53, 155, 174, 179, 194–99, 243–44, 270–72, 273, 283, 304
Cronkite, Walter, 259
Crosby, Bing, 65
Cryptococci, 275
Cubans, FBI check on, 201

Darren, James, 327
Delaware River, at Philadelphia, 19
Delia, Tony, 318
Dempsey, Jack, 312
Derr, Dan, 170
Diarrhea, 136
Didi (go-go dancer), 16
Dietrich, Marlene, 318
Diseased Prostitute Theory, 135
Division of Bacteriology (Center for Disease Control), 279
DNA, of virus, 204
Dolan, James (Jimmy), xii, 8–10, 13, 14, 18, 34–35, 84–94, 96, 115, 122–23, 160–61, 165, 310, 343
  autopsy, 90–94, 115–16, 147, 223
  at the convention, 62–63, 64, 65, 68–69, 262
  death of, 89–90, 150, 169, 258, 294, 295, 311
  funeral of, 149, 168, 169, 170, 172, 177, 190, 211–12, 215, 216, 258, 295, 296
  hospitalized, 77–78, 80–81, 84–89
  illness of, 74–75, 77–78, 171
Dolan, Richard (Dicko), xii, 8, 9, 10, 11, 12–14, 17, 18, 34–35, 74, 77, 78, 81, 84–86, 87, 89, 96, 108, 160, 161, 168–72, 189–90, 210–17, 257–63, 295, 311, 313–14, 343
  background of, 14
  at the convention, 60–64, 65, 68, 69, 261–62, 263
  Legion Post 239 responsibilities, 13
Dolan, Mrs. Richard (Joyce), 168, 170, 258, 259, 260, 313
"Dolan's Hole," at Legion Post 239 (Williamstown, Pa.), 13, 263
Duke University, 15, 76

Eastern Airlines, 38, 303
Ebola fever, 253
EIS. See Epidemic Intelligence Service
Eisenhower, Dwight D., 318
Elevator Theory, 239, 243, 245, 247–48, 289, 324
Elizabeth II, Queen of Britain, 20
Elizabethville, Pa., 16, 17, 18
Elizabethville Echo, 16, 17, 210
Emergency Medical Services, Philadelphia Health Department, 73

Encephalitis, 144, 253
Enemy Within Theory, 196
England, xiii, 29, 344
    See also Great Britain
Entamoeba, 275
Enteric viruses, 275
Environmental Health Services,
    Philadelphia Health Department,
    73
Epidemic Intelligence Service (EIS),
    of Center for Disease Control,
    Atlanta, 6, 7, 27, 30, 31, 101,
    102, 104, 105, 106, 109, 119,
    124, 128, 134, 138, 150, 157,
    158, 159, 165, 175, 176, 177,
    178, 190, 195, 223, 225, 238,
    240, 242, 245, 246, 258, 272,
    275–76, 283, 299, 308
Epidemiology, 27–28, 102, 156, 167
    fundamental assumption of, 136
EPI-1 and EPI-2 documents, of
    Center for Disease Control, 28
Erythromycin, 83, 220, 276, 346
Escoffier, Auguste, 24
E-76-1 (specimen number), 140
E-76-19 (lung specimen), 174
E-76-21 (specimen number), 140
Ethylene glycol, 166, 275
Eucharistic Congress. *See*
    International Eucharistic Congress

Fairview Evangelical Cemetery
    (Williamstown, Pa.), J. B.
    Ralph's burial at, 216
False Teeth Theory, 135
Federal Bureau of Investigation
    (FBI), 35, 40, 103, 120, 145,
    153, 154, 157, 158, 159, 201,
    235, 239, 280
Federal Telephone System (FTS),
    102, 103
Fetterhoff, Charlie, 295
Fetterhoff, Doris, 8, 9–10, 11, 13, 14,
    18, 34, 35, 63, 74–75, 77–78,
    80–81, 84–86, 87–89, 96, 115–16,
    123, 160–62, 169, 170, 211–12,
    213, 259, 294–97, 310–12
Fetterhoff, Tommy, 295–96
Flame retardants, 275
Florida, 7
Fonda, Henry, 57
Food and Agriculture Organization, 30
Food poisoning, 144
Ford, Gerald R., 5, 20, 39, 40, 43, 46,
    65, 145, 154, 157, 173, 201, 233,
    322, 326, 334
Fort Detrick, Md., 146, 154, 257,
    316, 318
Fort Dix flu virus, 139, 154, 254
Fort Indiantown Gap, Pa., 9, 34, 296,
    311
France, 345–46
Franklin, Benjamin, 19
Franklin Institute, Philadelphia, 283
Fraser, Dr. David, xi, 3–7, 28–29, 30,
    31, 45–47, 72, 73, 96, 102, 121,
    188, 341, 342, 343, 344
    appearance of, 3
    background of, 3–4, 126, 238
    elevator hypothesis of, 239, 243,
        245, 247–48, 289, 324
    EPI-2 (end-of-investigation report)
        of, 336–37
    guinea pig exposure, 283, 307–8
    Lassa fever investigation, 29–30, 31,
        76
    legionnaires' disease investigation,
        125–35, 137, 151, 152–55, 156,
        158–60, 165, 166–67, 172, 173,
        175–82, 192, 195, 201, 205–7,
        208, 209, 222, 224, 237–48, 254,
        258, 270–78, 283–85, 302–6,
        307–9, 314–18, 321–22, 329,
        336–37
    move to Philadelphia, 273–78, 305
    Murphy congressional hearings, 329,
        330, 335–36
    Pennsylvania headquarters, 177,
        178–80
    relationship with Bachman, 158–60,
        177, 178, 244–45, 274–75, 276,
        277
    style of investigating, 28
Fraser, Mrs. David (Barbara), 3, 45,
    46, 125–26, 237, 330
Fraser, Evan, 3
Fraser, Leigh, 3
Friendly Sons of St. Patrick, 37
Friends of the Bellevue Committee,
    323
FTS. *See* Federal Telephone System

Gaudiosi, Albert, xii, 40, 58, 73, 104,
    118, 119, 143–47, 157, 172–75,
    224, 230, 244, 245, 265, 271,
    284–87, 327
    CBW suspicions, 144–47

George V Hotel (Paris), compared to Bellevue Stratford, 26
George M. Kriz School of Dance (Williamstown, Pa.), 170
Germany, xiii, 345–46
"Gnomish syndrome," 34, 149, 165
Goldberger, Dr. Mark, xi, 128, 137–39, 179, 189, 193, 194, 200, 225, 240, 247, 266, 274, 315, 324
Gonorrhea, 47
"Good Morning America" (television show), 155
Grace, Princess, of Monaco, 43, 113, 173
Graitcer, Dr. Philip, xi, 31, 76, 77, 104–6, 112–13, 314, 341–42
legionnaires' disease investigation, 121, 128, 135, 137 41, 149 50, 151, 179, 195, 199–204, 205, 225–28, 240, 243–44, 247, 263–69, 289, 292–93, 315
Grand Ballroom (Bellevue Stratford Hotel), 174, 328
Great Britain, xiii, 29, 344, 347
See also England; Scotland; Wales
Greater Philadelphia Community Development Corporation, 333
Great Salt Lake City Conspiracy Theory, 196
Green Berets, 286
Greene, Frederick, 95
Griffin, Merv, 259
Grubb, Mayor Arthur, 74, 170, 260
Guinness Book of World Records, 9

Hafer, Elmer, 96, 97
Hahnemann Medical College and Hospital (Philadelphia), 189, 324
Harmonicats, 313
Harrisburg, Pa., 32, 56, 76, 79, 81, 83, 95, 104, 106, 108, 112, 113, 121, 125, 126, 128, 129, 130, 136, 137, 155, 170, 172, 175, 176, 195, 200, 205–7, 208, 209, 212, 224, 244, 247, 251, 260, 271–73, 283, 285, 304
See also War Room
Harrisburg Hospital, 171
Hartman, William, 94–95
Harvard Medical School, 4
Harvard University, 76
Health Center (Philadelphia), 71
Health Department (City of Philadelphia), xi, 119.

See also Philadelphia Health Department War Room
Health Program Analysis Division, Philadelphia Health Department, 73
Hemingway, Ernest, 115
Hemorrhagic fever, 7
Hepatitis, 7
Herbicides, 275
Herpes virus, 275
Heston, Charlton, 59
Hilton Hotel chain, 39
Histoplasma, 275
Histoplasmosis, 236
History Committee (Williamstown, Pa.), 312
Hoak, Edward, xii, 54, 57, 81, 96–97, 107, 108, 109, 169, 212–13, 214, 216, 224, 261, 343
Holiday Inn, 62, 63–64, 238
air-conditioning unit, 171
Holland, 345–46
Holy Spirit Hospital (Camp Hill), 79, 97, 109, 110, 148
Hong Kong flu. See B/Hong Kong influenza strain
Hoover, Dale, 8, 33–34, 96, 112, 121–23, 147–49, 160, 161, 163–65, 168, 210, 215–16
Hoover Funeral Home (Williamstown, Pa.), 112, 121–23
Hope, Bob, 42
Hornack, Andrew, 153, 174, 271, 280, 297, 304, 307
Hospitality Room Survey, of CDC, 315
Hunt Room (Bellevue Stratford Hotel), 231, 282, 318, 333, 334
Hurricane Agnes, and Williamstown, Pa., 12
Hussein, King of Jordan, 318
Hypocapnia, 241
Hypoxemia, 241

IARC (World Health Organization agency), 47
"I Love the Bellevue" buttons, 323, 326
"I Love the Bellevue" charity gala, 325–29
Indiana, 323
Influenza, 253, 275

Partners Factory (Williamstown, Pa.) 170
Pellegrino, Joe, 327
Penicillin, 47, 264, 308
Penn, William, 48
Pennsylvania Department of Health (Harrisburg), xi, 76, 101, 114, 116, 178
Pennsylvania Hospital (Philadelphia) 226, 227
Pennsylvania Mutual Building (Philadelphia), 58
Pennsylvania Supreme Court, 327
Pentagon, 198, 199
Penthouse (magazine), 55
Pertussis, 274
Pesticides, 275
Philadelphia, 8, 10, 11, 13, 19–20, 22–27, 32, 33, 34, 70–73, 75, 80 83, 84, 103, 106, 108, 112–13, 121, 127, 128, 133, 135, 172–75 176, 179, 182–86, 195, 196, 200 218, 220–21, 224, 225–37, 241, 242, 255, 260, 272–92, 302–9
  campaign against street vendors, 58–59
  geographical situation of, 19
  measles epidemic, 72
  refuse collection slowdown, 22, 39, 48, 57–58, 70–71, 200
  rodents, 70
  swine flu immunization readiness, 71, 72, 73
  See also American Legion State Convention of 1976; Bellevue Stratford Hotel; Health Department
Philadelphia *Bulletin*, 319
Philadelphia Catholic Charities, 37
Philadelphia *Daily News*, 118, 119, 134, 142, 143, 151, 152, 207, 230–31, 267, 273, 275, 277, 28 313, 319
Philadelphia Free Library, 284
Philadelphia Health Department W Room, 273, 277, 302–6, 307–9
Philadelphia *Inquirer*, 59, 118, 142, 151, 152, 191, 233, 319, 324
Philadelphia Magazine, 287, 334
Philadelphia Museum of Art, 284
Philadelphia Phillies, 327
Philadelphia Police Department, 39, 199, 202

See also Pandemic of 1918–19; type of influenza
Influenza Surveillance Center (Center for Disease Control), 243–45
Inquirer Book and Author Luncheon, 333
International Eucharistic Congress, 43, 59, 66, 80, 113–15, 138, 157, 173, 232, 233, 247, 280, 304
International Hotel Greeters Association, 37
Iran, 47
Ireland, 113
Italy, xiii, 253, 345–46

Japan, 145
Jeannette Post 344, 60
Jewish Defense League, FBI check on, 201
Johnson, Lyndon, 65
John Trotman's Coal and Ice Company (Williamstown, Pa.), 312

Katz, Dr. Sheila Moriber, 189
  illness of, 323–25
Kelly family, 327
Kennedy, Mrs. Jacqueline, 65
Kennedy, John F., xiv, 65, 215, 318
Kent State University, xiv
Keystone Cadets band, 174, 271
Kimball family, 327
King, Martin Luther, xiv
Kipling, Rudyard, 21
Klebsiella pneumonia, 95
Korean War, 208
Kriz, George, 170

Laos, 145
Lassa fever, 6, 7, 28–29, 76, 109, 119, 136, 253, 274
  vaccine breakthrough, 29–30, 31
Legion convention. *See* American Legion State Convention of 1976 (Philadelphia)
Legion *Journal*, 10, 171
Legionnaires' disease
  age factor, 150
  Atlanta-based specialists involved in, 254
  case definition question, 129, 156, 178, 306
  casualties, xiii, 75, 78, 80, 81, 83, 89, 97, 103, 105, 109, 113, 114,
    117, 128, 130, 133, 142, 149, 152, 189, 205, 275, 280, 304, 333
  early hypotheses, 138–39
  elevator hypothesis, 239, 243, 245, 247–48, 289, 324
  EPI-2 report, 336–37
  incubation factor, 222, 270
  introduction to, xiii–xv
  investigation of, 125–209 *passim*
  laboratory analysis of, 140–42, 149–50, 175, 222–23, 241–42, 254, 256–57, 274, 275, 278–80, 303
  Murphy congressional hearings, 334–36
  number of cases (1981), 346
  public panic, 153
  questionnaire, 131, 136, 137, 151, 165, 237–38, 239–40, 258, 260–61, 263, 276, 315
  scrogroups, 346
  serum testing of, 140–41, 149–50
  spread of, 150, 151, 344–47
  symptoms of, 78, 346
  theories about, 135, 154, 166, 180, 196–99, 201, 316, 335
  total number of cases, 215, 275
  toxicological analysis of, 222–23, 254, 256
  typical pattern of illness, 241
  viral analysis of, 140–42, 149–50
  X-ray evidence, 178, 241, 279, 303
  See also American Legion State Convention of 1976; names of theories
Legionella pneumophila, 341–43, 344, 345, 346–47
Leprosy and Rickettsia Branch (Center for Disease Control), 256
Leptospirosis, 6, 275
Levy, Franklin, 170
Lewis, John L., 313
Lewisburg, Pa., 83, 136
Lin Piao, 28
Lock Haven Hospital, Pa., 95
Los Angeles legionnaires' disease outbreak of 1977, 344
Los Angeles Times, 151, 332–33
Lowell, Amy, 21
LSD, 145, 146
Lymphocytic choriomeningitis, 274

McCarthy, Joseph, xiv, 316

McDade, Dr. Joseph, xi,
  279–80, 321
  background of, 257
  laboratory research and
    297–98, 306–7, 325,
    342
McKay, Maxine, 94–95
McKeesport, Pa., 81
Macy's (New York City)
  air-conditioner cooling
Malaria, 7
Mallison, George, xi, 187
  231, 233–37, 239, 24
  279, 281, 287–92, 29
Manor Post 472, 81
Marburg fever, 253, 274
Martin, Marjorie, 94–95
Maryland, 40, 47, 146, 2
Maryland Health Depart
Mayo Graduate School o
Measles, 72, 275
Medical Center Hospital
  Vt.), 344
Meningitis, bacterial, 6
Meningococci, 275
Mercury, 166, 275
Michigan, 251
Midway (motion picture
Miller, Slup, 170
Morgan, J. Pierpont, 21
Muffley, Arlene, 94–95
Mumps, 275
Murphy, John M., xii, 3
  329, 330, 331, 341
  congressional hearings,
Mycoplasma, 275
Mycoplasmal pneumonia
Mylai massacre, xiv

Nader's Raiders, 76
National Broadcasting C
  (NBC), 164, 172, 2
National Enquirer, 151,
  158, 276, 277
National Guard, 40
National Influenza Imm
  Program. See Swine
  immunization and va
  campaign
NBC. See National Bro
  Company
New Jersey, 138, 139, 1
New Mexico, 7

Ts

Tu
Tv
Ty
Ty

Ur
Ur

Ur

Ur

Ur

Ur

Un

Un

Un

Un

Un
Un
Un
Un

Var

Vat
Ver
Ver

Vet

Vie

Vie
Vik
Vira

Viro

Viru